OXFORD MEDICAL PUBLICATIONS

Psychiatry

Oxford Core Texts

Clinical Dermatology

Clinical Skills

Endocrinology

Health and Illness in the Community

Human Physiology

Medical Genetics

Medical Imaging

Neurology

Oncology

Palliative Care

Psychiatry

Psychiatry

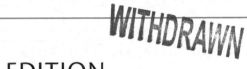

THIRD EDITION

Michael Gelder
Emeritus Professor of Psychiatry, University of Oxford

Richard Mayou
Professor of Psychiatry, University of Oxford

John Geddes
Professor of Epidemiological Psychiatry, University of Oxford

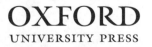

OXFORD
UNIVERSITY PRESS

OXFORD
UNIVERSITY PRESS

Great Clarendon Street, Oxford OX2 6DP

Oxford University Press is a department of the University of Oxford.
It furthers the University's objective of excellence in research, scholarship,
and education by publishing worldwide in

Oxford New York

Auckland Cape Town Dar es Salaam Hong Kong Karachi Kuala Lumpur
Madrid Melbourne Mexico City Nairobi New Delhi Shanghai Taipei Toronto

With offices in

Argentina Austria Brazil Chile Czech Republic France Greece
Guatemala Hungary Italy Japan South Korea Poland Portugal
Singapore Switzerland Thailand Turkey Ukraine Vietnam

Oxford is a registered trade mark of Oxford University Press
in the UK and in certain other countries

Published in the United States
by Oxford University Press Inc., New York

First edition published 2005

Reprinted 2006

A catalogue record for the this title is available from the British Library

Library of Congress Cataloging in Publication Data

Gelder, Michael G.
   Psychiatry/Michael Gelder, Richard Mayou, John Geddes. – 3rd ed.
     (Oxford medical publications) (Oxford core texts)
   Includes bibliographical references and index.
   1. Psychiatry.
   [DNLM: 1. Mental Disorders. WM 140 G315p 2005] I. Mayou, Richard. II. Geddes,
John, MD. III. Title. IV. Series V. Series: Oxford core texts
    RC454.G38 2005   616.89–dc22   2004019758

ISBN 13: 978-0-19-852863-0

ISBN 10: 0-19-852863-9

10 9 8 7 6 5 4 3

Typeset by EXPO Holdings Sdn Bhd., Malaysia
Printed in Great Britain
on acid-free paper by
Ashford Colour Press Ltd, Gosport, Hampshire

Preface

This third edition has been thoroughly revised to take account of recent advances in knowledge. We have made three changes in the arrangement of the chapters. Chapter 1 now deals not only with symptoms and signs (as in the last edition) but also with diagnosis (previously in a separate chapter). There are two new chapters: one brings together somatoform and dissociative disorders, which were previously separated; the other is concerned with disorders of eating and sleeping, which were previously within the chapter on psychiatry and medicine. Otherwise the layout resembles that of the second edition though with a rather greater use of lists and tables.

This book is one of a family of Oxford textbooks on psychiatry. The information and approach in this book has been chosen to meet the needs of students, primary care physicians, and others who need a general knowledge of psychiatry. The other two books are written for specialists but will be of use to readers of this book when they require more information, or who seek references to the literature (which we do not provide). They will find a fuller account of all the topics in this book in *The Shorter Oxford Textbook of Psychiatry* and more extensive information in the two-volume *New Oxford Textbook of Psychiatry*, which is a comprehensive work of reference. Some additional sources of information on the internet are considered in Chapter 3.

We are grateful to Drs Gillian Forrest, Karen Kearley, and Timothy Andrews for their most helpful advice; and to Wendy Swift and Philly White for secretarial assistance.

Oxford, September 2004   *MG, JG, RM*

Contents

1 Signs, symptoms, and diagnosis *1*

2 Assessment *15*

3 Aetiology and the scientific basis of psychiatry *39*

4 Personality and its disorders *49*

5 Reactions to stressful experiences *61*

6 Anxiety and obsessional disorders *73*

7 Physical symptoms not explained by organic pathology *89*

8 Mood disorders *97*

9 Schizophrenia and related disorders *119*

10 Delirium, dementia, and other cognitive disorders *137*

11 Psychiatry and medicine *149*

12 Eating and sleep disorders *161*

13 Suicide and deliberate self-harm *169*

14 Problems due to use of alcohol and other psychoactive substances *183*

15 Problems of sexuality and gender *205*

16 Psychiatry of the elderly *215*

17 Drugs and other physical treatments *231*

18 Psychological treatment *255*

19 Mental health care for the community *267*

20 Child and adolescent psychiatry *275*

21 Learning disability *303*

22 Psychiatry and the law *319*

Index *329*

CHAPTER 1

Signs, symptoms, and diagnosis

Chapter contents

Description of signs and symptoms 2

Abnormalities of mood 2
Depersonalization and derealization 3
Abnormalities of perception 3
Abnormalities of thinking 5
Motor signs and symptoms 10
Abnormalities of memory 10
Abnormalities of consciousness 11
Abnormalities of attention and
concentration 11
Insight 11

Diagnosis and classification 11

Syndrome, illness, disease, and disorder 11
Psychiatric disorder or deviant
behaviour? 12
Psychosis and neurosis 12
Some criticisms of the diagnostic
approach 12
Systems of classification 13
Reliability of diagnosis 14
Co-morbidity 14
Multiaxial classification 14

All doctors need to be able to detect and treat psychiatric problems because such problems are common in all kinds of medical practice. In primary care a quarter of the patients seen have a psychiatric problem, either alone or accompanying a physical illness, and in some branches of hospital practice, psychiatric problems are even more frequent. This chapter is concerned with the description of the symptoms and signs of psychiatric disorders and with making a diagnosis. Chapter 2 deals with the ways of eliciting these symptoms and signs as part of the assessment of patients.

The clinical skills required to elicit symptoms and signs and to make a diagnosis are similar to those used in other branches of medicine—careful history taking, systematic clinical examination, and sound clinical reasoning. The only substantial difference is that the clinical examination includes the mental as well as the physical state of the patient. As explained below, clinical examination and diagnosis are only part of the assessment of patients. They have to be accompanied by an understanding of each patient as a unique human being. This understanding cannot be acquired solely from books—it is learnt though listening to patients as they describe their lives. Some students are reluctant to do this, fearing that psychiatric patients may behave in odd, unpredictable, or alarming ways. In fact this is uncommon. Students should therefore take every opportunity of talking with patients because no textbook can replace this experience. (These and other aspects of the assessment of patients are described in Chapter 2.)

Form and content of symptoms

Many psychiatric symptoms have two aspects: **form** and **content**. The distinction can be explained with an example. A patient may say that, when alone and out of hearing distance of other people, he hears voices telling him that he is changing sex. The form of his experience is an auditory hallucination (a sensory perception in the absence of an external stimulus, see p. 4), and the content is the idea that he is changing sex. A second patient may hear voices saying that he is about to be killed by persecutors. The form of this symptom is again an auditory hallucination, but the content is different. A third person may experience repeated intrusive thoughts that he is changing sex but realizes that these thoughts are untrue. The content of this symptom is the same as that of the first patient, but the form is different—it is an obsessional thought (see p. 8). In making a diagnosis, the form of the symptom is important: delusions and obsessional symptoms have a different diagnostic significance. In helping patients, the content is important as a guide to how they may respond (for example, attack a supposed persecutor) and in understanding their experience of the illness.

Signs, symptoms, and the person

Although it is important to elicit the signs and symptoms of mental disorder, interviewers should never lose sight of their patients as unique individuals. They need to understand how the disorder affects how their patients feel about life, for example, making them feel hopeless, and how it affects their social roles, for example as the mother of small children. The more that interviewers gain insight into such personal experiences, the more they can help their patients. Because such understanding is equally important when caring for patients with physical illnesses, the experience gained during training in psychiatry is of value in every kind of clinical work.

Description of signs and symptoms

Abnormalities of mood (Table 1.1)

Changes in mood are the most common symptoms of psychiatric disorder. They are the prominent symptoms of depressive and anxiety disorders but they may occur in every kind of psychiatric disorder, during physical illness, and in healthy people encountering stressful events. (The term **affect** is sometimes used instead of mood, and the term affective disorder is an alternative name for mood disorder.)

TABLE 1.1 Abnormalities of mood
Abnormalities in the nature of mood
◆ depression
◆ elation
◆ anxiety
◆ anger
Abnormalities in the variability of mood
◆ blunting, flattening
◆ lability
◆ 'incontinence'
Inconsistency between mood and thinking
◆ incongruity of affect

As a technical term, mood includes depression, elation, anxiety, anger, and irritability (the state in which anger occurs more readily than is normal). Mood states are accompanied by characteristic facial expressions and postures (Box 1.1) and these can help to identify the mood of a patient who is denying emotion, for example that he is angry.

Abnormalities of the nature of mood

Pathological depression is a pervasive lowering of mood accompanied by feelings of sadness and a loss of the ability to experience pleasure (*anhedonia*).

BOX 1.1 ASSOCIATION BETWEEN MOOD AND APPEARANCE

Depression   The corners of the mouth are turned down and the centre of the brow has vertical furrows. The head is inclined forward with the gaze directed downwards, and shoulders are bent. The patient's gestures are reduced.

Elation   A lively, cheerful expression. Posture and expressive movements are normal.

Anxiety   The brow is furrowed horizontally, the posture is tense, and the person is restless and sometimes tremulous. Often there are accompanying signs of autonomic overactivity, such as pale skin and increased sweating of the hands, feet, and axillae.

Anger   The eyebrows are drawn down, with widening of the palpebral fissure, and a squaring of the corners of the mouth that may reveal the teeth. The shoulders are square and the body tense as if ready for action.

Pathological elation is a pervasive elevation of mood accompanied by excessive cheerfulness, which in extreme cases may be experienced as ecstasy.

Pathological anxiety is a feeling of apprehension that is out of proportion to the actual situation.

Autonomic changes accompany these mood states. The changes are especially evident in pathological anxiety in which they include pale skin and increased sweating of the hands, feet, and axillae (see p. 75 and Table 6.2).

The term **phobia** (or phobic anxiety) denotes anxiety that arises in relation to a *specific stimulus*. Phobia has two other characteristic features:

1. It is accompanied by a tendency to *avoid* the stimuli that evoke anxiety.

2. It is experienced when thinking about the stimulus as well as when in its presence—that is *anticipatory anxiety*.

The core symptoms are the same as those of other kinds of pathological anxiety; it is their occurrence in response to a particular object, event, or situation that defines phobia as a separate symptom. Phobias are common in healthy people; including phobias of spiders, snakes, thunderstorms, and high places. Phobias are the prominent symptoms of phobic disorders (see pp. 79–83) and they occur sometimes as a minor feature of other anxiety disorders and of depressive disorders.

(The reader may encounter the term **obsessional phobia**. It refers not to a phobia but to a special kind of obsessional symptom, see p. 9.)

Abnormalities in the variability of mood

In healthy people mood varies from day to day and hour to hour. In illness these normal fluctuations of mood may become abnormal in two ways. Normal emotional responsiveness may be: (i) reduced (a state called **blunting** or **flattening** of mood); or (ii) may be increased (a state called **lability of mood**). When the latter change is extreme it is sometimes called **emotional incontinence**—a symptom that may occur after a stroke or in dementia.

Abnormalities in the relation between mood and thinking

In healthy people, mood and thinking are related consistently: for example a person who recalls an unhappy event feels sad. In some psychiatric disorders, mood and thinking do not correspond, instead, for example, a patient may feel happy when thinking about a sad event. This symptom, which occurs mainly in schizo-phrenia, is called **incongruity of affect**. It has to be distinguished from apparent cheerfulness that hides embarrassment, and from the lack of outward show of emotion in people who feel it inwardly—a condition that occurs in some depressed patients.

Depersonalization and derealization

These symptoms are less easy to comprehend than are anxiety and depression because they are less often experienced by healthy people.

Depersonalization is the experience of being unreal, detached, and unable to feel emotion. Paradoxically, this lack of emotional responsiveness can be extremely distressing. People who experience depersonalization often have difficulty in describing it and use similes such as 'it feels as if I were cut off by a wall of glass'. An 'as if' description of this kind must not be confused with a delusion (see p. 6).

Derealization is a similar experience but occurs in relation to the environment rather than the self: for example the feeling that other people seem 'as if made of cardboard' or that things no longer evoke any emotional response.

Depersonalization and derealization are experienced occasionally by healthy people, sometimes when they are very tired. They occur as symptoms of many kinds of psychiatric disorder, especially anxiety disorders, depressive disorders, and schizophrenia. They occur also in temporal lobe epilepsy.

Abnormalities of perception

Before considering abnormalities of perception, it is necessary to explain two terms.

* **Perception** is the process of becoming aware of what is presented through the sense organs.

* **Imagery** is an experience originating within the mind that usually lacks the sense of reality that is part of perception.

We experience imagery when a face is remembered or when we think in pictures. Imagery differs from perception in that it can be called up and terminated at will. Almost always, imagery is obliterated when something is perceived in the same modality. A few people experience **idetic imagery**, that is imagery as vivid and detailed as perception.

Abnormalities of perception are of four kinds: (i) changes in intensity; (ii) changes in quality; (iii) illusions; and (iv) hallucinations. Each kind of abnormality will be described, but particular attention is paid to hallucinations as they are of most significance in diagnosis. (Sometimes, perception is normal in intensity and quality but has a changed meaning for the person who experiences it. This phenomenon is called **delusional perception**. Despite this name this is not a disorder of perception; rather, it is a disorder of thinking and is described with other disorders of thinking on p. 7.)

Changes in the intensity of perception

In mania perception seems more intense, and in depressive disorder less intense.

Changes in the quality of perception

In some disorders, especially schizophrenia, perceptions may seem distorted or unpleasant; for example, food tastes unpleasant or flowers smell acrid.

Illusions

An illusion is a *misperception of an external stimulus*. Illusions may occur in four circumstances:

1. When the level of *sensory stimulation is reduced* (e.g. at dusk the outline of a bush may be misperceived as a man).

2. When *attention is not focused* on the sensory modality (e.g. when a person whose attention is focused on a book may mistakenly identify a sound as a voice).

3. When the level of *consciousness is reduced* (see delirium, p. 138).

4. When there is a *state of intense emotion*, usually fear.

Healthy people sometimes experience illusions, particularly when more than one of the above circumstances occur together; for example, when a frightened person is in a badly lit street.

Hallucinations

A hallucination is a *perception experienced in the absence of an external stimulus to the corresponding sense organ*; for example, hearing a voice when no one is speaking within hearing distance. A hallucination has two qualities which distinguish it from imagery:

1. It is experienced as a true perception.

2. It seems to come from outside the head.

Unless the experience has these two qualities it is not a hallucination. (Experiences that possess one of these qualities, but not the other, are sometimes called **pseudohallucinations**.)

Although hallucinations are generally regarded as the hallmark of mental disorder, healthy people experience them occasionally, especially when falling asleep (**hypnagogic hallucinations**) or when waking (**hypn-**

opompic hallucinations). These two kinds of hallucinations are brief and usually of a simple kind, such as a bell ringing or a name being called. Usually the person wakes suddenly and immediately recognizes the nature of the experience. These two kinds of hallucination do not point to mental disorder.

Types of hallucination

Hallucinations can occur in all sensory modalities (Table 1.2) but those of hearing and seeing are the most frequent.

Auditory hallucinations may be experienced as voices, noises, or music. Hallucinatory voices may seem to speak words, phrases, or sentences. Some address the patient as 'you' (*second person hallucinations*). Others talk about the patient as 'he' or 'she' (*third person hallucinations*), and these latter are characteristic of schizophrenia (see p. 121). Sometimes, a voice seems to say what the patient is about to say; sometimes it seems to repeat what he has just been thinking (*thought echo*).

Visual hallucinations may be experienced as flashes of light or as complex images such as the figure of a man. Usually they are experienced as normal in size, but sometimes may seem unusually small or large. Visual hallucinations are associated particularly with organic mental disorders but can occur in other conditions.

Hallucinations of smell and taste are uncommon. The taste or smell may seem to be recognizable, but more often it is unlike any smell or flavour that has been experienced before, and have an unpleasant quality.

Tactile hallucinations are also uncommon. They may be experienced as superficial sensations of being touched, pricked, or strangled, or as sensations just below the skin, which may be attributed to insects or other small creatures burrowing through the tissues.

TABLE 1.2	Classification of hallucination
According to sensory modality	
◆ auditory	
◆ visual	
◆ smell or taste	
◆ tactile sensations	
◆ deep sensations	
Special kinds of auditory hallucination	
◆ second person	
◆ third person	
◆ echoing or repeating thoughts	

Hallucinations of deep sensation are also uncommon. They may be experienced as feelings of the viscera being pulled or distended, or as sexual stimulation.

Diagnostic associations of hallucinations

Hallucinations occur in severe affective disorders, schizophrenia, and organic disorders. Visual hallucinations occur particularly in organic psychiatric disorders, but also in severe mood disorders and schizophrenia. Although not specific to organic disorder, they should always prompt a thorough search for other symptoms of an organic disorder (see Chapter 10). Hallucinations of taste, smell, and deep sensation occur mainly in schizophrenia. Other associations between particular kinds of hallucination and individual disorders are described in the chapters on clinical syndromes.

Abnormalities of thinking

Disorders of thinking can be of several kinds:

1. An abnormality of the amount and speed of thought (the stream of thought).

2. An abnormality of the ways in which thoughts are linked together (the form of thought).

3. Delusions.

4. Overvalued ideas.

5. Obsessional and compulsive symptoms.

6. Intrusive thoughts.

Abnormalities of the stream of thought

In disorders of the stream of thought both the amount and the speed of thoughts are changed. There are three main abnormalities:

1. **Pressure of thought**. Thoughts are unusually rapid, abundant, and varied. The disorder is characteristic of mania but also occurs in schizophrenia.

2. **Poverty of thought**. Thoughts are unusually slow, few, and unvaried. The disorder is characteristic of severe depressive disorder but also occurs in schizophrenia.

3. **Thought blocking** refers to an experience in which the mind is suddenly empty of thoughts. The symptom of thought blocking should not be confused with the normal experiences of sudden distraction, the intrusion of a different line of thinking, or the experience of losing a particular word or train of thought while other thoughts continue. Thought blocking is the experience of an abrupt and complete emptying of the mind. It occurs especially in schizophrenic patients, who may interpret the experience in odd

ways—saying, for example, that their thoughts have been removed by another person.

Abnormalities of the form of thought

There are three main abnormalities of the ways in which thoughts are linked together:

1. **Flight of ideas**. In this abnormal state, thoughts and any accompanying spoken words move quickly from one topic to another, so that one train of thought is not completed before the next begins. Because topics change so rapidly, the links between one topic and the next may be difficult to follow. Nevertheless, understandable links are present, though not always in the form of logical connections. Instead the link may be through:

   ◆ *rhyme*, for example when an idea about chairs is followed by an idea about pears (rhyming links are sometimes called *clang associations*);

   ◆ *puns*, that is two words that have the same sound (e.g. male/mail);

   ◆ *distraction*, for example a new topic suggested by something in the interview room.

   Flight of ideas is characteristic of mania.

2. **Loosening of associations** is a lack of logical connection between a sequence of thoughts, not explicable by the processes described under flight of ideas. This lack of logical association is sometimes called *knight's move thinking* (referring to the indirect move of the knight in chess). Usually, the interviewer is alerted to the presence of loosening of associations because the patient's replies are hard to follow. This difficulty in understanding differs from that experienced when interviewing people who are very anxious or are of low intelligence. Anxious people become more coherent when put at ease, and people of low intelligence do so when questions are simplified. When there is loosening of associations, the links between ideas cannot be made more understandable in either of these ways. Instead, the interviewer has the experience that the more he tries to clarify the patient's thinking, the less he understands it. Loosening of associations occurs most often in schizophrenia. It is often difficult to distinguish loosening of associations from flight of ideas, and when this happens it is often helpful to tape-record a sample of speech and listen to it repeatedly.

3. **Perseveration** is the persistent and inappropriate repetition of the same sequence of thought, as shown either in speech or actions. It can be demonstrated by

asking a series of simple questions: the patient repeats his answer to the first question as his response to all subsequent questions even though these require different answers. Perseveration occurs most often in dementia but may occur in other disorders.

Delusions

A delusion is *a belief that is held firmly but on inadequate grounds, is not affected by rational argument or evidence to the contrary, and is not a conventional belief that the person might be expected to hold given his cultural background and level of education.* This rather lengthy definition is required to distinguish delusions, which are indicators of mental disorder, from other kinds of strongly held belief found among healthy people. A delusion is nearly always a false belief but not always so (see below). There are several problems surrounding the definition of delusions and these are considered briefly in Box 1.2.

Delusions and behaviour

Conviction in the truth of a delusion does not necessarily influence all the person's feelings and actions, especially when the delusion has been present for a long time, as in chronic schizophrenia. For example, such a patient may have the delusion that he is a member of the Royal Family and yet live contentedly in a hostel for discharged psychiatric patients.

Primary and secondary delusions

A **primary delusion** is one that *occurs suddenly without any other abnormal mental event leading to it.* For example, a patient may suddenly develop the unshakable conviction that he is changing sex, without ever having thought of this before and without any reason to do so at the time. Primary delusions are rare; when they occur they strongly suggest schizophrenia. However, the point is not very useful in practice because few patients can give a reliable account of the way in which they first had a delusional idea.

A **secondary delusion** *arises from some previous abnormal idea or experience,* which may be: (i) a *hallucination*: for example, a person hears a voice and believes he is being followed; (ii) a *mood*: for example, a person with deep depression feels worthless and believes that other people think the same about him; or (iii) *another delusion*. Secondary delusions occur in a variety of severe psychiatric disorders.

When one delusion gives rise to another in a sequence, the resulting network of interrelated ideas is known as a **delusional system**.

BOX 1.2 SOME PROBLEMS SURROUNDING THE DEFINITION OF DELUSIONS

Delusions are arrived at through abnormal thought processes   This is the fundamental point that characterizes delusions but it cannot be observed directly. The various clauses in the definition of a delusion are intended to provide indirect criteria to establish the point but there are some problems with each of them.

Delusions are held firmly despite evidence to the contrary. This is the key to the definition and it is often revealed through the person's words and actions. For example, a person with the delusion that persecutors are in the next room will not alter his belief when shown that the room is empty; instead, he may say that the persecutors left before he arrived. However, not all beliefs that are impervious to contrary evidence are delusions: some non-delusional beliefs are of this kind. For example, a convinced spiritualist hangs on to his belief in spiritualism when presented with contrary evidence that would convince a non-believer. These strongly held non-delusional beliefs are called *overvalued ideas*. When deluded patients recover, either with treatment or spontaneously, they pass through a stage of increasing doubt in the truth of their delusions. This stage of partial conviction in a belief that was previously a full delusion is called a *partial delusion*.

Delusions are false beliefs   Some definitions of delusion include this point. It is not included in our definition because very occasionally a delusional belief is either true from the onset, or subsequently becomes true. For example, a man may develop the delusional belief that his wife is unfaithful despite a complete lack of evidence of infidelity or of any other rational reason for holding the belief. The belief has been arrived at in an abnormal way and is delusional even if, unbeknown to him, the wife is unfaithful. The point is of mainly theoretical importance but it is sometimes brought up in discussions of delusion since it highlights the fact that the essential criterion for delusion is that it was arrived at in an abnormal way.

Delusions are usually odd and improbable beliefs   However not all odd and improbable beliefs are delusional. Some people express seemingly improbable beliefs (e.g. that they are being poisoned by close relatives), which are subsequently proved to be true. Apparently odd beliefs should be investigated most carefully before they are accepted as delusional.

Delusional mood, delusional perception, and delusional memory

These terms describe three special kinds of experience, none of which, despite their names, is a delusion though all are closely related to delusions.

Delusional mood is an inexplicable feeling of apprehension that is followed before long by a delusion that explains it. For example, the delusion that someone is following the patient with the intent to harm him.

Delusional perception is the misinterpretation of the significance of something perceived normally. For example, a patient may suddenly be convinced that the particular arrangement of objects on a desk indicates that his life is threatened.

Delusional memory is the retrospective delusional misinterpretation of memories of actual events. For example, the conviction that on a previous occasion when the patient felt ill his food had been poisoned by persecutors, though previously and at the time of the illness he did not believe this.

Shared delusions

Usually, other people recognize delusional beliefs as false and they argue with the deluded persons in an attempt to correct them. Occasionally, a person who lives with a deluded patient comes to share the delusional beliefs. This person is then said to have shared delusions or *folie à deux* (see p. 134). The affected person's conviction may be unshakable while they remain with the patient, but usually weakens quickly when the two are separated.

Delusional themes

Delusions are usually grouped according to their main themes (Table 1.3). Since there is some correspondence between delusional theme and type of disorder, and

TABLE 1.3 Delusional themes
◆ Persecutory (paranoid) themes
◆ Themes of reference
◆ Grandiose and expansive themes
◆ Themes of guilt and worthlessness
◆ Nihilistic themes
◆ Hypochondriacal themes
◆ Themes of jealousy
◆ Sexual or amorous themes
◆ Themes of control
◆ Religious themes
◆ Themes concerning the possession of thoughts

since this is helpful in diagnosis, the main themes will be described briefly and will be related to the disorders in which they occur most often. The associations are described more fully in the chapters concerned with these disorders.

1. **Persecutory delusions** are often called **paranoid delusions**. (Used strictly, 'paranoid' refers not only to persecutory but also to grandiose, jealous, and amorous delusions; however this strict usage is seldom adopted.) Paranoid delusions are ideas that people or organizations are trying to inflict harm on the patient, damage his reputation, or make him insane. It is important to remember that it is normal in some cultures to ascribe misfortunes to the malign activities of other people, for example through witchcraft. Such ideas are not delusions. Persecutory delusions are common in *schizophrenia*, and occur also in *organic states* and *severe depressive disorders*. When the delusions are part of a depressive disorder, the patient characteristically accepts that the supposed actions of his persecutors are justified by his own wickedness; in schizophrenia, however, he characteristically resents them.

2. **Delusions of reference** are concerned with the idea that objects, events, or the actions of other people have a special significance for the patient. For example, a remark heard on television is believed to be directed specifically to the patient; or a gesture by a stranger is believed to convey something about the patient. Delusions of this kind are associated with *schizophrenia*.

3. **Grandiose and expansive delusions** are beliefs of exaggerated self-importance. Patients may think themselves wealthy, endowed with unusual abilities, or in other ways special. Such ideas occur mainly in *mania* and sometimes in *schizophrenia*.

4. **Delusions of guilt and worthlessness** are beliefs that the person has done something shameful or sinful. Usually the belief concerns an innocent error that caused no guilt at the time, for example a small error in an income tax return, which the patient now fears will be discovered and lead to prosecution. This kind of delusion occurs most often in *severe depressive disorders*.

5. **Nihilistic delusions** include beliefs that the patient's career is finished, that he is about to die or has no money, or that the world is doomed. Nihilistic delusions occur most often in *severe depressive disorders*.

6. **Hypochondriacal delusions** are false beliefs about disease. The patient believes, in the face of convincing medical evidence to the contrary, that he has an as yet undiscovered disease. Such delusions are more common among the elderly, reflecting the increasing concerns about ill health in later life. Related delusions are concerned with the appearance of parts of the body, for example the belief that the person's (normally shaped) nose is seriously misshapen. Patients with delusions about their appearance may seek the help of plastic surgeons. Hypochondriacal delusions occur in *depressive disorders* and *schizophrenia*. (Hypochondriacal ideas are discussed further in Chapter 7).

7. **Delusions of jealousy** are more common among men. They may lead to dangerously aggressive behaviour towards the person who is believed to be unfaithful (see pathological jealousy, p. 133).

8. **Sexual or amorous delusions** are more frequent among women. Usually, the woman believes that she is loved by a man who has never spoken to her and who is inaccessible—for example, an eminent public figure.

9. **Delusions of control** are beliefs that personal actions, impulses, or thoughts are controlled by an outside agency. This experience has to be distinguished from: (i) voluntary obedience to commands given by hallucinatory voices; and (ii) culturally normal beliefs that human actions are under divine control. Delusions of control strongly suggest *schizophrenia*.

10. **Religious delusions** may be concerned with guilt (for example, divine punishment for minor sins) or with special powers. Before deciding that such beliefs are delusional, it is important to determine whether they held by other members of the patient's religious or cultural group.

11. **Delusions concerning the possession of thoughts**. Healthy people have no doubt that their thoughts are their own and that other people can know them only if they are spoken aloud or revealed through actions. Delusions concerning the possession of thoughts are ideas that:

    ◆ some of the person's thoughts have been implanted by an outside agency—the **delusion of thought insertion**;

    ◆ some of their thoughts have been taken away—the **delusion of thought withdrawal**;

    ◆ some of their their thoughts are known to other people through telepathy, radio, or some other unusual way—the **delusion of thought broadcasting**.

All three symptoms are found most often in schizophrenia.

Overvalued ideas

An overvalued idea is an *isolated, preoccupying, and strongly held belief that dominates a person's life and may affect his or her actions but which (unlike a delusion) has been derived through normal mental processes*. For example, someone whose parents developed cancer within a short time of one another may be convinced that cancer is contagious however many times he has been presented with evidence to the contrary. It is sometimes difficult to distinguish between overvalued ideas and delusions since the two may be equally strongly held, and the differentiation depends on a judgement of the way in which the idea developed. In practice, this difficulty seldom causes problems since diagnosis does not depend on a single symptom.

Obsessional and compulsive symptoms

Obsessions are *recurrent and persistent thoughts, impulses, or images that enter the mind despite efforts to exclude them*. The person recognizes that the ideas are senseless. The obsessions usually concern matters that the person finds distressing or unpleasant, and often feels ashamed to tell others about them. The person has no doubt that the intruding thoughts are the product of his own mind (contrast the deluded person who may believe that ideas have been implanted from outside.

A sense of struggling to resist the intrusions is part of an obsessional symptom. **Resistance** distinguishes obsessions (in which it is present) from delusions (in which it is absent). However, when obsessions have been present for a long time, resistance may decrease so that this distinction becomes difficult to make. In practice, this decrease seldom leads to diagnostic problems because it takes place late in the course of the disorder, when the diagnosis has already been made.

Obsessions have to be distinguished from:

1. Ordinary preoccupations of healthy people.

2. Intrusive concerns of anxious or depressed patients (see p. 75 and 99).

3. Recurring thoughts and images associated with disorders of sexual preference (see p. 211).

4. Recurring thoughts and images associated with drug dependency.

5. Delusions.

Patients with these non-obsessional ideas do not regard them as unreasonable, and do not resist them. Obsessional symptoms are essential features of **obsessive-compulsive disorder**. They occur also in other psychiatric disorders, especially anxiety and depressive disorders.

Types of obsessional symptoms (Table 1.4)

Obsessional thoughts are repeated, intrusive words or phrases, which take many forms including obscenities, blasphemies; and thoughts about distressing occurrences (e.g. that the patient's hands are contaminated with bacteria that will spread disease).

Obsessional ruminations are repeated sequences of such thoughts (e.g. about the ending of the world).

Obsessional doubts are recurrent uncertainties about a previous action (e.g. whether or not the person has switched off an electrical appliance that could cause a fire).

Obsessional impulses are urges to carry out actions that are usually aggressive, dangerous, or socially embarrassing (e.g. using a knife to stab someone, jumping in front of a moving train, or shouting obscenities in church). Whatever the urge, the person recognizes that it is irrational and does not wish to carry it out. This is an important point of distinction from delusions, which are regarded as rational by the patient and which may lead to action, such as aggression against a supposed persecutor.

Obsessional phobia is the term sometimes applied to obsessional thoughts with a fearful content (e.g. 'I may have cancer') or to obsessional impulses that arouse anxiety (e.g. the urge to stab another person). The term

---

BOX 1.3 THEMES OF OBSESSIONAL THOUGHTS

- **Dirt and contamination**, for example the idea that the hands are contaminated with bacteria
- **Aggressive actions**, for example the idea that the person may harm another person, or shout angry remarks
- **Orderliness**, for example the idea that objects have to be arranged in a special way, or clothes put on in a particular order
- **Disease**, for example the idea that the person may have cancer (some ideas of contamination refer to illness, e.g. ideas of contamination with harmful bacteria)
- **Sex**, usually thoughts or images of practices that the person finds disgusting
- **Religion**, for example blasphemous thoughts, or doubts about the fundamentals of belief (e.g 'does God exist?') or about the adequacy or completeness of a religious practice such as confession

---

is confusing and is best avoided by using one of the preceding four terms.

Themes of obsessional thoughts

Obsessional thoughts can be about any topic but, for unknown reasons, most are centred around the six themes shown in Box 1.3.

Compulsions

Although compulsions are actions not thoughts, it is convenient to describe them here because most compulsions are associated with obsessions. Compulsions are *repeated, stereotyped, and seemingly purposeful actions that the person feels compelled to carry out but resists, recognizing that they are irrational*. Compulsions are also known as **compulsive rituals**. Sometimes the association between the action and the thought seems understandable, as when handwashing is associated with the idea that the hands are contaminated. In other cases there is no meaningful connection between the actions and the thoughts, as when checking the position of objects is associated with aggressive ideas. Most compulsions are followed by an immediate lessening of the distress associated with the corresponding obsessional thoughts. However, the long-term consequence is that the thoughts persist for longer (see p. 87). Compulsions are sometimes accompanied by obsessional thoughts concerned with doubt that the compulsive behaviours have been

TABLE 1.4	Obsessional and compulsive symptoms
Obsessions	
◆ thoughts	
◆ ruminations	
◆ doubts	
◆ impulses	
◆ phobias	
Compulsions (rituals)	
◆ checking	
◆ cleaning	
◆ counting	
◆ dressing	

executed correctly, and this can lead to further repetitions, which may last for hours.

Compulsions can be of any kind but there are four common themes (Table 1.4):

1. **Checking rituals**, which are often concerned with safety (e.g. checking repeatedly that a gas tap has been turned off).
2. **Cleaning rituals** such as repeated handwashing or domestic cleaning.
3. **Counting rituals** such as counting to a particular number or counting in threes.
4. **Dressing rituals** in which the clothes are always set out or put on in a particular way.

Intrusive thoughts

Intrusive thoughts appear spontaneously, and interrupt the train of thought. According to their content they may provoke anxiety, depression, anger, or sexual arousal. The latter may be experienced as pleasurable and encouraged but the rest are resisted. Intrusive thoughts can usually be terminated by an effort of will—though they may return later—and are not, therefore, associated with the sense of struggle and resistance that characterizes obsessional thoughts. Intrusive thoughts are an important feature of post-traumatic stress disorder (see p. 65), and may occur in many other disorders, including anxiety and depressive disorders, and disorders of sexual preference.

Motor symptoms and signs

Abnormalities of facial expression, posture, and social behaviour, which are common in mental disorders of all kinds, are considered in subsequent chapters. Motor abnormalities such as mannerisms, sterotypies, and catatonic symptoms are briefly described in the chapter on schizophrenia (see p. 122) and more extensively in *The Shorter Oxford Textbook of Psychiatry*. Here we define three movement disorders:

1. **Tics** are *irregular repeated movements involving a group of muscles* (e.g. a sideways movement of the head).
2. **Choreiform movements** are *brief involuntary movements that are co-ordinated but purposeless*, such as grimacing or movements of the arms.
3. **Dystonia** is a *muscle spasm*, which is often painful and may lead to contortions.

Abnormalities of memory

Several kinds of memory abnormality occur in psychiatric disorders and it is usual to describe them in terms of the following three stages of memory (which though useful in practice, do not correspond exactly with the stages of memory identified through research):

1. **Immediate memory** is retention over a few minutes. It is tested by asking the patient to remember a name and address (which they did not know before the test) and to recall it after 5 minutes.
2. **Recent memory** concerns events in the last few days. It is tested by asking about recent events in the patient's daily life that are known—directly or via an informant—to interviewer, for example what the patient ate yesterday; or by asking about items of recent news.
3. **Long-term memory** concerns events over much longer periods of time. It is tested by asking about events that took place before the onset of any possible memory disorder.

In testing for memory, a distinction is made between spontaneous recall and the recognition of information. Some patients cannot recall information but can recognize it as correct, indicating that their problem is, at least in part, with retrieval.

Memory loss caused by organic conditions usually affects recent memory more than remote memory. Total loss of memory, including memory for personal identity, occurs very rarely in organic conditions and strongly suggests psychogenic causes (see p. 94) or malingering. Some organic causes lead to an *amnesic syndrome* in which short-term memory is severely impaired but longer term memory is retained (see p. 143).

The following terms describe other abnormalities of memory:

- **Anterograde amnesia** occurs after a period of unconsciousness. It is the impairment of memory for events between the ending of complete unconsciousness and the restoration of full consciousness.
- **Retrograde amnesia** is the loss of memory for events before the onset of unconsciousness. It occurs after head injury or electroconvulsive therapy (ECT).
- *Jamais vu* is a failure to recognize events that have been encountered before, and *déjà vu* is the recognition of events as familiar when they have never been encountered. Both abnormalities may occur in neurological disorders.
- **Confabulation** is the reporting as 'memories' of events that did not take place at the time in question. It occurs in some patients with severe disorders of recent memory (see amnesic syndrome, p. 143).

Memory is affected in several kinds of psychiatric disorder. In *organic disorder* all aspects of long-term memory are usually affected, although the memory of earlier events is impaired less than that of more recent memory. In *depressive disorder* memory is not impaired in any of the ways described so far, but unhappy memories are recalled more readily than other kinds of memory.

False memory syndrome

The recall of highly unpleasant events are sometimes blocked by the psychological mechanism of repression (see Box 5.1, p. 63). After a time, this repression usually decreases and recall becomes possible. It is uncertain how complete repression can be and for long it can last. These two uncertainties are important in relation to reported recalls during psychotherapy or counselling, carried out many years after the events, of memories of sexual abuse of which the person previously had no recollection. Often the reported abuse is strongly denied, not only by the supposed abuser but also by others present at the time. The possibility then arises that these experiences are not memories but ideas suggested during overzealous questioning or discussion during therapy. Although the matter is still undecided, it seems that it is, at the least, very uncommon for memories to be repressed completely for years and then appear suddenly. If this conclusion is correct, it follows that only a minority of 'recovered memories' are likely to be true memories and that great care should be taken, when enquiring about past abuse, to avoid suggesting that it has taken place.

Abnormalities of consciousness

Consciousness is awareness of self and the environment. Its level varies between the extremes of coma and alertness. Several terms are used for the intervening states of consciousness:

1. **Clouding of consciousness** refers to a state of drowsiness with incomplete reaction to stimuli; impaired attention, concentration, and memory; and slow, muddled thinking.

2. **Stupor** refers to a state in which the person is mute, immobile, and unresponsive, but appears to be conscious because the eyes are open and follow external objects. (This is the usage in psychiatry; in neurology the same term is often used when there is some impairment of consciousness.)

3. **Confusion** refers to muddled thinking. The term **confusional state** is sometimes applied to the state in which muddled thinking is associated with impairment of consciousness, illusions, hallucinations, delusions, and anxiety (see p. 138). **Delirium** is a better term for this state.

Abnormalities of attention and concentration

Attention is the ability to focus on the matter in hand. Concentration is the ability to maintain that focus. Attention and concentration can be impaired in many kinds of psychiatric disorder but especially in anxiety disorder, depressive disorder, mania, schizophrenia, and organic disorder. Detection of impaired attention or concentration does not help in diagnosis but is important in assessing the patient's disability; for example, poor concentration may prevent a person from working effectively in an office.

Insight

As a technical term insight means a *correct awareness of one's own mental condition*. Insight is not simply present or absent, but is a matter of degree. It is described best in terms of four criteria:

1. Awareness of oneself as presenting phenomena that other people consider abnormal (e.g. being unusually active and elated).

2. Recognition that these phenomena are abnormal.

3. Acceptance that these abnormal phenomena are caused by mental illness (rather than, for example, substances administered by a persecutor).

4. Awareness that treatment is required.

In general, insight is lost to a greater extent in psychotic (see p. 12) than in non-psychotic disorders. Assessment of insight is extremely important in determining a patient's likely cooperation with treatment. For example, a patient who believes that he is being persecuted and does not accept that his beliefs are a sign of illness, is unlikely to accept treatment readily. None the less he may be aware that he feels distressed and is sleeping badly, and may agree to accept help with these problems (which he ascribes to the persecution).

Diagnosis and classification

Syndrome, illness, disease, and disorder

In psychiatry, as in the rest of medicine, signs and symptoms often occur together in recognizable patterns known as **syndromes**. As in other branches of medicine it is important to identify syndromes (which in psychiatry are the basis of diagnosis) because they are a better guide to treatment and prognosis than are individual signs or symptoms. For example, the symptom of depressed mood occurs in the syndromes of depressive disorder, dementia, and schizophrenia, each of which differs from the others in terms of prognosis and treatment. Depressed mood is also experienced by healthy people, for example after bereavement. This distinction between depressed mood and depressive disorder is highly relevant in the practice of general medicine. A doctor may have to decide, for example, whether the depressed mood of a patient with cancer is a normal response to the prospect of dying, or instead part of a depressive disorder that would respond to antidepressant treatment.

Two other terms are widely used to describe a patient's condition. While the terms are often used interchangeably in everyday speech, as technical terms they have distinct meanings. **Illness** denotes the patient's experience of distress; **disease** denotes the presence of physical pathology. Disease and illness usually occur together but not always. Some patients have a disease but not an illness (e.g. the earliest stage of a carcinoma). Some patients have illness but no disease—they have medically unexplained symptoms (see Chapter 7).

In general medicine, the entries in a classification system are called diseases. In psychiatry, the term **disorder** is preferred because few conditions have the established physical pathology that is implied by the term disease. However, where physical pathology has been demonstrated, the term disease is used, as in Alzheimer's disease.

Psychiatric disorder or deviant behaviour?

Although some psychiatric disorders are characterized by deviant behaviour, not all deviant behaviour is caused by psychiatric disorder. Despite this, it is sometimes proposed that a person who shows extreme deviations of behaviour (e.g. commits multiple murders) must have a psychiatric disorder (must be 'mad' or 'sick'). In fact, people whose behaviour is grossly deviant may have no psychiatric disorder. Less extreme deviant behaviour is also sometimes thought of in the same way, for example in some countries extremes of political dissent have been considered evidence of mental disorder. Deviant behaviour should be ascribed to psychiatric disorder only when there is clear independent evidence that the necessary diagnostic criteria have been met.

Psychosis and neurosis

Psychiatric disorders are sometimes grouped into psychoses and neuroses. The terms should be avoided

although the reader should understand how others use them.

Psychosis is a collective term for the more severe forms of psychiatric disorder in which hallucinations and delusions may occur and insight is impaired. Schizophrenia, manic-depressive disorder, and the dementias are psychoses. The term is unsatisfactory because it groups together disorders that have little in common, and is less useful than a specific diagnosis such as schizophrenia. Nevertheless, some clinicians still use the term psychosis as a provisional diagnosis when the precise diagnosis is uncertain.

Neurosis is a collective term for psychiatric disorders in which, irrespective of severity, there are no hallucinations or delusions and no loss of insight. The objections to the term neurosis are the same as those for psychosis: it embraces conditions that have little in common, and is less informative than a specific diagnosis such as anxiety disorder. Like psychosis, the term neurosis is sometimes used to denote a disorder that cannot yet be assigned a more precise diagnosis.

Some criticisms of the diagnostic approach

Classifying disorders and understanding patients

Psychiatric diagnosis is sometimes criticized on the grounds that it fails to recognize the uniqueness of the individual patient. This criticism fails to understand the purpose of diagnosis, which is to identify features of the patient's problems that have been observed regularly in other patients. When these common features have been identified and summarized in a diagnosis, the clinician goes on to consider the individual features of the patient—he seeks to understand the person who is ill. These individual factors determine how the patient is likely to react to the disorder and the plan of treatment.

It might appear that the diagnosis of personality disorder is an exception to this line of reasoning. However, even this diagnosis is concerned with aspects of the person that are observed regularly in other people. When these have been identified, there remain the other aspects of personality that characterize the individual patient.

Diagnosis and stigma

It has been said that diagnosis stigmatizes patients, and that for this reason diagnoses should not be made. It is true that a diagnosis such as schizophrenia may cause social stigma, as do some medical diagnoses such as AIDS. However, this is not a reason to stop making diagnoses but a reason to inform the public about the true nature of the psychiatric disorders so that unrealistic beliefs (e.g. that all schizophrenic patients are violent) can be corrected. Failure to make a psychiatric diagnosis deprives patients of the guidance about effective treatment and prognosis that diagnosis provides.

Systems of classification

Classifications can be more or less detailed, depending on their purpose. We first present a basic classification, useful for gaining an initial broad understanding of the scope of the subject. After this we describe the two main systems of classification used in psychiatry, followed by a simpler one developed for use in primary care. Details of the two main classifications are of interest mainly to psychiatrists; readers who require further information will find this in *The Shorter Oxford Textbook of Psychiatry*.

Basic classification

The basic classification has the following three categories, each of which is divided further in the more detailed classifications. These subdivisions are described in subsequent chapters. For convenience, the subdivisions of the category mental disorders are shown in Table 1.5.

1. **Mental disorders**: abnormalities of behaviour or psychological experience with a recognizable onset after a period of normal functioning.

2. **Personality disorder**: dispositions to behave in certain abnormal ways that have been present continuously from early adult life.

3. **Learning disability** (also called **mental retardation**): impairment of intellectual functioning present continuously from early life.

TABLE 1.5	Classification of mental disorders

- Delirium, dementia, and related disorders
- Psychoactive substance use disorders
- Anxiety and obsessional disorders
- Mood disorder
- Schizophrenia and related disorders
- Somatoform disorders
- Dissociative disorders
- Factitious disorders
- Disorders starting in childhood
- Developmental disorders
- Conduct disorders

The International Classification of Diseases (ICD)

This system of classification, developed by the World Health Organization, is now in its tenth edition known as **ICD-10**. It is a comprensive list of all diseases, of which psychiatric disorders constitute one section. The diagnostic criteria exist in two versions: one for clinical practice, the other—more restrictive—one for research. In the clinical version diagnoses are made by comparing the features of a case with descriptions of the features of typical cases. In the research version diagnoses are made using operational criteria, that is lists of features that must be present (or absent) for the diagnosis to be made. In practice only the clinical version is much used; the alternative DSM system being generally preferred for research (see below).

The Diagnostic and Statistical Manual (DSM)

This classification, developed by the American Psychiatric Association, is now in its fourth edition known as **DSM-IV**. Although originally developed as the US National Classification, DSM is now used internationally, especially for research. It differs from ICD-10 mainly in the use of operational criteria for clinical work as well as for research. Most of these criteria are the same as those in the research version of ICD-10 and the few differences are mainly of concern only to psychiatrists. Since most research uses DSM criteria, the use of the same classification in clinical work has the advantage that research evidence can be related more directly to clinical problems than it can be when diagnoses are made with ICD.

Classification for primary care

The World Health Organization has published a simplified classification of the disorders that are most frequent in primary care (Table 1.6). The classification is not used widely but the categories are, nevertheless, a useful guide to the disorders that are most frequently found in primary care. (Although tobacco use disorder is not generally thought of as a psychiatric disorder, it is included because it is frequent in primary care.) Schizophrenia and related disorders are not shown separately, but are recorded under chronic psychotic disorders, presumably because a more precise diagnosis is usually made after referral to a specialist. Mood disorders are divided into bipolar disorders and depression for reasons that will be explained in Chapter 8. Anxiety disorders, which are common in primary care, are divided into phobic disorders, panic disorder, generalized anxiety, and mixed anxiety and depression (see Chapter 6). Obsessional disorders are not listed, presumably because they are uncommon. Disorders starting in childhood are not

TABLE 1.6 Classification for primary care

- Dementia
- Delirium
- Alcohol use disorders
- Drug use disorders
- Tobacco use disorders
- Chronic psychotic disorders
- Bipolar disorders
- Depression
- Phobic disorders
- Panic disorder
- Generalized anxiety
- Mixed anxiety and depression
- Adjustment disorder
- Dissociative (conversion) disorder
- Unexplained somatic complaint
- Eating disorders
- Sleep problems
- Sexual problems

included even though they are common in primary care, but eating disorders, sleep problems, and sexual problems are listed, though not in detail.

Reliability of diagnosis

Diagnosis is of little value unless interviewers agree with one another about the same patient. Good agreement depends on:

1. **Interviewing technique**. Interviewers vary in the information they elicit from the same patient, and they may interpret the information differently. These variations can be reduced by using standardized interviews in which predetermined questions are asked, and rules can be used to define whether particular symptoms are present. Standardized interviews are used mainly in research.

2. **Diagnostic criteria**. Reliability can be increased by providing a clear definition for each diagnosis, and by specifying what symptoms need to be present—or absent. Operational criteria (as used in DSM and the research version of ICD) lead to more agreement in diagnosis but they also leave more patients without a diagnosis because they narrowly fail to meet the criteria.

The symptoms that are included in the criteria are not necessarily the most distressing for the patient or the most relevant when planning treatment. For example, thoughts of suicide do not help in diagnosis because they occur in several kinds of disorder, but they are very distressing to patients and highly important when planning care.

Co-morbidity

Some patients have symptoms that meet the criteria for more that one diagnosis (co-morbidity). When this happens the clinician has a choice of approaches:

1. A hierarchy can be established, in which some diagnoses take precedence over others. For example, when symptoms of schizophrenia and dementia occur together, only the latter would be diagnosed since the brain disorders that caused dementia can also cause schizophrenia-like symptoms.

2. The clinician can diagnose all the conditions that meet the diagnostic criteria; in the foregoing example, both dementia and schizophrenia. This is the approach used in the American classification DSM-IV.

3. The clinician can make the minimum number of diagnoses needed to describe the case completely. This the approach adopted in ICD-10.

Multiaxial classification

In a multiaxial classification several kinds of problem are noted in every case and recorded on 'axes'. The usual axes are: *clinical syndrome*, *personality disorder*, *physical disease*, *severity of stressors*, and *disability*. In everyday practice only the first three axes are used commonly—psychiatric disorder, personality, and physical disease. These three can, of course, be recorded without the use of separate axes, but the axial system ensures that they are considered in every case. Multiaxial classification is used more often in child than in adult psychiatry, with intelligence taking the place of personality.

Further reading

Sims, A. C. P. (2002). *Symptoms in the Mind*, 2nd edn. W. B. Saunders, London.
A comprehensive account of the symptoms and signs of psychiatric disorder.
World Health Organization (1996). *Diagnostic and Management Guidelines for Mental Disorders in Primary Care ICD-10*. Chapter V, Primary care version. WHO/Hogrefe and Huber Publishers, Göttingen.

CHAPTER 2

Assessment

Chapter contents

Collecting information 16

Assessment 30

Recording information 32

Communicating with the patient and others 36

Appendix: Mini Mental State Examination 37

Assessment prepares the way for action. The form and detail of an assessment depends therefore on the action that is likely to be needed, and this depends in turn on the nature of the problem. Thus, after assessing a severely depressed patient, the general practitioner will either treat the patient or seek specialist help. After assessing a disturbed patient in an emergency department, the doctor's first action will be to calm the patient and ensure the safety of others. After assessing an elderly inpatient with severe memory loss, a physician will need to arrange appropriate aftercare. The length and focus of the assessment will differ in each case, although the basic structure will be the same.

Assessment begins as soon as the presenting problem is known—it does not wait until all the relevant data have been collected. From the start of the interview, the assessor begins to think what disorders could account for the presenting problem and what data will be required to decide. As the patient's personality and circumstances become known, further ideas will be generated about the plan of management that is most likely to succeed. Thus interviewing is not a fixed procedure, carried out in the same way with every patient, but a dynamic process in which interviewers make, test, and modify hypotheses as they gather information.

Although the details of the interview vary in this way, the *general aims* are always the same. These are to:

1. Understand the problem and the symptoms, and how much these affect the patient's life.

2. Understand the patient's concerns.

3. Compare the present condition of the patient with the former state, including any previous illnesses.

4. Enquire about current and past medication and other drug use.

5. Learn about the patient's family and other circumstances, including sources of support.

Whenever possible, information from the patient is supplemented by information from another informant. The interview is followed by an examination of the mental and physical state and, in some cases, by special investigations. These enquiries lead from the presenting problem to the assessment, which may be complete or provisional depending on the complexity of the problem, the time available, and the information immediately accessible. The assessment will include the diagnosis, an understanding of the ill person, an evaluation of the causes of the disorder, its effects on the patient and others, a plan of management, and a prognosis. When the assessment has been made, the results are discussed with the patient and often with a relative.

This chapter is concerned with the general assessment of adult patients. The assessment of children is described in Chapter 20, and of people with learning disability in Chapter 21. Assessment of suicide risk is on p. 179, of alcohol problems on pp. 189–92, of sexual dysfunction on p. 207, and of medicolegal problems on p. 327.

Summarizing the assessment: the formulation

The results of an assessment are sometimes summarized in a **formulation**, and this type of summary is often used in teaching and in examining students. For this reason, and because it may help readers to see, at this stage, an example of an assessment, a formulation is shown in Box 2.1. Formulations are organized under the headings: *presenting problem*, *diagnosis and differential diagnosis*, *aetiology*, *management*, and *prognosis*. The example in Box 2.1 concerns a young mother with children who was depressed. The diagnosis of depressive disorder was made and this led directly to the choice of medication. Other aspects of the problem were important for the overall plan of management. The risk of suicide was judged to be low, but it was thought necessary to reassess this risk after starting medication. Severely depressed mothers occasionally have thoughts of harming their children. This patient did not and so it was judged appropriate for her to continue caring for her children, with help from her sister. The immediate cause of the depressive disorder appeared to be the husband's infidelity but the family history of depres-

sive disorder suggested genetic predisposition (see Chapter 8). The prognosis was based partly on these opinions about causation, but also on an understanding of the ill person, and on the likelihood of further stressful events. This example shows how a written formulation can assist other clinicians who may be called upon to treat the patient, for example in an emergency.

Disablement

The case in the formulation shown in Box 2.1 illustrates the importance of the effects of psychiatric disorder on a patient's functioning—in this case her ability to care for her children. Interference with functioning is called **disablement**. Disablement can be thought of as taking three forms:

1. **Impairment**: interference with the functioning of a psychological or physical *system*, e.g. impairment of memory.

2. **Disability**: interference in the functioning and activities of the *whole person*, e.g. inability to dress or cook.

3. **Handicap**: the *social disadvantage* consequent upon impairment and disability, e.g. inability to work or care for children.

Usually both symptoms and disablement are the direct consequence of psychiatric disorder but this is not always the case. Sometimes symptoms result from disablement, for example when a person with schizophrenia cannot get a job and becomes depressed. Sometimes disablement results from other people's *stigmatizing attitudes*. Thus a person with schizophrenia may be unable to work, not because of the direct effects of the disorder, but because potential employers think, erroneously, that people with schizophrenia are unpredictable and dangerous.

Collecting information

Technique of interviewing

The interview serves not only to collect information, but also to establish a therapeutic relationship. Hence details of the approach to the patient are important. These details are described next, but they can only guide readers, who should take every opportunity to watch experienced interviewers at work and to practice under supervision.

Preparing for the interview

Interviews are carried out in many different settings including patients' homes and the wards of a general hospital. The advice that follows cannot be followed completely in every setting but it is, nevertheless, im-

BOX 2.1 **EXAMPLE OF A FORMULATION**

The problem

Mrs AB is a 30-year-old married woman who has been feeling increasingly depressed for 6 weeks and is now unable to cope adequately with the care of her children.

Diagnosis

Depressive disorder   Mrs AB has several typical symptoms of depressive disorder: she wakes unusually early, feels worse in the morning than in the evening, and has lost appetite and libido. She blames herself unreasonably, feels guilty, and does not think that she can recover, though she has no ideas of suicide or of harming the children. None of the findings is incompatible with this diagnosis.

Adjustment disorder   Although Mrs AB has experienced several stressful events, including her husband's recent infidelity, the presence of clear symptoms of a depressive disorder overrule the diagnosis of adjustment disorder.

Personality disorder   There is no evidence for personality disorder. Mrs AB is normally a resilient, caring, and sociable person who is a good mother. Although she experiences premenstrual mood change, she does not have a depressive or cyclothymic personality.

Conclusion   Depressive disorder. Severity, moderate. Suicide risk and risk of harm to the children, both low.

Aetiology

The symptoms were *precipitated* by her husband's infidelity. Although she has not been depressed before, both her mother and sister have had depressive disorders, so it is possible that she is *predisposed* to develop a depressive disorder. The disorder may be *maintained* by continuing quarrels with her husband and concerns about her mother's health.

Management

The pattern of symptoms indicates that Mrs AB should respond to an SSRI antidepressant. Although Mrs AB denies any suicidal ideas or ideas of harming her children, her mental state should be monitored regularly especially during the first few days of treatment because SSRIs occasionally cause increased agitation at this time. Her sister has offered to provide short-term help with the care of the children and Mrs AB is normally a good mother and should be able to take full care of her children when she improves. Her husband regrets his infidelity and is now supportive to his wife. Joint interviews may help to reduce any remaining marital problems. The management plan should be reviewed after a week, and regularly thereafter. To prevent relapse, medication should be continued for about 6 months.

Prognosis

Provided that the marital problems and her mother's health improve, Mrs AB should recover. The possible predisposing factors indicate that she may develop further depressive disorder.

portant to do everything possible to ensure privacy, put the patient at ease, and ensure safety.

Putting the patient at ease

The interview should be carried out in a place where it cannot be overheard and is, as far as possible, free from interruptions. If these requirements are difficult to meet, as in a medical ward, the interview should, if possible, be moved—for example to a side room. Patients should be seated comfortably, with the chairs arranged so that the interviewer sits at an angle to, and no higher than, the patient. Right-handed interviewers generally finds it easier to attend to the patient while making notes if they seat the patient on their left.

Arranging to take notes

Whenever possible, notes should be taken during the interview because attempts to memorize the history and make notes later are time consuming and liable to error. (Exceptions may have to be made when patients are very restless or agitated.) However, at the start of the interview, note taking should be deferred for a few minutes so that patients can feel that they have the undivided attention of the interviewer.

Ensuring safety

Only a very small minority of patients are potentially dangerous. Nevertheless the need for precautions should be considered when there is any possibility of violent behaviour, for example when a disturbed patient is to be assessed in an accident and emergency department. When appropriate, precautions should be taken as described below in the section on special problems.

Starting the interview

Interviewers should welcome the patient, introduce themselves by name, and if necessary explain their role (e.g. medical student). They should greet anyone who is accompanying the patient, and explain how long they can expect to wait, and whether they too will be interviewed. It is usually better to see the patient first, on his own, and interview any accompanying person later. Exceptions are made if that person has to leave early, and when the patient is unable to give an account of the problems. Interviewers should explain briefly:

- how long the interview will last;
- in general terms, how it will procede;
- the need to take notes;
- the confidentialty of these notes but the need to share certain information with others directly involved in treatment.

Interviews are more likely to be effective if the interviewer:

- appears relaxed and unhurried—even when time is short;
- maintains appropriate eye contact and does not appear engrossed in the case notes;
- is alert to non-verbal as well as to verbal cues of distress and shows an understanding of patients' feelings;
- attends to emotional problems and makes empathic responses to indications of distress, e.g. 'and that was very upsetting';

- intervenes appropriately when patients are over-talkative, have departed from or avoided the subject, or are unduly discursive;
- has a systematic but flexible plan.

The interviewer *begins with a general question* to encourage patients to express their problems in their own words: for example, 'tell me about your problem' or 'tell me what you have noticed wrong'.

During the reply, interviewers should notice whether their patients are calm, or distressed despite their efforts to put them at ease. If the latter, interviewers should try to find the nature of the difficulty and attempt to overcome it (see problems with interviewing, p. 20).

Continuing the interview

Having elicited the complaints, the next step is to enquire into them systematically. In doing this the interviewer should as far as possible *avoid closed and leading questions*. (A **closed question** allows only a brief answer, usually 'yes' or 'no'; a **leading question** suggests the answer. 'Do you wake early?' is a closed leading question: 'at what time do you wake?' is an open, non-leading question.) If there is no alternative to a leading question, it should be followed by a request for an example. Thus, the only way to ask about an important symptom of schizophrenia is to use the leading closed question 'have you ever felt that your actions were being controlled by another person?' If the answer is yes, the interviewer should ask for one or more examples of the experience, and should conclude that the symptom is present only if the examples are convincing. Leading questions can be avoided by prompting the patient indirectly by:

- repeating what the patient has said, but in a questioning tone, e.g. 'feeling low…?';
- restating the problem in other words, e.g. (after a patient has spoken of sadness) 'you say you have been feeling low';
- asking for clarification, e.g. 'could you say a little more about that?'

It is important to *establish when each symptom and problem began* as well as if and when it became worse or better. If a patient find it difficult to remember these dates, it may be possible to relate the events to others that are more easily remembered, such as a birthday or a public holiday.

As the interview progresses, the interviewer has a number of tasks:

1. *To help patients to talk freely* by nodding or saying, for example, 'go on' or 'tell me more about that' or 'is there more to say?'

2. *To keep patients to relevant topics* in part with non-verbal cues such as leaning forward or nodding to encourage the patient to continue with the topic.

3. *To make systematic enquiries* but without asking so many questions that other—unanticipated—aspects of the problem are not volunteered.

4. *To check understanding* by summarizing key points.

5. *To select questions according to the emerging possibilities* regarding diagnoses, causes, and plans of action. The choice of questions is modified progressively as additional information is gathered.

As explained above, *interviewing is an active and selective process, not the asking of the same set of questions to every patient.* The shorter the time available for the interview, the more important it is to proceed in this way. Occasionally the patient is so disturbed that it is impossible to follow an orderly sequence of questioning. In such cases it is even more important to keep the diagnostic possibilities in mind so that the most relevant questions are selected and the most relevant observations carried out.

Ending the interview

Before ending the interview, the interviewer should summarize the main points and ask whether the patient has anything to add to the account that he has given.

Interviewing relatives and other informants

What informants can contribute In every case informants can provide useful information about the patient's personality. Their information is essential when the patient is unable or unwilling to reveal important information, for example when the patient:

◆ is unaware of the extent of his abnormality (e.g. a demented patient);

◆ knows the extent of the problem but is unwilling to reveal it (e.g. a patient with an alcohol problem);

◆ cannot say reliably when the disorder started.

The need for consent With few exceptions, the patient's consent should be obtained before interviewing informants. The interviewer should explain that the interview is to obtain information that will help to decide how best to help the patient, and that information given to the interviewer by the patient will not be revealed to the informant unless the patient has agreed. The *exceptions to the need for consent* are when patients cannot provide an adequate history because they are: (i) confused, stuporose, extremely retarded, or mute; or (ii) extremely agitated or violent (A further exception is made for children, see p. 277.)

Arranging the interview It is generally better to interview relatives or other informants after the interview with the patient. It is usually better to see them away from the patient so that they can speak freely: for example a wife may be reluctant to talk in her husband's presence about his heavy drinking. The purpose of the interview should be explained because relatives sometimes expect that they are about to be blamed for the patient's problems, or asked to give help that they are not prepared to provide.

Confidentiality Unless informants have agreed to disclosure, the interviewer should not tell the patient what they have said. This rule applies even when the relative has spoken of something that the interviewer needs to discuss with the patient, such as heavy drinking that has been denied. If the relative has refused permission for the information to be disclosed, the interviewer can only try to help the patient reveal the information himself. In view of this and because patients may ask to see their case notes, it is better to record the interview with the informant on a separate sheet.

The informants' concerns As well as asking for information about the patient, the interviewer should find out how the informants view the problem, how it affects them, and what help they are seeking.

Helping the informants When the interview with informants reveals that they too have emotional problems, either as a result of the patient's illness or for other reasons, the interviewer should either offer help or assist them to obtain help from another professional.

Intreviewing patients from another culture

If the patient and the interviewer do not speak a common language, it is obvious that an interpreter will be needed. However, language is not the only problem in such cases, cultural differences are also important and interpreters may share the patient's language but not their culture. Information about culture is important for several reasons.

1. *Cultural beliefs* may explain why certain events are experienced as more stressful or shameful than they would be in the host culture.

2. *Roles* within the family may differ from those in the host culture.

3. *Distress may be shown in different symptoms*. In some cultures, distress is often expressed in physical rather than mental symptoms.

4. *Distress may be shown in different behaviours*. In some cultures, unrestrained displays of emotion that would suggest illness in the host culture, are socially acceptable ways of expressing distress.

5. *Cultural beliefs* may include ideas that would suggest delusional thinking in the host culture, such as being under the influence of spells cast by neighbours.

6. *Expectations about treatment* may be based on experiences of very different traditions of medical care.

These and other differences can be understood best by talking with someone from the patient's cultural group.

Choosing the interpreter Ideally the interpreter should be a member of a health profession who knows both the language and the culture of the patient. This ideal arrangement is not easy to achieve and often the only available interpreter is a family member. Although a family member will know both the language and the culture, patients may not talk freely about personal matters through such a person, especially when the patient is female and the interpreter is male, and when there are problems within the family.

Some problems with interviewing

Patients who appear anxious or angry

The first step is to discover the reason for the anxiety or anger. The cause might be, for example, that the patient has come to the interview reluctantly, and at the insistence of another person (e.g. when there is an alcohol problem). Some patients are worried that their employers could learn about the interview. Once the problem is understood, appropriate reassurance usually reduces the distress enough for the interview to proceed.

Patients who appear confused

Sometimes the patient's initial responses are muddled and confused. This problem can be caused by *anxiety*, *low intelligence*, or *cognitive impairment*—the latter due to delirium or dementia. If cognitive impairment seems possible, brief tests of concentration and memory should be carried out (see p. 28). If the results are abnormal, it is usually better to interview an informant before continuing with the patient.

Patients who could be violent

If the risk of violence seems low, it may be enough to make sure that someone else is available to help and knows where and when the interview is taking place, and how long it is expected to last. If the risk is thought to be greater, the interviewer should:

◆ *identify a way of calling help*—check for an alarm button in the interview room and if there is none, arrange another way of calling for help;

◆ *ensure an escape route*—arrange that neither the patient nor any physical obstruction is between them and the exit;

◆ remove anything that could be used as a weapon or hide it.

And while the interview is taking place the interviewer should:

◆ watch for signs of increasing anger (see p. 25);

◆ *avoid any actions that might provoke anger*, such as approaching too close, prolonging eye contact, or avoiding eye contact altogether;

◆ stay calm.

Psychiatric history

Basic structure of the psychiatric history

As explained above (see p. 15), the amount of detail and the focus of the psychiatric history varies from case to case but the basic aims are the same—it is not necessary to learn a separate interview for each condition. These common aims are reflected in the basic structure of the interview shown in Table 2.1. When time is short, background and personality can be covered only in outline but even a little information can be useful when planning immediate management.

Brief history for screening

In primary care and general hospital medicine, when a patient complains of symptoms of physical illness it is often appropriate to check for evidence of a psychiatric

TABLE 2.1   The basic psychiatric history
The problem
Other symptoms or abnormal behaviours
Previous psychiatric disorder
Any current medication
Use of alcohol and drugs
Background and present circumstances of the patient
Personality

disorder since this may be present as the cause or a consequence of the symptoms. For this purpose, a brief screening interview is required to detect any symptoms and problems that have not been complained of spontaneously. The usual screening questions deal with: general well-being, anxiety, depression, memory, and the use of alcohol and drugs. The following points are considered under each heading:

1. **Well-being**: fatigue, irritability, poor concentration, poor sleep, and a feeling of being under pressure.

2. **Anxiety**: tension, sweating frequency, palpitations, and repeated worrying thoughts. If replies are positive, go on to systematic questions about anxiety disorders (p. 75).

3. **Depression**: persistent low mood, low energy, loss of interest, loss of confidence, and hopelessness. If these questions are answered positively, go on to questions concerning depressive disorder (including suicidal ideas) (see p. 108).

4. **Memory**: difficulty in recalling recent events; if difficulties are reported or suspected, use simple tests of memory (see p. 37).

5. **Alcohol and drugs**: the extent of use of alcohol and drugs is noted, and in appropriate cases the CAGE (see p. 192) or Alcohol Use Disorders Identification Test (see p. 190) are used.

If symptoms or problems are revealed by this screening, the interviewer goes on to take an appropriate history.

History taking in an emergency

When urgent action is required, the interview has to be brief, focused on the basic points set out above, and effective in leading to a provisional diagnosis and a plan of immediate action. The information needed includes, at the least, the following points:

- the *presenting problem* in terms of symptoms or behaviours, together with their onset, course, and present severity;

- *other relevant symptoms*, with their onset, course, and severity;

- *stressful circumstances* around the time of onset and at the present time;

- *previous and current physical or mental disorders* and how the patient coped with them;

- current medication;

- the *use of alcohol and drugs*;

- *family and personal history*, covered with a few salient questions;

- *social circumstances*, and the possibilities of support;

- *personality*—this is valuable although it may be difficult to obtain this information in the circumstances of an emergency.

Throughout, the interviewer should think which questions need to be answered at the time and which can be deferred. If the patient has had previous treatment, efforts should be made to contact a professional who knows the patient. However short the time, the patient should feel that he has the interviewer's undivided attention and an opportunity to say everything that is important.

Items in a full psychiatric history

The structure of the full psychiatric history is shown in Box 2.2. Readers may find it helpful to copy this page and refer to it when they interview their first patients. As explained already, the amount of detail required in a particular case varies with the diagnostic possibilities of the case and the time available. Experienced interviewers focus on the most relevant items but students should practice the full history until they are confident in its use, before they learn the more selective approach. The following account explains some important points concerning the items in Box 2.2.

History of the presenting condition
The problems
The interviewer should allow patients adequate time to talk spontaneously before asking questions, otherwise they may not reveal all their problems. For example, a patient who begins by describing depression may also have a marital problem that she is hesitant to reveal. If the interviewer asks further questions about depression as soon as this is mentioned, the marital problem may not be revealed. To avoid overlooking problems, when patients have finished speaking spontaneously the interviewer should summarize the problems that have been revealed, and ask if there are any others. The interviewer's subsequent questions are designed to determine a number of points:

1. The **nature of the problem**. For example, a patient who complains of worrying excessively could be describing anxiety, obsessional symptoms, or intrusive thoughts occurring in a depressive disorder.

2. The **severity of the problem**.

3. The **distress** caused by the problem.

BOX 2.2   THE PSYCHIATRIC HISTORY

Name, age, and address of the patient; name of any informants, and their relationship to the patient.

History of present condition

- Patient's description of the problem
- Details of the problem including its severity
- Other relevant problems and symptoms
- Onset and course of problems and symptoms

Family history

- Parents: age (now or at death), occupation, personality, and relationship with the patient
- Similar information about siblings
- Social position; atmosphere of the home
- Mental disorder in other members of the (extended) family, and abuse of alcohol and drugs

Personal history

- Mother's pregnancy and the birth
- Early development
- Childhood separations, emotional problems, and illnesses
- Schooling and higher education
- Occupations

- Sexual relationships
- Menstrual history
- Marriage and other partnerships
- Children
- Social circumstances
- Forensic history

Past illness

- Past medical history
- Past psychiatric history

Personality

- Relationships
- Leisure activities
- Prevailing mood
- Character
- Attitudes and standards
- Habits

Drugs, alcohol, tobacco

---

4. The **interference with day-to-day activities** (relevant to disablement).

5. The **onset** and **course**, whether unchanging, progressing, fluctuating, or improving.

6. Any **factors making it worse or better**.

Problems and symptoms may start suddenly or gradually, and may appear spontaneously or be in reponse to stressful events. Their course may be continuous or intermittent; and severity may change gradually or stepwise.

Other problems and symptoms

The interviewer should now enquire about the symptoms and problems that he judges relevant and that have not yet been volunteered by the patient. These further enquiries are guided by the interviewer's knowledge of the disorders in which the presenting symptoms and problems can occur (this information will be found in subsequent chapters). For example, if the presenting problem is poor sleep, the interviewer would ask about the symptoms of depressive and anxiety disorders, and about pain, all of which can cause insomnia. The *date of onset* and *sequence* of the various symptoms should be noted, for example whether obsessional symptoms began before or after depressive symptoms (this information is relevant to diagnosis and treatment, see pp. 86–7). The sequence of problems is similarly important; for example, whether abuse of alcohol began before or after marital difficulties. A note should be made of any *treatment already received*.

Family history

This part of the history concerns the patient's father, mother, siblings, and other relatives. Enquiries about the patient's spouse or partner, and children are made later. The family history is important for four reasons:

1. Psychiatric disorder in other family members may point to *genetic causes*.

2. Past events in the family, such as the divorce of parents, are the background to the patient's *psychological development*.

3. Past events in the family may help to *explain the patient's concerns*. For example the discovery that a brother died of a brain tumour may help to explain a patient's seemingly excessive concerns about headaches.

4. Current events in the family may be *stressful*.

A useful introduction to this part of the enquiry is: 'I would like to ask about the family into which you were born. Let us start with your father—is he still alive?' If the father is alive, his age, state of health, and job are recorded. (The latter is of interest mainly as a guide to the circumstances of the family, see below.) If the father has died, the cause of death, and his age and that of the patient at the time of the death should be determined. The father's personality and relationship with the patient can be elicited by asking 'what was your father like when you were a child?', 'what is he like now?', 'how did you get on when you were a child?', and 'how do you get on now?' Similar enquiries are made about the mother, siblings, and other important figures in the patient's early life, such as a stepfather or a grandmother living with the patient.

The amount of detail required varies from case to case. It is unlikely to be profitable to spend time in detailed enquiries about the childhood of an elderly patient seeking help for poor memory, but it could be highly relevant to obtain this information about a young adult whose behaviour is unusual.

Personal history

The aims in taking the personal history are to describe and understand the following:

1. Any *stressful circumstances*, and to find out how the patient reacted to them.

2. The *life story* including any influences that help to explain the patient's personality, concerns, and preferences. For example, sexual abuse in childhood may partly explain a woman's sexual difficulties in adult life; and being the unwanted child of an unaffectionate mother may partly explain a man's fear of rejection.

3. The *present circumstances* of the patient.

The amount of detail required to achieve these aims varies from patient to patient.

Maternal health during pregnancy and the circumstances of the patient's delivery

For adult patients, this information is relevant mainly to learning disability. (For history taking in child psychiatry, see pp. 277–8.) Information from the patient is often unreliable and should be checked whenever possible with the mother or with hospital records made at the time of the event. In most other cases, it is necessary to enquire only about any major deviations from the normal.

Early development

The comments above about the relevance and reliability of information about pregnancy and delivery apply equally to developmental milestones, which are seldom important except when the patient is a child or an adult with learning disability. A note should be made of any *prolonged separation* from either parent for whatever reason. Since the effects of separation vary considerably, it is important to find out whether the patient was distressed at the time and for how long. If possible, this information should be checked with the parents. Serious and prolonged *childhood illnesses* may have affected the patient's emotional development. Diseases of the central nervous system in this period may be relevant to learning disability.

Educational history

The history of school and, if applicable, university education gives a general indication of intelligence and achievements, and contributes to an understanding of personality. As well as academic achievement, enquiries are made about friendships, sociability, aggressive behaviour, bullying, leadership, and relationships with fellow students and with teachers.

Occupational history

The occupational history throws light on abilities and achievements, and on personality. Frequent changes of job, failure to gain promotion, or arguments with senior staff, may reflect aspects of personality (there are, of course, many other reasons for these events).

Sexual relationships

This part of the history includes the success and failure of relationships, as well as sexual preferences and behaviour. Detailed enquiries are not needed in every case, but when they are relevant the interviewer should be able to make them sympathetically, objectively, and without embarrassment. Common sense judgement and a knowledge of clinical syndromes will indicate how much to ask. If the patient is sexually active, questions about contraception may be relevant. Detailed questions about sexual preferences and behaviour may be relevant when one of the problems is a sexual one; in other cases it is usually enough to ask more generally whether there are any sexual problems.

Women should be asked about *menstrual problems* appropriate to their age, including symptoms of the premenstrual syndrome and the menopause.

History of marriage and other partnerships

The interviewer should asks whether the partnership is happy; how long it has lasted; about the partner's work and personality; and about the sex, age, parentage, health, and development of any children. Similar enquiries are made about any previous partnership(s). If the partnership is unhappy, further questions should be asked about the nature and causes of this unhappiness; how the couple came together; and any periods of separation or plans for future separation or divorce. These enquiries may also throw light on the patient's personality which may be relevant to the management plan

Social circumstances

Questions should be asked about *living arrangements.* Potentially relevant enquiries include the size and quality of the patient's home; whether it is owned or rented; who else lives with the patient; and how these people relate to one another, and to the patient. Ask also whether the patient has any *financial problems.*

Forensic history

The forensic history concerns behaviour that breaks the law. It is important in all cases of alcohol or drug misuse; in other cases common sense should be used to judge its relevance. If the patient has a criminal record, note the charges and the penalties, and find out whether other such acts have gone undetected.

Past illnesses

Medical and psychiatric illnesses should be asked about in every case.

Personality

Personality assessment is discussed more fully in Chapter 4 and only salient points will be mentioned here. Enquiries should begin by asking patients to describe their personality. Subsequent questions are concerned with education, work, social relationships, leisure activities, prevailing mood, character, attitudes and standards, and habits. Whenever possible, an informant should be interviewed since few people can give a wholly objective account of their own personality. Sometimes, the interviewer's impressions of the patient formed during the interview are useful, but these impressions can be misleading especially when the patient is very distressed or suffering from a psychiatric disorder. General practitioners are able to build up a picture of their patients' personalities over years of occasional medical contacts. This information is valuable and should be passed on if the patient is referred to a psychiatrist.

Alcohol and drug use

These items are sometimes recorded under 'habits' in the section on personality but it is more logical to note them separately.

Mental state examination

In taking the history, the interviewer will have learnt about the patient's symptoms up to the time of the consultation. The components of the mental state examination are listed in Box 2.3, and are explained further in this section. Often the symptoms on the day of the interview are no different from those described in the recent past, in which case the mental state overlaps with the history. However, the symptom enquiry in the mental state examination is generally more systematic than in the history. Also, it is important to have a record of the mental state at the time of the interview to compare with that recorded after treatment has been started.

Students should at first carry out a complete mental state examination with every patient. With increasing experience, they will become able to focus on items judged from the history to be of particular relevance. Readers may find it useful to refer to the descriptions of symptoms in Chapter 1 while reading about the mental state examination. (The few uncommon signs and symptoms not described there are described in the corresponding chapter of *The Shorter Oxford Textbook of Psychiatry*—most are uncommon symptoms of schizophrenia.) Mental state examination is a practical skill that can be learnt only by observing experienced interviewers and by practising under supervision. The following account can assist the reader with this training but cannot replace it.

Appearance and behaviour

Much can be learnt from general appearance, facial expression, posture, voluntary or involuntary movements, and social behaviour.

General appearance includes physique, hair, make-up, and clothing. Manic patients may dress incongruously in brightly coloured or oddly assorted clothes. Signs of *self-neglect* include a dirty unkempt appearance and stained, crumpled clothing. Self-neglect suggests alco-

BOX 2.3 EXAMINATION OF MENTAL

Appearance and behaviour

+ General appearance
+ Facial expression
+ Posture
+ Movements
+ Social behaviour

Speech

+ Rate
+ Amount
+ Continuity

Mood

+ Prevailing mood and associated symptoms
+ Variations of mood
+ Appropriateness of mood

Depersonalization and derealization

Thinking

+ Preoccupations
+ Obsessional and compulsive symptoms
+ Delusions

Perception

+ Illusions
+ Hallucinations

Cognitive function

+ Orientation (time, place, person)
+ Attention and concentration (digit span, serial 7s)
+ Memory (name and address, remote personal events)
+ Estimate of intelligence

Insight

holism, drug addiction, dementia, or schizophrenia. An appearance of *weight loss* is important in psychiatry as in general medicine, suggesting especially physical illness, anorexia nervosa, depressive disorder, or chronic anxiety.

Facial expression Turning down of the corners of the mouth and vertical furrows in the brow suggest *depression*. Horizontal furrows on the brow, wide palpebral fissures, and dilated pupils suggest *anxiety*. An unchanging 'wooden' expression may result from a *parkinsonian syndrome*, either primary or caused by antipsychotic drugs.

Posture may also give indications of prevailing mood. A depressed patient characteristically sits with shoulders hunched, and with the head and eyes cast downwards. An anxious patient typically sits upright, with the head erect and the hands gripping the chair.

Movement Manic patients are overactive, restless, and move rapidly. Depressed patients are inactive and move slowly. Rarely, a depressed patient becomes completely immobile and mute, a condition known as *stupor*. Anxious or agitated patients are restless, and sometimes tremulous. Any involuntary movements should be noted, including tics, choreiform movements, dystonia, or tardive dyskinesia.

Social behaviour Manic patients are disinhibited, and may break social conventions, for example by being unduly familiar. Some demented and some schizophrenic patients are disinhibited, while others are withdrawn and preoccupied. In describing these behaviours, a clear description of what is done or not done is more useful than general terms like 'disinhibited' or 'bizarre'.

Signs of impending violence include restlessness, clenched fists, intrusion into the interviewer's 'personal space', and a raised voice. Only a small minority of psychiatric patients are violent, but interviewers should be alert to the possibility, for example among intoxicated patients in an accident and emergency department.

Summary Relevant features should be summarized in a few phrases that give a clear picture to someone who has not met the patient. For example, 'a tall, gaunt, stooping, and dishevelled man with a sad countenance who looks much older than his 40 years'.

Speech

How patients speak comes under this heading; the thoughts they express are recorded later. Depressed patients speak more slowly than usual; manic patients speak faster. Depressed patients speak less than usual; manic patients speak more. Occasionally a patient does not speak at all (**mutism**). Abnormalities of the *continuity* of speech should be noted, including any sudden interruptions, rapid shifts of topic, and lack of logical thread (pointers to thought disorders are discussed below).

Mood
Prevailing mood

As noted above, the first clues to mood are often in expression and posture. Questions should be asked about the prevailing mood and the symptoms associated with particular mood states. Questioning begins with an enquiry such as: 'how are your spirits?' or 'what is your mood like?' If a **depressed** mood is reported, the associated symptoms may include a feeling of being ready to cry, lack of interest and enjoyment, and pessimistic thoughts, including thoughts of suicide.

When **anxiety** is reported, associated symptoms include palpitations, dry mouth, tremor, sweating, and worrying thoughts (see pp. 75–6 for a full list).

When **elevated mood** is reported, associated symptoms include excessive self-confidence, grandiose plans, and an inflated assessment of the person's own ability (see p. 101 for a full list). These symptoms have, of course, to be elicited indirectly, for example by asking the patient about his plans and his assessment of his abilities.

Thoughts of suicide should be asked about in stages, for example: 'have you felt that you have lost hope for the future?', 'have you thought life is not worth living?', 'have you wished you could die?', 'have you thought of ending your life?', 'have you thought how you might do this?' Some interviewers are reluctant to ask about suicide, in case the questions should suggest the idea. Questions of this kind do not suggest suicide to people who have no suicidal inclination, and they should be asked whenever relevant.

Variations in mood

Fluctuations of mood may be greater than normal—**labile** mood—with dejection giving way quickly to normal mood or elation, and vice versa; or less than normal—that is **blunted** or **flattened**.

Appropriateness of mood

Normally mood and thinking go together: a sad person thinks of sad things, and an elated person thinks of happy or grandiose things. Sometimes this linkage is lost, so that, for example, a person appears cheerful while describing sad events. This phenomenon, which is called **incongruity of mood**, is sometimes observed in schizophrenia (see p. 121).

Depersonalization and derealization
These symptoms are described on p. 3.

Thinking
Preoccupations
Preoccupations are thoughts that recur frequently but can be put out of mind by an effort of will. Some preoccupations are noticed during history taking; others may be revealed by asking 'what sort of things do you worry about?', 'what sort of thoughts occupy your mind?' Preoccupations are particularly important in three conditions: (i) **depressive disorders**, where preoccupations about suicide should be explored carefully (see p. 172); (ii) **anxiety disorders**, where preoccupations may prolong the disorder (see p. 74); and (iii) **sexual disorders** where preoccupations may influence behaviour (see p. 74).

Obsessional and compulsive symptoms
Obsessional thoughts can be asked about with the question 'do any thoughts keep coming repeatedly into your mind, even when you try hard to get rid of them?' Patients who reply yes, should be asked for examples. Patients are often ashamed of their obsessional thoughts (e.g. those with aggressive or sexual themes), so questioning needs to be sympathetic and patient. The interviewer should make certain that patients regard the thoughts as their own, because some schizophrenic patients have similar intrusive thoughts that they believe to have been implanted from outside (thought insertion, see p. 8).

Compulsive rituals Although not disorders of thinking, rituals are usually recorded with obsessional phenomena. The following questions are useful: 'do you ever have to repeat actions over and over, which most people would do only once?' or 'do you have to go on repeating the same action when you know this is unnecessary?'

Delusions

Often the first indication of the presence of delusions is during history taking, either from the patient or from an informant. When there is no such indication, judgement should be used about whether to enquire about delusions, because the questions may antagonize patients who have come for help for another problem. Questions should be asked whenever there is evidence of a *severe depressive disorder*, when *schizophrenia* enters the differential diagnosis, or in cases of doubt. It is often difficult to elicit delusions during mental state examination because the patient does not regard them as abnormal. A good way of starting the enquiry is to ask for for an explanation of any unusual statements, unpleasant experiences, or unusual events that the patient has mentioned. For example, a patient may say that his headaches started when his neighbours caused him trouble; when asked why the neighbours should do this, he may say they are conspiring to harm him. Patients often hide delusions, and the interviewer needs to be alert to evasions, vague replies, or other hints that information is being withheld.

Having discovered an unusual belief, the interviewer has to decide a number of things:

1. *Is the belief true.* Some beliefs are clearly false; for example, that persecutors are damaging the patient's brain by beaming radiowaves on him. Other beliefs need to be checked—for example, that neighbours are mounting a whispering campaign against the patient.

2. *How strongly beliefs are held.* Considerable tact is required when finding out. The patient should feel that he is having a fair hearing, and that the interviewer's response is enquiring, not argumentative or dismissive. The interviewer should question the reasons for the beliefs gently but persistently.

3. *Whether the beliefs are culturally determined*, and accepted by others sharing the patient's cultural background or religious beliefs. In some cultures belief in evil forces or witchcraft are widespread. Any doubt can usually be resolved by finding another person from the same religion or culture, and asking whether the patient's ideas are held by others from the same background.

Delusions of *thought broadcasting*, *thought insertion*, *thought withdrawal*, or *control* can usually be elicited only by asking direct questions. Since their presence strongly suggests schizophrenia, it is essential to check any positive answer by asking for examples. Appropriate questions include: 'do you ever think that other people can tell what you are thinking, even though you have not told them?' or 'do you ever think that thoughts have been put into your mind?' Other kinds of delusion are described on pp. 7–8.

Perception
Illusions

Illusions may come to notice when the history is taken, or when the patient is being observed, for example in a medical ward. Visual illusions can be elicited with a question such as 'have you seen anything unusual?' (or frightening if the patient seems afraid). If the answer is positive, the interviewer should attempt to find out whether the experience is based on an actual visual stimulus (e.g. mistaking a shadow for a threatening person).

Hallucinations

Hallucinations occur in any sensory modality but visual and auditory hallucinations are the most common (see p. 4). Enquiries about hallucinations should be made tactfully, lest patients take offence. With experience, the interviewer will be able to judge when it is safe to omit these enquiries. If enquiry is indicated, questions can be introduced by saying: 'when their nerves are upset some people have unusual experiences'. Questions can then be asked about hearing voices or sounds when there is nobody within earshot, or about seeing unusual things. If patients say yes to either of these questions, they should be asked whether the voice, sound, or vision appeared to be inside or outside the head. When the history makes it relevant, similar questions should be asked about other kinds of hallucinations. If the patients describe **auditory hallucinations**, further questions should be asked, to determine whether they are of a kind which is characteristic of schizophrenia (see p. 123). They should be asked whether they hear sounds or voices; if the latter, whether one voice or more, and whether the voices talk to them or to each other. Hallucinations of voices discussing patients (**third person hallucinations**, see p. 4) should be distinguished from the delusion that people at a distance are discussing them (**delusion of reference**, see p. 7). If the hallucinatory voices talk to the patient (**second person hallucinations**, see p. 4), the interviewer should find out whether they give commands, and if so, what kind of commands, and whether the patient feels impelled to obey them. The reasons for these distinctions are explained in Chapter 9. Other kinds of hallucinations, found mainly in schizophrenia, are described on pp. 4–5.

Orientation

Orientation is assessed by asking about awareness of time, place, and personal identity. Questions begin with the time, day, month, year, and season. In assessing responses to questions about time, the interviewer should remember that many people do not know the exact time of day (although they usually know it to the nearest hour) or the exact date (though they are usually accurate to a few days). Orientation in place is assessed by asking the name of the place in which the interview is being held. If the answer is inaccurate, further questions are asked about the kind of place (e.g. his home, a hospital ward, or a home for the elderly), and the name of the town.

Personal orientation is assessed by asking about other people present (e.g. relatives in the home, or the staff in a hospital ward). If patients give wrong answers, they should be asked about their own identity—their name, occupation, and role in life.

Disorientation is an important symptom that indicates impairment of consciousness.

Attention and concentration

Attention is the ability to focus on the matter in hand. Concentration is the ability to sustain that focus. While taking the history, the interviewer should look out for evidence of impaired attention and concentration. In the mental state examination, specific tests are given. It is usual to begin with the '**serial 7s test**'. The patient is asked to subtract 7 from 100 and then to take 7 from the remainder repeatedly until it is less than 7. The interviewer assesses whether the patient can concentrate on this task. If it seems that poor performance could be due to lack of skill in arithmetic, the patient should be asked to do a simpler subtraction, or to say the months of the year in reverse order. If mistakes are made with these tests, he can be given the less demanding task of naming the days of the week in reverse order. Tests of attention are given before tests of memory because poor attention can lead to poor performance on memory tasks, even when there is no memory defect.

Memory

Difficulties in remembering may come to light during history taking. During the examination of mental state, tests are given to assess immediate, recent, and remote memory. None of these tests is wholly satisfactory and the results should be assessed cautiously and in relation to other information about the patient's ability to remember. If there is doubt, standardized psychological tests can be given by a clinical psychologist.

Assessment of short-term memory Short-term memory is assessed by asking patients to repeat sequences of digits immediately after they have been spoken slowly enough for them to register the digits (the 'digit span test'). An easy sequence of three digits is given first to make sure that patients understand the task. Then a new sequence of four digits is presented. If patients can repeat four digits correctly, sequences of five, six, and seven are given. When patients reach a level at which they cannot repeat the digits, a different sequence of

the same length is given to confirm the finding. Healthy people of average intelligence can repeat seven digits correctly; five or less suggests impairment. (The test involves concentration and therefore—as noted above—cannot be used to assess memory when tests of concentration are abnormal.)

Ability to take in and remember new information is usually assessed by asking the patient to remember a name, an address, and the name of a flower. Common names and addresses likely to be familiar to a patient should be avoided. Patients are asked to reproduce the task straight away to make sure it has been registered correctly, and then asked to remember the information. If the material has not been registered correctly, the task is repeated until there is accurate immediate recall. Other topics are then discussed for 5 minutes, after which recall is tested. Responses should be recorded verbatim and the number of errors noted. A healthy person of average intelligence makes only minor errors in this task.

Memory for recent events is assessed by asking about news items from the last day or two, or about recent events in the patient's life that are known with certainty to the interviewer (do not ask the commonly used question about what the patient had for breakfast unless you know the answer). Questions about news items should be adapted to the patient's interests, and should have been widely reported in the media.

Assessment of long-term memory This can be assessed by asking the patient to recall personal events or well-known public events from some years before. Personal events could be the birth dates of the patient's children or grandchildren (provided these dates are known to the interviewer); public events could be the names of well-known political leaders, sportsmen, or musicians. Awareness of the sequence of events is as important as the recall of individual items.

Observations suggesting memory disorder When a patient is in a general hospital, important information about memory is available from observations made by nurses or other staff. These observations include how rapidly patients learn the daily routine of the ward, and the names of staff and other patients, and whether they forget where they have put things, or cannot find their way about (though the latter may indicate spatial disorientation rather than poor memory). When the patient is at home, relatives may report comparable observations about the patient's ability to learn and remember.

Special tests Among elderly patients, questions about memory do not distinguish well between those who have cerebral pathology and those who do not. For cases of doubt there are standardized ratings of memory for recent personal events, past personal events, and general events, which allow a better assessment of severity. Standardized tests of learning and memory can help also in the diagnosis of organic mental disorder, and can be used for quantitative assessments of the progression of memory disorder. These tests are usually administered by a clinical psychologist (see also Chapter 10). A useful short test of memory and other cognitive functions, the *Mini Mental State Examination*, is given in Appendix 2.1.

Intelligence

During history taking, the interviewer should be alert to the possibility that the person is of low intelligence. If this seems possible and the impression is confirmed during mental state examination, a test of intelligence can be arranged.

Insight

By the end of the history taking and mental state examination, the interviewer should have a provisional estimate of the patient's awareness of the morbid nature of their experiences. Insight is assessed further by asking the patient: (i) about their awareness of the nature of individual symptoms, for example whether extreme feelings of guilt are justified; (ii) whether they believe that they are ill (rather than, say, persecuted by enemies); and (iii) if so, whether they think that the illness is physical or mental, and (iv) whether they think that they need treatment. The answers are important because they suggest how far patients are likely to collaborate with treatment. The answers to all questions should be noted; a summary statement such as 'partial insight' is of little value.

Some difficulties in mental state examination

Apart from the obvious problem of examining patients who speak little or no English—a problem that requires the help of an interpreter—difficulties can arise with patients who are unresponsive, overactive, or confused.

Unresponsive patients

When patients are mute or stuporous (conscious but not speaking or responding in any other way) it is possible only to make observations of behaviour. Nevertheless, these observations can be informative.

Since stuporous patients can sometimes become suddenly violent, it is prudent to be accompanied when examining such a patient. Before deciding that the patient is mute, it is important that the interviewer:

♦ establishes that he is speaking a language that the patient understands;

♦ has allowed adequate time for reply;

♦ has tried a variety of topics;

♦ has found out whether the patient will communicate in writing.

As well as making the observations of behaviour described on pp. 24-5, the interviewer should note whether the patient's eyes are open or closed. If they are open, he should note whether they follow objects, move apparently without purpose, or are fixed. If the eyes are closed, the interviewer should note whether they are opened on request and, if not, whether attempts at opening them are resisted.

Physical examination, including neurological assessment, is essential in all such cases, which should be seen, whenever possible, by a specialist who will look for certain additional, uncommon signs found in catatonic schizophrenia (**waxy flexibility** of muscles and **negativism**, see p. 122). In all such cases it is essential to interview an informant to discover the onset and course of the condition.

Overactive patients

When the patient is overactive (e.g. because of mania) questions have to be limited to a few that seem particularly important, and conclusions have to be based mainly on observations of behaviour and on spontaneous utterances. Sometimes the overactivity has been made worse by attempts at physical restraint. A quiet confident approach by the interviewer may calm the patient enough to allow a more adequate examination.

Patients who appear confused

When patients give the history in a muddled way, and especially when they appear perplexed or frightened, cognitive functions should be tested early in the interview. If consciousness is impaired, try to orientate patients and reassure them, and then start the interview again in a simplified form. In such cases every effort should be made to interview another informant.

Physical examination and special investigations

The extent of the physical examination is decided by considering diagnostic possibilities in the individual case. When there is doubt, a systematic physical examination should be performed. When an organic disorder is suspected, a neurological examination is essential. In selected cases this examination should include assessment of language, constructional apraxias, and agnosias. The methods of examination are described in textbooks of neurology, and are learnt during neurology training. Readers who have not had this training are advised to study the summary of salient points in chapter 2 of *The Shorter Oxford Textbook of Psychiatry*, to consult a textbook of neurology, and to obtain supervised practice of the relevant clinical skills.

Special investigations are chosen according to the patient's symptoms and the diagnostic possibilities. There is no single set of routine investigations appropriate for every patient. Relevant special investigations are discussed in subsequent chapters.

Psychological tests

Psychological assessment requires special training and it is carried out by clinical psychologists.

Tests of intelligence

In most cases it is not necessary to have a precise assessment of intelligence. If a patient seems to be of low intelligence, or if his psychological symptoms could be a reaction to work beyond his intellectual capacity, intelligence tests are essential. In child psychiatry, tests of intelligence are often supplemented by tests of *reading ability*.

Neuropsychological tests

Such tests are available for assessing dysfunction of the frontal or parietal cortex. Although brain imaging methods are generally more useful in diagnosis, neuropsychological tests may be used to follow the progress of the disorder.

Personality tests

These tests are of little value in the assessment of an individual patient, where more can be learnt from the clinical assessment described earlier in this chapter. Personality tests are more often used in research to compare groups of patients.

Rating-scales of behaviour

Rating scales are used in certain cases to follow the progress of a disorder, especially during behavioural treatment (see Chapter 18).

Assessment

Stages of assessment

The stages of a full assessment are shown in Table 2.2. Not every item in the table applies to every case but interviewers should keep all of them in mind as the

TABLE 2.2	Stages of assessment
The problem	
◆ diagnosis	
◆ severity	
◆ disablement	
◆ effects on others	
The risks	
◆ risk of suicide or self-harm	
◆ risk of dangerousness to others	
The person	
◆ personality and life story	
◆ social circumstances	
Aetiology	
Prognosis	
Management	
Ethical issues	

interview progresses. Assessment of disablement may require information that is not available at the first interview, but usually a provisional assessment can be made.

The problem The assessment begins with a summary statement of the problem, for example: a 35-year-old mother of three children complains of depression and is drinking excessively.

Diagnosis and differential diagnosis are considered next. The evidence for and against each diagnosis is assessed and the most likely one is chosen. (The diagnosis of particular disorders is considered in the chapters on clinical syndromes.)

Severity is usually assessed using the broad categories, mild, moderate and severe, though more precise methods are sometimes used, for example the Beck Inventory for depression.

Disablement is assessed in terms of impairment, disability, and handicap (see p. 16).

Effects on others include, for example, the effect of patients' problems on their children, or spouses, as well as the possibility of violence.

Risk of suicide and self-harm is considered in Chapter 13.

Risk to others is considered separately below. (Risk to the interviewer during the assessment was considered on p. 18.)

The ill person

Personality and life story The assessment of personality is described on p. 24. The patient's 'life story' is assessed much as a biographer would do, making commonsense links between previous experiences and present ways of thinking or behaving. For example, a serious suicide attempt following a minor set-back may become understandable as the last stage in a sequence of failures and frustrated hopes.

Assessing the circumstances This part of the assessment is concerned with the patient's way of life, including the available support from family, friends, and neighbours.

Aetiology Possible causes are divided into predisposing, precipitating, and maintaining factors (see pp. 40–1). Of these, maintaining factors, such as stressful events, are usually the most relevant to the plan of management since it may be possible to modify them. A life chart is a useful way of assessing the causal role of stressful events (see recording information, p. 32).

Management and prognosis The assessment of prognosis and management of particular disorders are described in subsequent chapters on clinical syndromes. The management plan should assess the likely value of drug treatment, psychological treatment, and social measures. It should also consider the needs of others, especially any children cared for by the patient.

Assessment of risk of harm to others

Few psychiatric patients present a risk to other people. Nevertheless it is important to be prepared to assess such problems. The assessment of risk of harm to others is based on four kinds of information:

1. Personal factors.

2. Factors related to the disorder and its treatment.

3. Factors in the mental state.

4. Situational factors.

The first and last of these categories are relevant also to the assessment of patients who do not have a psychiatric disorder but may be dangerous, for example some patients attending emergency departments.

It is important to obtain information not only from the patient but also, whenever possible, from other sources such as from friends and relatives, medical records, and social services. Also, as well as factors that increase risk, account is taken of any obvious *protective factors* that could decrease risk such as a supportive relationship. Several factors are considered under each heading (Table 2.3).

TABLE 2.3 Risk factors for harm to others

Personal factors
- Previous violence to others***
- Antisocial, impulsive, or irritable personality traits
- Male and young
- Recent life crisis
- Poor social network
- Divorced/separated
- Unemployed
- Social instability

Illness-related risk factors
- Substance abuse*
- Treatment resistance
- Stopped treatment recently
- Poor compliance or engagement with services

Factors in the mental state
- Specific threats to a person to whom the patient has access**
- Planning violence**
- Thoughts of violence to others
- Hallucinations commanding violence to others
- Suicidal ideas in a severely depressed patient (see p. 100)
- Paranoid delusions
- Delusional jealousy
- Irritability, anger, hostility, suspiciousness

Situational factors
- Ready availability of weapons**
- Confrontataion or provocation by others
- Repeat of situations that provoked previous violence

The starred entries on Table 2.3 are considered to be the *strongest predictors of dangerousness*. Of these the most powerful is a record of *past violence*. The entry concerning *suicidal ideas* refers to the occasional killing, usually of one or more members of the close family, by a person with a severe depressive disorder (see p. 100). *Situational factors* are highly important. Actual or perceived confrontation by others may trigger violence, and so may the return to a situation where violence has been expressed in the past. The predictors listed in the table are usually thought of as acting cumulatively but there is no reliable mathematical formula into which they can be entered, and the final judgement depends on clinical experience. For this reason, when risk is judged to be increased it is often appropriate to discuss the case with an experienced colleague.

Risk management plans

Risk assessment is the first stage of a risk management plan, which includes any steps that can be taken to reduce the risk or to contain it. Possible interventions depend on the nature of the risk factors that have been identified. They include case monitoring, treatment of psychiatric disorder, provision of extra support in the community, compulsory admission to hospital, and, in some cases, involvement of the police.

The risk management plan should be agreed with any others involved in the patient's management. If a person is identified as being at high risk of being harmed by the patient, the need to warn this person must be considered carefully because the need to warn that person may override patient confidentiality. In such a case the advice of an experienced colleague and medicolegal advice should be sought. Risk management plans should be *reviewed frequently*.

Ethical issues

Ethical issues should be considered in the course of every assessment. In the brief account that follows, we assume that readers are already familiar with the general approach to medical ethics. Those who are not should consult a textbook of medical ethics. The ethical problems encountered in psychiatry are assessed, as in other branches of medicine, using three general principles: (i) the patient's right for autonomy; (ii) the doctor's duty to do good and avoid harm; and (iii) the requirement to act fairly and justly (particularly relevant to the allocation of resources). These principles are applied to individual problems in three ways:

1. **Utilitarian reasoning**: that is by examining the consequences to the patient and to others of different courses of action.

2. **Casuistry**: that is by comparing the current problem with others that appear similar.

3. **Rules**: a few problems are decided by applying absolute rules, for example the rule that therapists shall not exploit their patients sexually or in other ways.

Table 2.4 lists some ethical issues that are encountered commonly by non-specialists when dealing with psychiatric problems. The problems are considered on the pages given in the table. Issues of confidentiality, which are particularly relevant to assessment, are summarized in this chapter—see Box 2.4.

TABLE 2.4   Some ethical problems in psychiatry
Confidentiality
◆ Confidentiality (see p. 33)
◆ Confidentiality in group psychotherapy (see p. 265)
◆ Confidentiality in community psychiatry (see p. 268)
Conflicts of interest
◆ Assessment of risk to others (see p. 32)
◆ Conflict of interest in care in the community (see p. 268)
Consent to treatment
◆ Consent (see p. 154)
◆ Advance directives (see p. 218)
◆ Involuntary treatment (see p. 129)
Problems of psychiatry and medicine
◆ Patients who refuse essential medical treatment (see p. 154)
◆ Genetic counselling (see p. 157)
◆ Problems related to factitious disorder (see p. 96)
Problems of resource allocation (see p. 268)
Special problems
◆ Problems related to the care of the elderly (see p. 218)
◆ Problems related to disorders of sexuality and gender (see p. 206)
◆ Imposing values in psychotherapy (see p. 263)
◆ Problems in the treatment of children and adolescents (see p. 299)
◆ Problems in the care of people with learning disability (see p. 315)

Recording information

Case notes

Good case notes are important in psychiatry, as in other branches of medicine, for both clinical and medicolegal reasons. Case notes are not only an *aide-mémoire* for the writer but are also an essential source of information for any other person called to help the patient in an emergency. The results of the assessment and the progress notes should be recorded with this purpose in mind. Since patients may ask to read their notes, any information that informants have refused to make available to the patient should be recorded on a separate sheet.

Problem lists

A problem list is a useful way of summarizing a complicated case. It is particularly useful in cases with both medical and psychiatric aspects, and is therefore suitable for use in primary care and in general hospital

BOX 2.4 ETHICAL ISSUES OF CONFIDENTIALITY

General rule   Confidentiality is important in psychiatry because patients often reveal highly personal information. Doctors have a general duty to maintain confidentiality unless the patient gives informed consent to disclosure.

Exceptions to the rule   This general duty is overridden in two circumstances: (i) in response to a court order; or (ii) when disclosure may assist the prevention, detection, or prosecution of a major crime such as a serious assault or the abuse of children. In both circumstances every effort should be made to obtain the patient's informed consent to disclosure. If despite this consent is withheld, the case should be discussed with an experienced colleague and the need for medicolegal advice should be considered.

Confidentiality and the treatment team   Psychiatric treatment often involves not only the interviewer but also other members of a treatment team. To do their job effectively, these members need at least a part of the information given by the patient to the interviewer. Interviewers should explain the need to share information and seek the patient's agreement to this way of working. The other members of the team must, of course, respect the confidence of the information. The sharing of information with other members of the team for the purpose of providing best treatment is not generally viewed by the law as a breach of confidence. Problems may arise when the treatment plan involves other professions whose members may have slightly different practices about confidentiality. If these problems seem possible, they should be discussed with the patient and appropriate consent should be sought.

Consent to obtaining further information   Generally, patients' consent should be obtained before eliciting information from other people. The exception to this rule is when patients who are unable to give an account of themselves are unable to give consent to seeking information from others, and the information is needed to assist them. The same considerations apply when information is given to relatives or others, concerning a patient who is unable to give consent.

medical practice. The problem list makes the stages of treatment clear to anyone who sees the patient when the original doctor is not available. It is also a reminder of times when progress should be reviewed.

An example of a problem list is shown in Table 2.5, together with a vignette of the case to which the list refers. In the example, the patient's response to antide- pressants is to be checked weekly for 3 weeks by the family doctor, and then reviewed; the mother's progress is to be reviewed in 3 weeks and future man- agement is to be discussed with the geriatrician. An appointment is to be made with a clinical psychologist for treatment of agoraphobia, and the progress of this arrangement is to be checked in 3 months. The

TABLE 2.5   Case study and problem list

Case study

A 54-year-old woman consulted her general practitioner because of mixed anxiety and depressive symptoms. The diagnosis was depressive disorder, and the immediate cause appeared to be the stress of caring for an elderly debilitated mother (also the general practitioner's patient), whose condition had worsened in the last 2 months. Important contributory factors were menorrhagia and chronic agoraphobia, which prevented the patient from visiting friends and relatives. The immediate plan was to treat the patient's depressive disorder with amitriptyline, and to obtain respite care for her mother. In the longer term, the agoraphobia would be treated with behaviour therapy, and a gynaecological opinion would be obtained about the menorrhagia

Problem list

Problem	Action	Agent	Review
Anxiety and depression	Amitriptyline rising to 150 mg at night	GP	Check reponse weekly for 3 weeks then review
Caring for elderly mother	Obtain respite care for mother	Geriatrician	3 weeks
Chronic agoraphobia	Behaviour therapy	Clinical psychologist	3 months
Menorrhagia	Gynaecological opinion	GP	1 month

TABLE 2.6	Example of a life chart			
Year	Age (years)	Events	Physical illness	Psychiatric disorder
1958	Born			
1959	1			
1960	2			
1961	3			
1962	4			
1963	5	Started school	Bed-wetting	
1964	6			
1965	7			
1966	8			
1967	9			
1968	10	Grandmother died		School refusal
1969	11			
1970	12			
1971	13	Father's illness	Unexplained abdominal pain	
1972	14			
1973	15			
1974	16			
1975	17			
1976	18	Started at university		Adjustment disorder
1977	19			
1978	20			
1979	21			
1980	22	Married		
1981	23			
1982	24	First child born		
1983	25			
1984	26	Second child born (Caesarean section)		
1985	27			
1986	28			
1987	29		Cone biopsy	
1988	30			
1989	31			
1990	32			
1991	33			
1992	34	Mother died		Depressive disorder
1993	35			
1994	36	Intestinal obstruction		
1995	37			
1996	38			
1997	39	Husband's illness		Depressive disorder
1998	40			
1999	41	Son started university		(Depressed)
2000	42			
2001	43			
2002	44	Husband died		
2003	45			Depressive disorder

BOX 2.5 COMMUNICATING WITH PATIENTS AND RELATIVES

When giving information to patients and their relatives, it is useful to keep in mind relevant questions from the following list.

The diagnosis

- What is the diagnosis—if it is uncertain, what are the possibilities?
- Is further information or special investigation required?
- What may have caused the condition?
- What are the implications of the diagnosis for this patient's life?

The care plan

- What is the plan, and how far is it likely to help the patient and the family?
- If medication is included:

  What is its name, and why has it been chosen?

  What is the dosage schedule?

  What are the effects, side effects, and possible toxic effects—and what should be done if the latter are experienced?

  When should improvement be expected?

  Has the patient any concerns (e.g. that antidepressants are addictive)?

  How long is the planned course of treatment?

- If psychological treatment is included:

  What is involved?

  How often will it take place and how long will it last?

  When should improvement be expected?

Who does what?

- Will the general practitioner carry out the treatment alone, or will another person be involved (e.g. practice nurse, consultant psychiatrist, member of community health team)?
- If others are involved, what is their role?
- What can the family do to help the patient?

Emergencies

- Are they likely and how can they be avoided?
- Are there possible warning signs of a crisis?
- Who should be approached in an emergency, and how can they be found urgently?

progress of the gynaecological referral is to be checked in 1 month and the results incorporated into the treatment plan.

Life charts

A life chart is a way of relating stressful events to the occurrence of medical and psychiatric illness. The chart has five columns: the year, patient's age, life events, physical illness, and psychiatric disorder. The example in Table 2.6 is of a woman with a depressive disorder. She has had two episodes of emotional disorder in childhood (bed-wetting and school refusal), a third at the age of 18 (adjustment disorder), and a depressive disorder at age 34. The chart shows that the episodes of emotional disturbance were related in time to separations (starting school and going to university) and loss (the deaths of her grandmother and mother). The present illness is related in time to the death of her husband. None of the episodes were related to physical illness or childbirth.

Formulations

A formulation is another way of recording the results of an assessment. Formulations were considered at the beginning of this chapter (see p. 16 and Box 2.1).

Communicating with the patient and others

Confidentiality

Interviewers should be aware of the ethical and legal principles that govern the giving of information to people other than the patient. These principles are summarized in Box 2.4. Sometimes a relative or another person telephones the interviewer to ask for information about the patient. As a general rule, no information should be given over the telephone. Instead the patient should be told of the request. If he agrees that the information should be given to the enquirer, an interview should be arranged with that person. The clinician should never allow a conspiratorial atmosphere to develop in which he conceals from the patient conversations with family, friends, or others.

Explaining the diagnosis and management plan

Patients and relatives need to know more than the diagnosis and the basic facts about treatment. It is useful to begin by finding out what they know already, and what help they are expecting. This information makes it easier to meet their requirements, help with their concerns, and explain the treatment plan. It is useful to keep in mind the list of frequently asked questions shown in Box 2.5. The plan should be explained in an unhurried way, avoiding jargon, checking from time to time that the patient (or relative) has understood, and seeking questions. If, after a full discussion, the patient does not accept some part of the plan, or the relatives do not accept the role proposed for them, a compromise should be negotiated. Sometimes it is appropriate to write down the plan so that the patient and relatives can consider it further, and refer to it later.

Letters of referral to psychiatrists

A referral letter should include as a minimum:

1. The *course and development* of the disorder, with the dates at which problems began or changed.

2. The *mental state* at the time of writing.

3. Any *abnormal behaviour that may be concealed or denied* by the patient when interviewed by the psychiatrist (e.g. excessive use of alcohol) or not recognized by the patient (e.g. lapses of memory).

4. Relevant points in the *medical history*.

5. Details of any *treatment*, together with a note of the therapeutic response and side effects.

6. *Family relationships*, including marital problems and difficulties between parents and children.

7. *Personality* as known to the referring doctor from previous contacts with the patient.

Further reading

Goldberg, D. (ed.) (1997). *The Maudsley Handbook of Practical Psychiatry*. Oxford University Press, Oxford.
A practical guide to psychiatric examination in a range of clinical situations—including advice on managing difficult interviews.

Appendix 2.1 Mini Mental State Examination*

			Score	Points
(Add points for each corrrect response)				
Orientation				
1.	What is the:	Year?	—	1
		Season?	—	1
		Date?	—	1
		Day?	—	1
		Month?	—	1
2.	Where is the:	State?	—	1
		Country?	—	1
		Town or city?	—	1
		Hospital?	—	1
		Floor?	—	1
Registration				
3.	Name three objects taking 1 second to say each. Then ask the patient all three after you have said them (give one point for each correct answer)		—	3
	Repeat the answers until the patient learns all three		—	3
Attention and calculation				
4.	Serial 7s (give one point for each correct answer) Stop after five answers Alternative: spell 'WORLD' backwards		—	5
Recall				
5.	Ask for names of three objects learned in Q3 (give one point for each correct answer)		—	3
Language				
6.	Point to a pencil and a watch. Have the patient name them as you point		—	2
7.	Have the patient repeat 'No ifs, ands, and buts'		—	1
8.	Have the patient follow a three-stage command: 'Take a paper in your right hand. Fold the paper in half. Put the paper on the floor'		—	3
9.	Have the patient read and obey the following: 'CLOSE YOUR EYES' (write it in large letters)		—	1
10.	Have the patient write a sentence of his or her choice (this sentence should contain a subject and an object, and should make sense; ignore spelling errors when scoring)		—	1
11.	Enlarge the design printed below to 1.5 cm per side, and have the patient copy it. (Give one point if all sides and angles are preserved and if the intersecting sides form a quadrangle.)		—	1
				= Total 30

* Reprinted from Anthony, J. C., Le Resche, L., Niaz, U., Von Korf, M. R. & Folstein, M. F. (1982). Limits of the 'Mini Mental State' as a screening test for dementia and delirium among hospital patients. *Psychological Medicine* 12, 397–408.

CHAPTER 3

Aetiology and the scientific basis of psychiatry

Chapter contents

Aetiology and the individual patient 39

Methodological approaches 42

Keeping up-to-date: evidence-based medicine 47

Doctors need to be able to combine scientific knowledge with an empathic understanding of the patient to form a coherent account of their patients, their illnesses, and their predicaments. In this chapter, we will initially describe how this can be achieved for the aetiological formulation. We will then review ways of finding out the most up-to-date evidence for all kinds of clinical questions (but particularly methods of identifying the best treatments for specific clinical situations) by using the strategies of evidence-based medicine.

A knowledge of the causes of psychiatric disorders is important for two main reasons. First, in everyday clinical work it helps the doctor to evaluate possible causes of an individual patient's psychiatric disorder. Second, it adds to the general understanding of psychiatric disorders, which may contribute to advances in diagnosis, treatment, or prognosis. In this section we will only deal with the first of these—the *assessment of the causes of disorder* in the individual patient. The aetiology of specific disorders is considered when these conditions are reviewed in subsequent chapters.

Aetiology and the individual patient

The causes of psychiatric disorder in an individual patient can be assessed properly only if certain conceptual problems are understood. These problems are illustrated in Case study 3.1 (below).

In assessing the causal significance of these events, the clinician can draw first on his knowledge of scientific studies of depressive disorders. Genetic investigations have shown that a predisposition to depressive

CASE STUDY 3.1 **CAUSES OF PSYCHIATRIC DISORDER**

For 4 weeks a 38-year-old married man became increasingly depressed. His symptoms had started soon after his wife left him to live with another man. The following points in the history were potentially relevant to aetiology. The patient's mother had received psychiatric treatment on two past occasions, once for a severe depressive disorder and once for mania; on neither occasion was there any apparent environmental cause for the illness. When the patient was 14 years old, his mother went to live with another man, leaving her children with their father. For several years afterwards the patient felt rejected and unhappy but eventually settled down. He married and had two children, aged 13 and 10 at the time of his illness. Two weeks after leaving home, the patient's wife returned saying that she had made a mistake and really loved her husband. Despite her return the patient's symptoms persisted and worsened. He began to wake early, gave up his usual activities, and spoke at times of suicide.

disorder is probably genetically transmitted (see p. 105). It is possible, therefore, that this patient inherited this kind of predisposition from his mother. Is the separation from his mother likely to have been significant? There have been several studies of the long-term effects of separating children from their parents, but they refer to people who were separated when younger than the patient was at separation. So this body of knowledge does not help here. Nonetheless, extrapolation from this evidence and clinical experience suggests that his mother's departure is likely to have been important. It is also understandable that a man should feel depressed when his wife leaves him; this particular man is likely to be especially affected by the experience because the event recapitulates the similar distressing separation in his own childhood. Empathy and common sense would also suggest that the patient should have felt better when his wife came back, but he did not. This lack of improvement can be explained, however, by evidence that distressing events can induce a depressive disorder, which then runs an independent course and requires treatment.

This case study illustrates several important issues concerning aetiology in psychiatry: the interaction of different causes in a single case; the need to distinguish different kinds of cause; the concept of stress and of psy-

chological reactions to it; and the roles of scientific evidence and of evaluation based on empathy and common sense.

Explaining and understanding

There are two ways of trying to make sense of the causes of a patient's problems. Both are useful, but it is important to distinguish between them. The first approach is quantitative and based on research findings; for example, a person's aggressive behaviour may be explained as the result of an injury to the frontal cortex sustained in a road accident. This statement draws on the results of scientific studies of the behaviour of patients with damage to various areas of the brain. It is conventional to refer to this kind of statement as **explaining** the behaviour.

The second approach is qualitative and is based on an empathic understanding of human behaviour. We use this approach when we decide, for example, that a person was aggressive because his wife was insulted by a neighbour. The connection between these two events makes sense; it is convincing even though no quantitative study has shown a statistical association between aggression and this kind of insult. It is conventional to refer to this kind of statement as **understanding** the cause of the behaviour.

In every branch of medicine doctors need to explain and to understand their patients' problems. In psychiatry understanding is often a particularly important part of the investigation of aetiology.

Remote causes and multiple causes

In psychiatry, certain events in childhood are associated with psychiatric disorder in adult life. For example, subjects who develop schizophrenia are more likely than controls to have been exposed to complications of pregnancy and labour.

One cause can lead to *several effects*; for example, lack of parental affection in childhood has been reported to predispose to suicide, antisocial behaviour, and depressive disorder. Conversely, a *single effect* can have *several causes*, which act singly or in combination. For example, learning disability can be caused by any one of several distinct genetic abnormalities, whilst a depressive disorder can be caused by the combined effects of genetic factors and recent stressful events.

Classification of causes

When there are multiple causes it is useful to group them into predisposing, precipitating, and perpetuating factors (Fig. 3.1; Table 3.1).

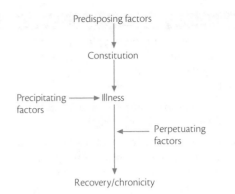

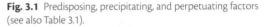

Fig. 3.1 Predisposing, precipitating, and perpetuating factors (see also Table 3.1).

TABLE 3.1 Predisposing, precipitating, and perpetuating factors in psychiatric disorder
◆ Predisposing factors
◆ Genetic endowment
◆ Environment *in utero*
◆ Trauma at birth
◆ Social/psychological factors in development
◆ Precipitating factors
◆ Physical diseases, drugs
◆ Psychological stressors
◆ Social changes
◆ Perpetuating factors
◆ Intrinsic to the disorder
◆ Social circumstances

Predisposing factors determine vulnerability to other causes that act close to the time of the illness. Many predisposing factors act early in life, for example: genetic endowment; the environment *in utero*; trauma at birth; and social and psychological factors in infancy and childhood.

Precipitating factors are events that occur shortly before the onset of a disorder and appear to have induced it. They may be physical, psychological, or social. Physical precipitating causes include diseases such as cerebral tumour, and the effects of drugs taken for treatment or used illegally. An example of a *psychological cause* is bereavement; while moving home is a *social cause*. Some causes may act in more than one way; for example, a head injury may induce a psychiatric disorder through physical changes in the brain and through psychological effects.

Perpetuating factors prolong a disorder after it has begun. Sometimes a feature of a disorder makes it self-perpetuating (e.g. some ways of thinking commonly prolong anxiety disorders, see p. 77). Social factors are also important (e.g. overprotective attitudes of relatives). Awareness of perpetuating factors is particularly important in planning treatment because they may be modifiable even when little can be done about predisposing and precipitating factors.

Models in aetiology

In discussions of aetiology the word 'model' is often used to mean a way of ordering information. Like a theory, a model seeks to explain certain phenomena and to show the relationships between them. Unlike a theory, it does so in a broad and comprehensive way that cannot be proved wrong by carrying out an experiment. Darwin's ideas of natural selection are an example of a successful model in the biological sciences. Freudian theory is an example of a model that was widely used in the past in psychiatry.

Reductionist models seek to understand causation by tracing back to simpler, earlier stages. This kind of model, which is familiar in science, is exemplified in psychiatry by the supposition that schizophrenia is caused by disordered neurotransmission in certain areas of the brain.

Non-reductionist models seek to understand causation in terms of a wider (rather than a narrower) set of issues. This kind of model, which is familiar in the social sciences, is exemplified in psychiatry by the supposition that the cause of a patient's neurosis is in his family, and that his symptoms are only one aspect of a disordered family life.

The **medical model** is an approach to research in which psychiatric disorders are investigated in ways that have proved useful in general medicine. For example, by identifying regularly occurring patterns of symptoms (syndromes) and relating them to pathological findings. This model has proved particularly useful in investigating organic psychiatric disorders, and in studying schizophrenia and severe affective disorders. It is less useful, although not without value, in the study of neuroses and personality disorders.

The **behavioural model** refers to an approach to research in which psychiatric disorders are explained in terms of factors that determine normal behaviour; for example drives and reinforcements, attitudes and beliefs, and cultural influences. This model has been most useful in investigating neuroses and personality disorders. Behavioural models can be either reductionist (e.g. explanations in terms of conditioning) or non-reductionist (e.g. explanations in terms of social influences).

Methodological approaches

In this section it is not our intention to provide an extensive review of the aetiology of psychiatric disorders. Current knowledge about the causes of specific disorders is presented in the relevant chapters. Here, we provide a brief summary of the kinds of approach that have been, and are being, used in investigating the causes of psychiatric disorder. We suggest that the reader first reads the aetiology sections in the following chapters, using this section as a guide to allow them to keep up to date with advances in knowledge.

Epidemiology

Epidemiology is the study of the distribution of diseases in space and time within a population, and of the factors that influence this distribution. In psychiatry, epidemiology is used to provide information about prevalence (which is useful for planning services) and about causation. Information about the epidemiology of particular psychiatric disorders is given in other chapters in this book. Some terms used in epidemiology are defined in Box 3.1.

In psychiatry, the best method of *case definition* is usually by reference to the definitions in a standard system of classification, such as DSM-IV or ICD-10 (see

---

BOX 3.1   EPIDEMIOLOGY: DEFINITIONS

Case   A person in the population or study group identified as having the disorder. In psychiatry, the *case definition* is usually a set of agreed criteria or a cut-off point on a continuous scale.

Rate   The ratio of the number of cases to the number of people in a defined population.

Prevalence   The rate for all cases, new and old. Prevalence may be determined on a particular occasion (*point prevalence*) or over a period of time (e.g. 1-year prevalence).

Incidence   The rate for *new* cases. *Inception rates* represent the number of people who were healthy at the beginning of a defined period but became ill during it. *Lifetime expectation* represents the number of people who could be expected to develop a particular illness in the course of their whole life.

Chapter 1). The main types of study designs used in psychiatric epidemiology are shown in Box 3.2.

Genetics

Genetic studies in psychiatry are concerned with three issues:

1. The relative contributions of genetic and environmental factors to aetiology.

BOX 3.2   STUDY DESIGNS USED IN PSYCHIATRIC EPIDEMIOLOGY

Case–control study   This is an observational study comparing the frequency of an exposure in a group of persons with the disease of interest (*cases*) with a group of persons without the disease (*controls*). Case–control studies are commonly used to look for *risk factors* for psychiatric disorders. For example, a finding that a group of patients with schizophrenia had a higher rate of exposure to birth complications than a non-schizophrenic control group could be interpreted as meaning that birth complications predisposed to schizophrenia. Case–control studies are quick to do and relatively cheap, but are susceptible to bias.

Cohort study   This is an observational study in which a group of persons without the disorder are followed up to see which of them get the disorder. For example, a cohort of newly delivered babies could be followed through childhood and adolescence to see which of them developed schizophrenia—and if any birth characteristics are associated with a higher risk for the disorder. Cohort studies are potentially less susceptible to bias, but take a long time to do and are expensive.

Prevalence (or cross-sectional) study   This is an observational study in which the presence or absence of a disorder and any other variable of interest is measured in a defined population. For example, a sample of homeless people could be surveyed to estimate the prevalence of schizophrenia.

Ecological studies   These studies examine the rates of disorder in the population and relate them to other population rates of factors in the environment. For example, in the UK, it was observed that there was a reduction in the suicide rate following the change from coal gas to natural gas. This was interpreted as showing that reducing the availability of methods could prevent suicide.

2. The mode of inheritance of disorders that have a genetic basis.

3. Biochemical mechanisms involved in hereditary disease.

Some progress has been made with answering the first two questions, but little with the third.

Three methods have been used to study these problems. **Epidemiological methods** of studying populations and families can evaluate the contribution of genetic factors to aetiology, and throw light on the mode of inheritance (e.g. whether dominant or recessive). The main study designs are shown in Box 3.3. **Cytogenetics** and **molecular genetics** provide information about chromosomal and genetic abnormalities and the mechanisms of inheritance (Box 3.4).

Biochemical studies

Biochemical studies in psychiatry are difficult to carry out for three main reasons.

1. The living brain is inaccessible to direct study and post-mortem tissue is not often available (since most psychiatric disorders do not lead to death). To overcome this problem, indirect approaches have been made through more accessible sites. Their value has been limited because concentrations of substances in cerebrospinal fluid, blood, and urine (especially in the latter two), have uncertain relationships to their concentrations in the brain.

2. Animal studies are of limited use because there are no obvious parallels in animals to the mental disorders found in man. (Animal studies are useful, however, in the study of the actions of drugs on the brain.)

3. It is difficult to prove that any biochemical abnormalities detected are causal and not secondary either to changes in diet or in activity induced by the mental disorder, or to the effects of drugs used in treatment.

BOX 3.3 EPIDEMIOLOGICAL STUDY DESIGNS USED IN GENETICS

Family risk studies   The affected people (*probands*) are identified, rates of disorder are determined among various classes of relatives, and these rates are compared with those in the general population. From the observed prevalence, estimates are computed of the numbers of people likely to develop the condition subsequently. These corrected figures are called *expectancy rates* or *morbid risks*. Rates higher than those expected in the general population show that a familial cause is likely. Family studies can show whether a condition is familial but they do not distinguish between the effects of inheritance and those of family environment.

Twin studies   Comparisons are made between concordance rates in uniovular (monozygotic, or MZ) twins and in binovular (dizygotic, or DZ) twins. If concordance is significantly greater among uniovular twins than among binovular twins, a significant genetic component is inferred. A more precise estimate of the contributions of heredity and environment can be made by comparing the rates of disorder among the rare cases of MZ twins reared apart, with the rates among MZ twins reared together. If the rates are the same in those reared apart and those reared together, this indicates an important genetic component to aetiology.

Adoption studies   Children who, since early infancy, have been reared by unrelated adoptive parents are studied. Two comparisons can be made. The first is between adopted persons with a biological parent who had the disorder under investigation, and adopted persons with biological parents free from the disorder. A higher rate of the disorder among the former indicates a genetic cause. The second comparison is between the biological parents and the adoptive parents of adopted persons who have the disorder. A higher rate of the disorder among the biological parents indicates a genetic cause. Such studies can be affected by several biases; for example, adoptees may be assigned to adoptive parents on the basis of the socioeconomic status of the biological parents. In psychiatry, adoption studies have been applied to schizophrenia (see p. 126) and affective disorder (see p. 105), and the findings point to genetic causes in both conditions.

Mode of inheritance   This is assessed by using statistical methods to test the closeness of fit between the rates of disorder in various classes of relatives of the probands, and the rates predicted by various models of inheritance (e.g. dominant, recessive, sex-linked). When applied to psychiatric disorders, such studies have generally given equivocal results, suggesting that the mode of inheritance is not simple.

BOX 3.4 STUDY DESIGNS USED IN CELLULAR AND MOLECULAR GENETICS

Cytogenetic studies   These aim to identify abnormalities in the structure or number of chromosomes. *Karyotyping* is a commonly used technique in which chromosomal spreads are examined with a microscope. Cytogenetic abnormalities have been identified as causes of learning disabilities (e.g. Down's syndrome, in which there is a trisomy of chromosome 21). Chromosomal abnormalities have not been identified as a primary cause of functional psychiatric disorders although, occasionally, such abnormalities may give indirect clues to the aetiology of some disorders. For example, subjects with the *velo-cardio-facial syndrome* (associated with a deletion on chromosome 22) have a high incidence of bipolar affective disorder.

Linkage studies   These studies seek to identify the chromosomal region likely to be carrying the genes responsible for a disorder in a family or group of families. Linkage studies have been successful in identifying the genes causing Huntington's disease and familial Alzheimer's syndrome. Their role is limited in disorders that are not due to single major genes, such as most psychiatric disorders. There are also problems in using linkage studies in psychiatric disorders due to uncertain phenotypes and statistical complexities. To date, no confirmed linkage has been found between a common psychiatric disorder and a single specific chromosomal region.

Association studies   These are case–control studies (see Box 3.2) in which the frequency of a genetic variant (or polymorphism/allelic variant) in a group of subjects with a disorder is compared to the frequency of the variant in a group of subjects without the disorder. The *advantages* of association studies compared to linkage studies are that they are easier to perform in complex disorders, they do not need familial samples, and they make fewer statististical assumptions. The *disadvantages* are that they require a *candidate gene* (a genetic marker that is close to or part of a gene that is suspected of being involved in the disorder) and that they are susceptible to *confounding* (a situation when an observed association with a gene or other cause is simply due to other differences between the cases and controls). So far, although encouraging, association studies have not produced unequivocal results in psychiatric disorders.

TABLE 3.2 Brain-imaging techniques

Structural imaging techniques

Computerized tomography (CT scan)	X-rays taken of the brain from many different angles combined to produce a series of images or 'slices' through the brain. It has demonstrated lateral ventricular enlargement in schizophrenia
Magnetic resonance imaging	Non-ionizing radio-waves directed at the brain (MRI scan) in the presence of a strong magnetic field. Asymmetrical nuclei align and resonate, producing signals which are converted into an image by a computer. It has demonstrated more subtle brain abnormalities in schizophrenia

Functional imaging techniques

Positron emission tomography (PET scan)	Radiolabelled short-living isotopes (produced in a cyclotron) are injected and emit radiation, which is detected by a scanner and converted to an image by a computer. It is used to measure regional cerebral blood flow and ligand binding
Single photon emission tomography (SPET scan)	This is simpler than PET and does not require a cyclotron. Photons emitted by injected radiochemicals are detected by a rotating gamma camera. It is used to measure regional cerebral blood flow and ligand binding
Functional magnetic resonance imaging (fMRI)	This is based on the sensitivity of MRI to magnetic effects caused by variations in the oxygenation of haemoglobin, which is induced by local changes in blood flow during task activation. Because it does not involve radiation, it may be used repeatedly in the same subject

Despite these problems, *biochemical studies of post-mortem brain* tissue have been moderately informative in Alzheimer's disease, schizophrenia, and affective disorder. In Alzheimer's disease there is a widespread decline of transmitter function; however, this decline could be no more than a consequence of the loss of cells in this disorder. In schizophrenia, the density of dopamine receptors is increased in the caudate nucleus and nucleus accumbens, but this increase could be the result of treatment with antipsychotic drugs, which block dopamine receptors and so might lead to a compensatory increase in their density. In severe affective disorder, some studies have found reduced 5-HT (serotonin) function in the brainstem, but these findings were based on patients who had died by suicide, and they could result from terminal anoxia or the drugs used for suicide.

More recently, *brain-imaging methods* have been used to study biochemical function in living brain tissue (Table 3.2).

Pharmacology

If a drug alleviates a disorder, and if the mode of action of the drug is known, then it might be possible to infer the biochemical abnormality underlying the disorder. This line of argument must be pursued cautiously, however, since effective drugs do not always act directly on the biochemical abnormality underlying the disorder. For example, anticholinergic drugs are effective in Parkinson's disease but the symptoms of this disorder are caused by a defect in dopaminergic transmission, not by an excess of cholinergic transmission.

Endocrinology

In psychiatric patients tests of endocrine function have been used to study the following:

* Tests have been used to determine how hormonal activity changes in psychiatric disorder. For example, it has been shown that cortisol is produced at an increased rate in depressed patients.

* Changes in endocrine function have been used as indirect measures of other processes. This usage is possible because many endocrine functions are controlled through neurotransmitters that could be involved in causing psychiatric disorder. Thus, if an abnormality in endocrine function is due to the disordered function of a particular neurotransmitter in one brain system, it is possible that the same neurotransmitter could be functioning abnormally in another brain system, and that this second mal-

functioning could be the cause of the psychiatric disorder. For example, endocrine abnormalities indicating reduced 5-HT function have been found in depressive disorder, and it has been proposed that more widespread reduction of 5-HT is a cause of this disorder.

Neuropathology

Post-mortem brain studies have been carried out for over a century, yielding useful information about dementias and other organic disorders, but until recently they have shown no consistent abnormalities in the functional psychoses. Modern quantitative methods have demonstrated abnormalities in the medial temporal lobes and other brain areas of patients with schizophrenia, and these abnormalities could be relevant to the aetiology of this disorder. Advances in brain-imaging techniques have provided a method of investigating the structure and function of the brain before death (Table 3.2).

Electrophysiology

Electrophysiological recordings made with electrodes on the skull surface (as in electroencephalography) do not give precise information about the nature and site of abnormal brain activity and have contributed little to the understanding of psychiatric disorders, except for those related to epilepsy.

Psychology

Psychology is the study of normal behaviour, and is therefore highly relevant to the study of abnormal behaviour in mental disorders. Psychological studies have contributed to the understanding of causes of anxiety disorders (p. 84), but their main importance is not in relation to the onset of psychiatric disorder but to the factors that maintain the disorders once started. The most relevant psychological mechanisms concern conditioning, social learning, and cognitive processing. (Readers who are unfamiliar with these concepts should consult a textbook of psychology or behavioural science.)

Classic conditioning Learning through association explains, for example, the development of situational anxiety in phobic patients following an initial attack of anxiety in the situation (see p. 80).

Operant conditioning The reinforcement of behaviour by its consequences explains, for example, the maintenance of disruptive behaviour in some patients by the extra attention that is provided by staff or relatives when this behaviour occurs.

Cognitive processes are concerned with aspects of the ways in which patients select, interpret, and act on the information from the sense organs and memory stores. Some disorders are maintained, in part, by the ways that patients think about the physical symptoms associated with emotional arousal. For example, patients with panic disorder think that palpitations are a precursor of a heart attack and so become more anxious (see pp. 83–4). Knowledge of these psychological mechanisms led to the development of the cognitive-behaviour therapies (see Chapter 18).

Coping mechanisms are ways in which people attempt to deal with stressors. The term is used in both a wide and narrow sense. The *wide sense* includes any way of responding to stressors, whether or not the response reduces the stress reaction. The *narrow sense* refers only to ways of responding that reduce the stress reaction. To avoid confusion it is useful to apply the terms *maladaptive* or *ineffective* to responses that fail to reduce the stress reaction, or do so but cause other problems (e.g. taking an excessive amount of alcohol). Coping mechanisms have two components: (i) internal processes; and (ii) observable behaviour. For example, after bereavement, a person's coping mechanisms might include thinking about religious beliefs (an internal process) and joining a social club to combat loneliness (observable behaviour). Another internal coping mechanism is to change the meaning attached to an event; for example, an imposed alteration of job may be regarded at first as a threat but later as a challenging opportunity. Examples of maladaptive coping mechanisms are avoiding the problem or consuming alcohol to relieve distress.

Ethology

Ethology, which is concerned with the observation and description of behaviour, has contributed usefully to research into behaviour disorders of children. The methods provide quantitative observations that allow comparisons of an individual's behaviour with that of other people, and with relevant behaviour in animals. Thus, the effects of separating human infants and infant monkeys from their mothers have been shown to be similar in certain ways; for example, infants of both kinds are distressed and active at first, and then call less and adopt a hunched posture. Such parallels help to distinguish between innate and culturally determined aspects of behaviour.

Sociology

Clinical observations indicate that psychiatric disorder may be provoked or influenced by factors in the social environment. Sociology, the study of human society, is therefore a potentially valuable source of information about the causes of psychiatric disorder. The main sociological concepts that have been applied to psychiatric disorders are listed below.

Social role Behaviour that develops as a result of other people's expectations of, or demands on, a person. Each individual takes more than one role (e.g. as worker, father, husband, and so on).

Sick role Behaviour expected and required of an ill person. It includes exemption from some responsibilities, the right to expect help from others, the expectation of a wish to recover, and an obligation to seek treatment.

Illness behaviour The behaviour of the person in the sick role. It includes seeking help, consulting doctors, taking medicines, and giving up responsibilities. A person may adopt the sick role and show illness behaviour without having any illness, or may show illness behaviour that is out of proportion to the degree of ill health (see Chapter 11).

Social class Status within society, determined usually on the basis of job or income. There is an association between schizophrenia and low social class (see Chapter 9).

Life event A stressful aspect of living that may be associated with changes in health status. Life events have been shown to contribute to the onset and maintenance of schizophrenia, affective disorder, and some other psychiatric disorders.

Culture The way of life shared by a group of human beings. A *subculture* is the way of life shared by a subgroup within a wider cultural group. Culture affects the ways people behave when ill (the sick role and illness behaviour mentioned above), as well as the routines and values of carers and families. The presentation and course of mental disorders may be influenced by cultural factors.

Social mobility A change of role or status in a society. Schizophrenia may lead to downward social mobility (decline to a lower social class), while upward mobility may be a stressful experience provoking an adjustment disorder.

Migration Movement between societies. Migration can be a stressful experience and it has been suggested as a cause of mental disorder.

Social institution An established social organization (e.g. the family, school, or hospital). The roles taken by the mother and father, and in the relationships between the 'nuclear' family of parents and children, and the 'extended' family of grandparents, aunts, and uncles may differ between cultures. These family differences are important in understanding the impact of one member's illness on other family members.

Total institution An institution in which the inmates spend all their time in the one place and have little freedom to choose their way of life: long-stay psychiatric hospitals can be total institutions. If life in the institution is unduly ordered, repetitive, and restrictive, the people living there may lose initiative, withdraw into fantasy, or rebel. In this way, institutional living can add further handicaps ('institutionalization') to those of the mental disorder.

Keeping up-to-date: evidence-based medicine

Although every effort is made to ensure that textbooks (including this one!) are accurate, comprehensive, and up to date, inevitably as knowledge increases, they become out of date. For example, questions about treatment arise frequently in clinical practice. Although the doctor will have learned about treatments during his training, it is in this area of practice that the most rapid advances occur and so it is the most difficult aspect to keep up to date. New drugs, other kinds of treatment,

and other clinical procedures are being introduced all the time and it can be difficult for a doctor to find unbiased information about them.

The doctor needs a way of quickly accessing the best available information—and also needs to know how to combine it with his understanding of the patient and their preferences. In the past, the doctor had to rely on potentially out-of-date or biased sources of information such as textbooks, authoritative reviews, promotional materials, or, most commonly, the opinions of colleagues. Recently, a number of techniques derived from advances in clinical epidemiology and information science have been introduced. Collectively, these strategies are often called **evidence-based medicine** (EBM) and they are helpful for answering frequently arising clinical questions and keeping up to date.

It is sometimes thought that there is little evidence on which to base treatment decisions in psychiatry—and that psychiatry is too complex to be susceptible to this approach. Both of these assumptions are wrong. In fact, there is a great deal of evidence in psychiatry, probably as much as in any other branch of medicine. The aim of EBM is to allow the doctor to access the best available evidence as quickly as possible and to integrate it with his clinical expertise to best help a particular patient. EBM also helps answer questions regarding diagnosis, prognosis, and aetiology (Table 3.3). Details of some of the most useful sources of evidence are provided in Box 3.5.

TABLE 3.3 Types of clinical question and best study design

Type of question	Form of the question	Best study design
Diagnosis	How likely is a patient who has a particular a specific disorder?	A *cross-sectional study* of patients suspected of having the symptom, sign, or diagnostic test result to have disorder, comparing the proportion of patients who really have the disorder and who have a positive test with the proportion of patients who do not have the disorder and who have a positive test result
Treatment	Is the treatment of interest more effective in producing a desired outcome than an alternative treatment (including no treatment)?	A *randomized controlled trial* (RCT) in which the patients are randomly allocated to receive either the treatment of interest or the alternative
Prognosis	How likely is a specific outcome in this patient?	A study in which an *inception cohort* (patients at a common stage in the development of the illness, especially first onset) are followed up for an adequate length of time
Aetiology	What has caused the disorder?	A study that compares the frequency of an exposure in a group of persons with the disease (*cases*) of interest with a group of persons without the disease (*controls*)—this may be an RCT, a case–control study, or a cohort study (see Box 3.1)

BOX 3.5 **SOURCES OF EVIDENCE**

The National Electronic Library for Health (http://www.nelh.nhs.uk/) and **The National Electronic Library for Mental Health** (http://www.nelmh.org/) Web resources that act as portals to any other sources of high quality evidence, including several of those listed below.

The Cochrane Library   This is published quarterly on CD-ROM, floppy disk, and the world wide web (http://www.cochrane.org/reviews/index.htm). It contains:

◆ *The Cochrane Database of Systematic Reviews (CDSR).* This is a continually updated database of high quality systematic reviews maintained by the Cochrane Collaboration. The reviews are published in a uniform format. The CDSR is probably the best place to start searching.

◆ *The Database of Abstracts of Reviews of Effectiveness (DARE).* This is a database of critically appraised non-Cochrane reviews maintained by the UK National Health Service Centre for Reviews and Dissemination.

◆ *The Cochrane Controlled Trials Register.* This is a database of controlled clinical trials identified by the Cochrane Collaboration. Many of them are not indexed on MEDLINE or other bibliographic databases.

◆ *The Cochrane Review Methodology Database.* This is a comprehensive database of methodological articles.

PubMed (http://www.ncbi.nlm.nih.gov/entrez/query.fcgi)   This is the online portal to MEDLINE, the computerized index of biomedical journals maintained by the National Library of Medicine in the USA. It contains about 45% of relevant articles and is best at covering articles published in English. PubMed has a number of search filters that allow rapid searching for the most relevant articles.

PsycLIT   An electronic database similar to MEDLINE, but maintained by the American Psychological Association and specifically covering psychology and psychiatry journals.

EMBASE   A European equivalent of MEDLINE, good for searching for drug trials.

Evidence-based Mental Health (http://ebmh.bmjjournals.com/)   This is a journal that publishes systematically selected abstracts of the best mental health evidence research as it is published

As we hope we have illustrated in this chapter, clinical decisions need to be based on other factors as well as sound scientific evidence. These factors involve an understanding of the patient and their circumstances and preferences. They also include an awareness of the costs of new treatments. Limited resources mean that there is an increasing requirement for new treatments to be at least as effective as existing treatments, but also to confer some additional added value, such as fewer adverse effects or reduced costs.

Further reading

Sackett, D. L., Straus, S., Richardson, S., Rosenberg, W. & Haynes, R. B. (2000). *Evidence-based Medicine: How to Practise and Teach EBM*, 2nd edn. Churchill Livingstone, Edinburgh.
How to search for, critically appraise, and use research evidence in everyday clinical practice.

Lawrie, S. M., McIntosh, A. & Rao, S. (2000). *Critical Appraisal for Psychiatrists*. Churchill Livingstone, Edinburgh. *Critical appraisal of scientific articles for evidence-based practice in psychiatry.*

CHAPTER 4

Personality and its disorders

Chapter contents

Assessment of personality *50*

Types of personality disorder *52*

Epidemiology *54*

Aetiology *55*

Prognosis of personality disorder *55*

Management of personality disorder *55*

Appendix: Specialist classifications of personality disorder *59*

The term **personality** refers to the enduring characteristics of an individual as shown in ways of behaving in a wide variety of circumstances. Every personality is unique but there are common features, called traits that are observed in different degrees in different people. These traits provide a useful structure in which to describe personality: for example, sociability, aggressivity, and impulsivity. As these examples indicate, personalities have both favourable and unfavourable features and a textbook description necessarily devotes more space to the latter. In clinical work it is important to explore the favourable features of the personality as thoroughly as the unfavourable ones because it is usually easier to encourage the former than it is to discourage the latter.

Clinicians need to understand the personality of all their patients because this helps to predict their response to illness and its treatment. Clinicians also need to understand the minority of patients who have a personality disorder, that is a personality that causes problems for the patients or for those around them. People with a personality disorder may:

◆ *react in unusual ways to illness or to treatment*, for example by becoming overdependent or aggressive;

◆ *behave in unusual ways when mentally ill*, so that diagnosis is difficult;

◆ *react unusually to stressful events*, for example by becoming aggressive or histrionic instead of anxious. Sometimes these reactions are so unusual that they may be mistaken for a psychiatric disorder;

- *behave in ways that are stressful or dangerous* to themselves or other people;
- *develop other psychiatric disorders* more often than other people.

All clinicians need to be able to: (i) evaluate personality and determine when it is abnormal; (ii) distinguish personality disorder from psychiatric disorder; (iii) manage the effects of abnormal personality as it affects their own practice; and (iv) know when to refer to a specialist.

What is personality disorder?

It not difficult to agree that extreme deviations of personality should be classified as disorders, but it is difficult to draw a line between normal personality and personality disorder. If personality could be measured like intelligence, a statistical cut-off could be used (e.g. two standard deviations from the population mean). However, although psychologists have devised measures of some traits, there are no reliable and valid measures of the aspects of personality that are most important in clinical practice. In the absence of such measures, a simple pragmatic criterion is used: *a personality is disordered when it causes suffering to the person or to other people*. This definition may appear simplistic and it is certainly subjective, but it is nevertheless useful in clinical practice and no better alternative has been devised.

Personality disorder versus psychiatric disorder

Personality disorder, like other kinds of personality, develops gradually from the early years through adolescence—there is no clear time of onset. Psychiatric disorder has a definable onset. Differential diagnosis therefore depends on a reliable history of the onset and course of the disorder, and on evidence of the presence or absence of the characteristic features of the various psychiatric disorders. Difficulties arise occasionally when schizophrenia develops slowly in adolescence, when it is difficult to distinguish it from personality disorder (see p. 125).

Personality change

By definition, personality is enduring and stable. Small changes often take place very gradually over many years; for example a person may become less impulsive and aggressive in middle or late life. The term personality change does not refer to these gradual modifications but to the more abrupt changes that result sometimes from:

- *injury to, or organic disease of, the brain*;
- *residual effects of severe mental disorder*, usually schizophrenia;
- *exceptionally severe stressful experiences* such as those experienced by hostages or victims of severe torture.

Assessment of personality

The assessment of personality was described briefly in Chapter 2. The reader may find it useful to refer to this account again before continuing with the more detailed description given below.

Sources of information

In everyday life we learn about the personalities of people we know by observing how they respond in various circumstances over the time that we have known them. Clinicians get to know some of their patients in the same way but they also have to be able to assess the personality of patients whom they have not known for long. To do this they can draw on four sources of information:

1. A description by someone who knows the patient well. Provided that person is observant and reliable, this is usually the best source.

2. A patient's own account of their past behaviour in a variety of circumstances. This is less objective but potentially more complete.

3. A patient's self-description of personality. This is also subjective and sometimes influenced by the wish to create a good impression, or by depression or elation.

4. The patient's behaviour in the interview. This is often unreliable because it is influenced by temporary factors such as anxiety, depression, or elation.

The evaluation of personality formed from the last two of these items should be checked by comparing it with an objective record of past achievements and difficulties and, whenever possible, with the accounts of people who know the patient well.

Describing normal personality

Unless there is a personality disorder (see below), personality can be described without using technical terms by listing relevant attributes, for example: pessimistic, overcautious, and prone to worry excessively; or precise and reliable but touchy and easily offended; or outgoing and generous but highly emotional. Such brief descriptions are sufficient in most clinical situations. Nevertheless it is important to employ a standard

TABLE 4.1	A scheme for assessing personality

◆ Relationships

◆ Habitual mood

◆ Other traits (see Table 4.2)

◆ Attitudes and standards

◆ Habits

TABLE 4.2	Common personality traits (for brevity, only negative attributes are listed; corresponding positive features should also be noted)

◆ Prone to worry

◆ Strict, fussy, rigid

◆ Lacking self-confidence

◆ Sensitive

◆ Suspicious, jealous

◆ Untrusting, resentful

◆ Impulsive

◆ Attention seeking

◆ Dependent

◆ Irritable, quarrelsome

◆ Aggressive

◆ Lacking concern for others

method of enquiry to ensure that all relevant aspects of personality have been considered. The usual scheme is shown in Table 4.1. Some useful words for describing personality are is listed in Table 4.2.

When a patient asks advice for a problem, personality assessment is at first concerned with traits that can lead to difficulties and with those could help to explain the presenting problem. It is, however, important to go on to assess traits that are actual or potential assets. Some traits are assets in one situation but cause problems in others. For example, to be orderly and precise may be an asset in certain kinds of work but a problem when faced with the uncertainties of physical illness.

Systematic enquiries about personality

As with other assessments, the amount of detail required in personality assessment varies with the problem and the situation. The following account indicates the full range of enquiries under each of the headings in the scheme for assessment. Students should practice the full scheme repeatedly before using a more selective approach as they gain experience. When time is short, as in an emergency, only a few points relevant to the immediate problem can be covered. Others, more relevant to further care, can be considered later.

Starting the enquiry

Before starting the specific enquiries listed below, it is useful to ask a general question; for example: 'How do you think your friends and family would describe your personality?'

Relationships

This section is concerned with *relationships at work* (with colleagues, people in authority, and juniors) *and with friends*, and with *intimate relationships*. The interviewer asks whether the patient makes friends easily, has few friends or many, has close friends in whom he or she can confide, and has lasting friendships. The interviewer also asks whether the patient is sociable and confident in company, or shy and reserved.

Habitual mood

The aim is to discover the person's habitual mood, not the present or recent mood. The interviewer asks whether mood is generally cheerful or gloomy, stable or changeable. If mood is changeable, the interviewer asks how long the changes last, and whether they occur spontaneously or in relation to events. Finally, the interviewer asks whether the person shows his feelings or hides them.

Other traits

When enquiring about other personality traits it is useful to keep in mind the list of qualities in Table 4.2. Each characteristic has a positive as well as a negative side and it is appropriate to ask patients where they lie between the extremes; for example, 'Some people are placid, others get into arguments—where do you fit in?' It is useful to check answers by asking for examples from the patient's recent life. Characteristics such as jealousy or lack of feeling for others may not be revealed because the person is ashamed of them or does not recognize their presence. When there is doubt, the patient's own account should be checked against those of informants. Observations should be recorded objectively, avoiding value judgements. Imprecise terms such as 'immature' or 'inadequate' should not be used: instead, the interviewer should record in what ways the person has difficulty in meeting the demands of adult life.

Attitudes, beliefs, and standards

Relevant points include attitudes to illness, religious beliefs, and moral standards. Usually, these become apparent when the personal history is being taken, but they can be explored further at this point in the interview.

Habits

Although not strictly part of personality, the use of tobacco, alcohol, and illicit drugs is sometimes included under personality, though it is generally better to record it separately (see p. 22).

Is there personality disorder?

Having built up a picture of the personality, the interviewer decides whether the personality is disordered. The criterion for disorder is suffering by the patient or by others as a result of the patient's personality (see above). The criterion requires a difficult judgement about the extent to which the patient's problems have been caused by personality and how much by circumstances. One source of error is that temporary modes of behaving due to a concurrent psychiatric disorder may be mistaken for life-long traits. These temporary behaviours are not always those that might be expected. For example, depressive disorder occasionally leads not to self-depreciating and restrained behaviour but to histrionic behaviour.

Types of personality disorder

Psychiatrists classify abnormal personalities according to one or other of the detailed schemes set out in ICD-10 and DSM-IV. For other doctors, who treat people with highly abnormal personalities less often, a simpler scheme is usually adequate. Such a scheme, which with one exception (see below) is compatible with the specialist classifications, is shown in Table 4.3. Each of the groups in this scheme will be described together with its relationship to the specialist classifications. The latter are shown in outline in Table 4.4 and summarized for reference on pp. 59–60.

Cyclothymic and **schizotypal personalities** are, by convention, not included in the formal or informal classifications. This is because cyclothymic personality is closely related to bipolar mood disorder and is therefore classified with it (see p. 102), and schizotypal personality disorder is closely related to schizophrenia and is classified with it (see p. 103).

TABLE 4.3 A simplified classification of personality

- Anxious, moody, and prone to worry
- Lacking self-esteem and confidence
- Sensitive and suspicious
- Dramatic and impulsive
- Aggressive and antisocial

TABLE 4.4 Classification of personality disorders in DSM-IV and ICD-10 (generally, the same terms are used in DSM-IV and ICD-10; where there are differences the ICD term is shown in parentheses)

Anxious, moody, and prone to worry
- Avoidant (ICD: anxious)
- Obsessive-compulsive (ICD: anankastic)
- Depressive
- Hyperthymic
- Cyclothymic

Sensitive and suspicious
- Paranoid
- Schizoid
- Schizotypal

Dramatic and impulsive
- Histrionic
- Borderline (ICD: impulsive)
- Dependent

Aggressive and antisocial
- Antisocial (ICD: dissocial)

Note that the category for personalities lacking self-esteem and self-confidence is not included in either DSM-IV or ICD-10.

Anxious, moody, and worry-prone personalities
(Table 4.5)

Some of these people are persistently anxious and fearful, some are persistently gloomy and pessimistic; others have fluctuating moods, in which periods of mild elation and overconfidence alternate with low mood and self-deprecation. Worries may be about everyday problems concerning the patient or the family, or may take the form of persistent concerns about illness (hypochondriasis, see p. 91). People with **obsessional traits** of inflexibility, obstinacy, and indecisiveness are included in this group. (This group corresponds with the dependent, anxious avoidant, and obsessive-

TABLE 4.5 Characteristics of anxious, moody, worry prone personalities

- Persistently anxious
- Worried about problems and health
- Inflexible and obstinate
- Indecisive
- Persistently gloomy *or*
- Unstable moods

TABLE 4.6 Characteristics of personalities lacking self-esteem
◆ Lack confidence
◆ Feel inferior
◆ Expect criticism
◆ Strive to please others

compulsive (anankastic) groups in the specialist classifications.)

Personalities lacking self-esteem and confidence (Table 4.6)

This group is common and important in primary care and general medical practice. These people lack confidence in their abilities, feel inferior to others, and expect criticism. These inner uncertainties may lead to shyness, social withdrawal, and failure to achieve, or to inappropriate efforts to please other people or forced attempts at sociability. These personality features are associated with recurrent depressive moods, eating disorders, and self-harm and are often seen among young people who seek help for these problems. (This group does not appear as a separate entity in the specialist classifications of personality disorder; these patients could appear under several of the headings.)

Sensitive and suspicious personalities (Table 4.7)

Some of these people see rebuffs where none exist and are suspicious, mistrustful, touchy, and irritable. Others are cold and detached, show little concern for others, and reject help when it is offered. Still others appear eccentric, with unusual ideas about topics such as telepathy and extrasensory perception. People in this group are difficult to engage in treatment and they may distrust their doctors. (This group corresponds with the paranoid, schizoid, and schizotypal groups in the specialist classifications (see p. 59).)

TABLE 4.7 Characteristics of sensitive and suspicious personalities
◆ Sensitive
◆ Suspicious
◆ Mistrustful
◆ Self-sufficient
◆ Lacking concern

TABLE 4.8 Characteristics of dramatic and impulsive personalities
◆ Vain, self-centred
◆ Demanding of others
◆ Acts a part; self-deceiving
◆ Impulsive; short-lived enthusiasms
◆ Unrestrained emotional display

Dramatic and impulsive personalities (Table 4.8)

These people seek the limelight and dramatize their problems. They make unreasonable demands on other people and may use 'emotional blackmail'. They have brief enthusiasms but lack persistence. Some have a great capacity for self-deception and a lack of awareness of the impression they make on others. They react impulsively, sometimes with ill-judged behaviour including self-harm. (This group corresponds with the histrionic, borderline, and dependent groups in the specialist classifications (see p. 60).)

Borderline personality disorder

This category from the specialist classification is described here because the term is used widely. It is a subgroup within the dramatic and impulsive personalities and is characterized by:

◆ intense but unstable relationships;

◆ persistent feelings of boredom and emptiness;

◆ self-damaging behaviours such as recklessness with money or sex, binge eating, or substance abuse;

◆ recurrent threats or acts of self-harm;

◆ unstable moods;

◆ unwarranted outbursts of anger;

◆ uncertainty about personal identity and fear of being abandoned;

◆ impulsivity and low tolerance of stress.

These features cause many problems for the people themselves and for others. A special treatment—**dialectical behaviour therapy**—has been developed for these patients. The treatment is not widely available and it is uncertain whether it is substantially better than the management described on p. 58 for dramatic and impulsive personalities.

TABLE 4.9	Characteristics of aggressive and antisocial personalities

- Impulsive behaviour
- Low tolerance of frustration
- Tendency to violence
- Lack of guilt
- Failure to learn from experience
- Failure to sustain relationships
- Disregard of the feelings of others

Aggressive and antisocial personalities

(Table 4.9)

These people have low tolerance of frustration, behave impulsively, and tend to be violent. They lack guilt and fail to learn from experience. They are unloving and unconcerned with the feelings of others. When severe, these features are referred to as **antisocial personality disorder** (Box 4.1) and the people are sometimes called 'psychopaths' (though it is better not to use this term because it is imprecise). Such people have an unstable work record and may be involved in violence, family problems, and offences against the law. The difficulties are often increased by abuse of alcohol or drugs. (This

---

BOX 4.1 ANTISOCIAL PERSONALITY DISORDER

'Antisocial' personality is the term used in DSM-IV; in ICD-10, the term is 'dissocial'. These people fail to sustain loving relationships and disregard the feelings of others. They may act callously, for example inflicting pain, cruelty, or degradation.on others. They may be superficially charming but lack tender feelings, and their relationships are shallow and unsustained. Marriage may be marked by violence towards the partner, or neglect of, or violence to, the children. Many marriages end in separation or divorce.

Impulsive behaviour and a lack of consistent striving towards a goal may be reflected in an unstable work record. Impulsivity, low tolerance of frustration, and tendency to violence often lead to repeated offences against the law. These offences may begin with petty acts of delinquency, but go on to callous and violent crime. Lack of guilt and failure to learn from experience results in behaviour that persists despite serious consequences and legal penalties.

---

group corresponds with the dissocial or antisocial groups in the specialist classifications; see p. 60.)

Dangerous severe personality disorder This term denotes to an administrative category rather than a clinical syndrome. It refers to a small number of people, mostly with antisocial personality disorder, who are dangerous to other people. In the United Kingdom, powers have been proposed to allow the detention of such people in a psychiatric unit in order to prevent future violence, and at the time of writing the proposal is under discussion. The proposal arises in part from public concern about reports of personality disordered persons who have committed serious acts of violence. Enquiries into such cases often trace a sequence of events that suggests that the violence could have been prevented had the person been detained in time.

There are several practical problems about proposals of this kind. The first is that retrospective enquiries, in which the outcome is already known, tend to overestimate the certainty with which predictions of violence could have been made at the time. In fact, such predictions are imprecise, producing both false positives and false negatives. There are two consequences:

1. Because there are false positives, some people who will not be violent will be detained.

2. Because there are false negatives, some people who will be violent will not be detained.

Thus attempts to detect and detain as many as possible of those who will be violent would inevitably result in the detention of some people who will not be violent, and even then some who will commit violence will remain free. Moreover, even when the prediction of future violence is accurate, it is seldom certain *when* the violence will take place, so that it is difficult to decide how long detention should last. Moreover, although violence in the community will be prevented as long as the person is detained, there is limited evidence that any kind of inpatient treatment is effective in the longer term. As well as these special problems, the proposal shares the more general ethical problems associated with any involuntary detention (see p. 129).

Epidemiology

The overall prevalence of personality disorder in community surveys is between about 5 and 10 per cent. Overall rates are higher in men than women and decrease with age. Antisocial personality disorder, which is present in about 1–3 per cent in community surveys, is more common in men. Histrionic personality disorder (about 2 per cent) and borderline personality disorder (about 1–2 per cent) are more common in women. Personality disorders often coexist with mental disorders. A particularly important association is between antisocial personality disorder and alcohol and substance abuse.

Aetiology

Personality and its disorders result from the interaction of genetic factors and upbringing. The relative contribution of these causes is uncertain and difficult to clarify because of the many factors involved in childhood upbringing and the difficulty of recording these accurately and relating them to personality features assessed many years later.

The little scientific knowledge that has been accumulated is mainly concerned with antisocial personality disorders and it is the only aspect that will be considered here. Despite this lack of scientific data concerning other kinds of personality disorder, it is sometimes possible to achieve an intuitive understanding (see p. 40) of the possible childhood origins of some aspects of personality. For example, when frequent criticism and lack of affection from parents are the antecedents of a personality marked by low self-esteem.

Causes of antisocial personality disorder

Genetic factors The children of parents with antisocial personality disorder have greater rates of antisocial behaviour than children of parents who do not have this kind personality. A similar excess has been reported also among adopted children whose biological parents have antisocial personality disorder and whose adoptive parents do not. These findings suggest a genetic contribution to aetiology.

Childhood experience Separation from parents in early childhood is more frequent among people with antisocial personality disorder than among controls. This association could be due to parental disharmony preceding the separation, rather than to the separation itself, or to one of the consequences of separation such as upbringing in an institution.

Injury to the brain at birth is sometimes followed by impulsive and aggressive behaviour. Such injury has been suggested as a cause of antisocial personality disorder but without convincing evidence. **Abnormal brain development** has been suggested as a cause. The only evidence, which is indirect, is that some adults with antisocial personality have non-specific abnormalities in the electroencephalogram (EEG) of a kind found normally in adolescents, not adults. This suggests that these findings might reflect delayed brain maturation among people with antisocial personality.

Serotonin Recent studies have found an association between aggressive behaviour and low levels of brain serotonin (5-HT), inferred from the results of neuroendocrine challenge tests. However, the association between serotonin and aggression is not confined to aggression in antisocial personality disorder.

Prognosis of personality disorder

Clinical experience indicates that some abnormal features of personality, such as aggressive traits, tend to become less abnormal as the person grows into middle age. There are, however, no reliable follow-up studies to confirm this observation. In old age, abnormal features of personality sometimes increase again, causing difficulties for patients and carers (see p. 227).

Management of personality disorder

Since personality is by its nature unchanging, it is not surprising that personality disorders are generally unresponsive to treatment. There are, nevertheless, other ways (described below) of helping patients with personality disorder, usually by dealing with any factors that exacerbate the problems. Since personality disorders lead to problems that may affect the management of any illness, all clinicians should be able to assess the problems and arrange appropriate management, either within their own clinical team or by referral to a psychiatric service.

Aims of management

Since personality cannot usually be changed by treatment, management focuses on ways of dealing with any recent exacerbations of the problems associated with the personality disorder. This can be done in five ways:

1. Identify and treat any co-morbid psychiatric disorder(s).

2. Treat any associated substance misuse.

3. Help the patient to deal with or avoid situations that provoke problem behaviours.

4. Provide general support to reduce tension and increase self-esteem.

5. Support the family.

Help may be needed over a long period, often many years, and therapists need patience and the ability to accept repeated set backs.

Assessment

Diagnose the personality disorder and identify positive features The diagnosis of personality disorder focuses on unfavourable features of personality. Management requires an assessment of the positive features as well because it may be possible to encourage and develop these. *Low self-esteem* is a frequent problem in all kinds of personality disorder. Self-esteem can sometimes be improved by identifying talents and skills, which can be developed by further education or training, leading to a greater sense of self-worth. This assessment of the negative and positive features of personality should be added to in five ways (Table 4.10).

Identify any co-morbid psychiatric disorder Treatment of a co-morbid disorder can lead to an improvement in the problem behaviours associated with the personality disorder. Depression should be considered whenever the personality problems have increased recently without another obvious cause, even when the patient does not complain spontaneously of depression.

Assess any substance misuse Alcohol or other substances may be used by people with personality disorder to relieve tension, unhappiness, or feelings of inadequacy. However, their disinhibiting effects can encourage histrionic or aggressive behaviour, or self-harm.

Identify provoking factors for problem behaviours by asking the patient to keep a *daily diary* of the behaviours and the situations in which they occur. Most patients co-operate with this practical approach and provoking factors can often be identified directly. Sometimes, however, the link between the provoking factor and the response is indirect. For example, aggression may be provoked by social rejection, which is the response of others to the patient's lack of social skills. Treatment would then include social skills training.

Assess the effects on the family, particularly the effects on any children living with the patient. Although these enquiries are particularly important when the person is aggressive, the problems of people who are persistently anxious, histrionic, or suspicious may also affect their families. The effects may come to light when another family member seeks help for physical symptoms for which no medical cause can be found.

Enquire about aggressive acts, including those that break the law, and *assess risk* (see Chapter 2) especially when the personality disorder is of an antisocial type.

General aspects of management (Table 4.11)

The plan should be realistic, focusing on specific problems and not attempting personality change. The aims should be clearly understood by the patient, and carried out consistently. The general approach is to help patients to:

* *take responsibility for their actions and be willing to solve their own problems*;

* *agree modest aims and work to achieve them over time.* Progress is usually by a series of small steps, punctuated by failures. Patience is needed in the management of personality disorders, which may have to be provided for many years;

* *gain confidence and learn from their mistakes.* Setbacks are viewed as opportunities to learn more about the problem, not as signs of failure.

The relationship between the patient and therapist is particularly important when treating personality disorder. The patient should feel valued as a person, and be able to trust and confide in the therapist. At the same time, the relationship should not be allowed to become too intense, nor should the patient become dependent or demanding. When more than one person is involved in treatment, their respective roles should be defined and made clear to the patient. Any attempt

---

TABLE 4.10 Assessment for the management of personality disorder

* Type of disorder and potential strengths
* Co-morbid psychiatric disorder
* Alcohol and drug use
* Provoking factors
* Effects on the family
* Antisocial behaviour

TABLE 4.11 Management of personality disorder

* Modest aims; achieved slowly
* Establish a relationship and set limits
* Assist responsibilty taking and learning from experience
* Build on strengths
* Deal with or avoid provoking factors
* Reduce alcohol/drug intake
* Help the family

to play one off against the other should be discussed between the professionals and with the patient.

Agreeing a care plan Some patients with personality disorder make unreasonable demands on those caring for them. They may seek help at inappropriate times, attempt to impose unrealistic conditions on treatment, behave in a seductive way, or threaten self-harm if their demands are not met. Such problems are met especially with overdependent, histrionic, or aggressive personalities. Once established, these behaviours can be very difficult to control, so clinicians should be alert for their first signs. The practical limits on the help that can be offered should be agreed by all those involved in the patient's care and explained to the patient.

Building on strengths Management should not focus exclusively on defects in the personality. Whenever possible patients should be encouraged to recognize and develop their talents and skills by obtaining further training, changing to a job better suited for their skills or interests, or by developing more satisfying leisure activities. As noted above, such actions improve low self-esteem and frustration which are frequent among people with all kinds of personality disorder.

Provoking factors The patient should be helped to identify and find new ways of dealing with or avoiding any situations that regularly cause problems. These changes may require patients to give up some of their previous goals and accept new ones more in keeping with the structure of their personalities.

Misuse of alcohol and drugs When abnormal behaviour is provoked or made worse by the misuse of alcohol or drugs, help should be given to limit the use of these substances. Among prescribed drugs, benzodiazepines can have disinhibiting effects similar to those of alcohol. They should be avoided when prescribing for patients with abnormal personalities.

Help for the family This may be needed, especially when the personality disorder is of the aggressive or antisocial kind. When a mother has a personality disorder, the health and development of the children should be assessed and appropriate steps taken to alleviate any problems.

Drug treatment has little general value in treating personality disorder but there are a few specific uses:

1. *Antipsychotic drugs* may be calming at a time of increased stress, especially for aggressive and antisocial personalities.

2. *Lithium carbonate* has been claimed to benefit some people with recurrent mood changes; a specialist opinion should be obtained before prescribing.

3. *Antidepressants* are of value when there is an associated depressive disorder. It has been claimed that, in the absence of a depressive disorder, specific serotonin reuptake inhibitors diminish impulsive behaviour and repeated self-harm, but their long-term value is uncertain at the time of writing.

4. *Carbamezapine* and some other antiepileptics have been claimed to reduce aggressive behaviour in some patients. The value is uncertain and, if real, applies to only a minority of patients. Specialist opinion should be sought before prescribing.

5. *Anxiolytic drugs should be avoided* because although they may improve immediate well-being they may produce disinhibition and dependency.

Role of the psychiatric services The general measures described above can be carried out by all clinicians, though it may be difficult for them to find time to deal with the more complex problems. Psychiatric services adopt the same general approach, supplemented at times by one or more of the special techniques described below. Referral to a psychiatrist is indicated: (i) for *assessment*; (ii) to *stabilize* the patient at times of crisis; and (iii) when there is *co-morbidity* with substance abuse or with another psychiatric disorder.

Psychotherapy may help some people with low self-esteem and difficulties in social relationships. *Cognitive-behaviour methods* are generally more appropriate than dynamic therapy since they focus on current behaviour and the patient's own role in changing this. Sensitive and suspicious, and antisocial and aggressive personalities seldom benefit from any form of psychotherapy.

Therapeutic community methods (see p. 265) have been used to assist people with antisocial personality to learn from experiences of their relationships within the community, and from the frequent and intensive discussion of problems that takes place. Good results have been claimed for a minority of such patients but these have not been supported by randomized controlled trials, and there are no agreed criteria for selecting the minority who may be helped.

Treatment according to personality type

Anxious, moody, and worrying types These patients are generally helped most by a cognitive-behaviour treatment designed to identify and change maladaptive ways of dealing with situations that the patient finds stressful, and to recognize the relation between thinking and emotion. In this group, patients with obsessional traits are least likely to change.

Sensitive and suspicious personalities These patients seldom benefit from any kind of psychological treatment. The aim is to establish a gradually greater degree of trust with the patient. These patients may provoke strong negative feelings in their carers, who should learn to recognize these reactions at an early stage and ensure that such feelings do not affect their clinical judgement.

Dramatic and impulsive personalities It is particularly important to set limits for this group. A problem-solving approach should be used to help the patient cope better with the stressful events that provoke abnormal behaviours. Dynamic psychotherapy is seldom effective and may lead to transference problems (see p. 257) that are difficult to manage.

Aggressive and antisocial behaviour Usually the most practical aim is to prevent the accumulation of secondary problems resulting from rash decisions, unintentional antagonism of potential helpers, and the abuse of drugs and alcohol. The approach should be practical and take account of the patient's sensitivities. Rude or aggressive behaviour has to be accepted tolerantly though, at times, much effort may be needed to restrain angry responses. Patients who are irritable and impatient should not be kept waiting without first explaining the reason. Potentially aggressive patients should be seen in a place where help can be called for (see p. 20).

A *problem-solving approach* should be taken to situations that regularly provoke aggressive and antisocial behaviour. *Anger management techniques* (a form of cognitive behaviour therapy) may help some patients to respond more appropriately. As noted above, limited time is sometimes spent most usefully in *helping the family*, especially any dependent children.

Low self-esteem and confidence These patients are helped by a trusting relationship in which they are encouraged to see the positive side of their personality and gain confidence. A cognitive-behaviour approach can help these patients understand the relationship between their unrealistic ways of thinking and their response to situations in which they feel defeated or inferior. Assertiveness training (p. 260) may help people who are unduly submissive.

Further reading

Tyrer, P. (ed.) (1996). *Personality Disorders: Diagnosis, Management and Course*. Wright/Butterworth Scientific, London. *Reviews the clinical features, diagnostic classification, treatment, and prognosis of personality disorders.*

Appendix 4.1 Specialist classifications of personality disorder

The scheme for personality disorders in the International Classification of Diseases, 10th edition (ICD-10), and the Diagnostic and Statistical Manual of the American Psychiatric Association, fourth edition (DSM-IV), are similar in all both but details. Most of the differences are in the terms used, rather than the concepts or the criteria for diagnosis. Where the terminology in DSM-IV and ICD-10 differs, the alternative term is shown in brackets: for example, 'obsessive-compulsive (ICD: anankastic)' indicates that the DSM term is obsessive-compulsive, the ICD term for the same personality is anankastic, and that we prefer the DSM term.

Group A: Anxious, moody, and prone to worry personalities

Anxious (DSM: avoidant) personality disorder

These people are persistently anxious, ill at ease in company, and fearful of disapproval or criticism. They feel inadequate and are timid. They avoid taking new responsibilities at work or new experiences generally. (This tendency to avoid is the basis of the DSM term.)

Obsessive-compulsive (ICD: anankastic) personality disorder

These people are inflexible, obstinate, and rigid in their opinions, and they focus on unimportant detail. They are indecisive and having made a decision they worry about its consequences. They are humourless and judgemental, while worrying about the opinions of others. Perfectionism, rigidity, and indecisiveness can make employment impossible. Such people appear outwardly controlled but may have violent feelings of anger, especially toward those who disturb their carefully ordered routine.

Dependent personality disorder

These people are passive and unduly compliant with the wishes of others. They lack vigour and self-reliance, and they avoid responsibility. Some achieve their aims by persuading other people to assist them, while protesting their own helplessness. Some are supported by a more self-reliant spouse; left to themselves, they have difficulty in dealing with the demands and responsibilities of everyday life.

Affective personality disorder

This category appears in both the DSM and ICD classifications, although not among the personality disorders; instead, it is grouped with the affective disorders because it is closely related. We describe affective personality disorder here for convenience.

These people have lifelong abnormalities of mood regulation which can take three forms:

1. **Depressed personality disorder**. The person is persistently gloomy and pessimistic with little capacity for enjoyment.

2. **Hyperthymic personality disorder**. The person is in a persistent state of mild elation, over-optimistic, and prone to making rash judgements.

3. **Cyclothymic (or cycloid) personality disorder**. In this disorder, which is the most important of the three, mood alternates between gloomy and elated states over periods of days to weeks with a characteristic frequency for each person. This instability is particularly disrupting to work and social relationships.

Group B: Sensitive and suspicious personalities

Paranoid personality disorder

These people are sensitive and suspicious; they mistrust others and suspect their motives, and are prone to jealousy. They are touchy, irritable, argumentative, and stubborn. Some of these people have a strong sense of self-importance and a powerful conviction of being unusually talented, though unable to fulfil their potential because let down or deceived by other people.

Schizoid personality

These people are emotionally cold, self-sufficient, and detached. They are introspective and may have a complex fantasy life. They show little concern for the opinions of others, and pursue a solitary course through life. When this personality disorder is extreme, the person is cold, callous, and insensitive.

Schizotypal personality disorder

These people are eccentric and have unusual ideas (e.g. about telepathy and clairvoyance) or ideas of reference. Their speech is abstract and vague, and their affect may be inappropriate to the circumstances. It has been suggested that this kind of personality is related to schizophrenia and in ICD it is classified with schizophrenia and not as one of the personality disorders.

Appendix 4.1 *Cont'd.*

Group C: Dramatic and impulsive personalities

Histrionic personality disorder

These people appear sociable, outgoing, and entertaining but at the same time they are self-centred, prone to short-lived enthusiasms, and lack persistence. Extreme displays of emotion may leave others exhausted while the person recovers quickly and without remorse. Sexually provocative behaviour is common but tender feelings are lacking. There may be astonishing capacity for self-deception and an ability to persist with elaborate lies long after others have seen the truth.

Borderline personality disorder

The term 'borderline' refers to a combination of features seen also in histrionic and antisocial personalities. The term originates in the now abandoned idea that the condition was related to (on the borderline with) schizophrenia. These people have a wide variety of problems, most of which can be part of other personality disorders. They include: inability to make stable relationships; persistent feelings of boredom; damaging behaviour such as reckless spending, uncontrolled gambling, or stealing; variable moods; unwarranted outbursts of anger; uncertainty about personal identity; and recurrent suicidal threats or behaviour. They are impulsive and unable to tolerate stressful events.

Narcissistic personality disorder (included only in DSM)

Narcissism is morbid self-admiration. Narcissistic people have a grandiose sense of self-importance and are preoccupied with fantasies of success, power, and intellectual brilliance. They crave attention, exploit others, and seek favours but do not return them.

Group D: Aggressive and antisocial personalities

Antisocial personality disorder

This disorder is described in Box 4.1 (p. 54).

CHAPTER 5

Reactions to stressful experiences

Chapter contents

Components of the stress response 62

Reactions to acute stress 62

Prolonged reactions to stress 65

Reactions to special kinds of acute stress 67

Long-term effects of sexual trauma in childhood 67

Normal and abnormal adjustment reactions 67

Adjustment to special situations 68

Stressful events are important causes of many kinds of psychiatric disorder including depressive disorders, anxiety disorders, and schizophrenia. In this chapter we consider three other kinds of response to stressful events: (i) disorders starting very soon after stressful events (acute stress disorder); (ii) disorders following exceptionally severe stress (post-traumatic stress disorder); and (iii) disorders occurring after a change in the circumstances of life (adjustment disorders).

All clinicians see patients with these three kinds of disorder because: (i) acute physical illness and its treatment are stressful; (ii) chronic illness or disability can result in substantial changes in life circumstances; and (iii) clinicians are called on to treat people involved in other kinds of stressful experiences. For these reasons, all clinicians should be able to diagnose and manage the conditions considered in this chapter.

The chapter begins with a description of the normal response to stressful events. This is followed by an account of the three types of reaction referred to above, and of the long-term effects of psychological trauma in childhood. Finally, we consider reactions to three special kinds of stressful event: serious physical illness, terminal illness, and bereavement. *Throughout the chapter, readers should remember that these are not the only reactions to stressful events.* Exceptionally severe stress is also followed by anxiety and depressive disorders: indeed after road accidents, anxiety disorders are almost as frequent as post-traumatic stress disorders. Similarly, changes in life circumstances do not only provoke adjustment disorder—anxiety and depressive disorders also follow these life changes.

Components of the stress response

The normal stress response has three components:

1. An emotional response with accompanying somatic changes.

2. Psychological responses that reduce the potential impact of the experience.

3. Ways of coping with the situation and the emotional response.

Emotional responses and accompanying somatic changes

Emotional responses to stressful events are of two kinds: responses to danger or threat, and responses to separation and loss (Table 5.1). The *emotional responses to danger and threat* are fear and anxiety, respectively. In both, the *accompanying somatic change* is autonomic arousal, with increases in heart rate, blood pressure, and muscle tension, and dry mouth. The *emotional response to separation or loss* is depression, and the *accompanying somatic change* is reduced physical activity.

Psychological changes that reduce the impact of stressful events

Difficulty in recall and numbing

People who have experienced stressful circumstances tend to have **difficulty in recalling** the details of the experiences. They may also experience an unexpected absence of feeling about the events (**numbing**). Freud suggested that both these responses are caused by an active but unconscious mental process, which he called **repression** (Box 5.1).

Coping strategies

People cope with anxiety in a variety of ways. Their actions are of two kinds (Table 5.2): adaptive strategies, which reduce distress in both the short and long term; and maladaptive strategies, which are effective in the short term but lead to difficulties in the longer term.

Adaptive coping strategies include the avoidance of situations that cause distress, working through problems, and coming to terms with situations. Avoidance ceases to be adaptive when it is continued for so long that it prevents working through and coming to terms with the situation.

Maladaptive coping strategies include the excessive use of alcohol or drugs, discharging emotion through histrionic or aggressive behaviour, and deliberate self-harm. Avoidance that is at first adaptive (see above) becomes maladaptive if it is continued for too long since this interferes with other adaptive responses (see above).

Culturally determined coping strategies In some cultures, open displays of extreme distress are a socially accepted and adaptive means of discharging emotion, for example after the sudden death of a loved one. In cultures where such displays are not the norm, they may be maladaptive because they seem excessive and thereby lose the sympathy of potential helpers.

Reactions to acute stress

Normal response to acute stress

As explained above, the normal response to sudden stressful events comprises an emotional response with accompanying physical symptoms, numbness and difficulty in recall, and coping strategies:

1. The *emotional response* to acute stress is anxiety (the normal response to threat): the person feels anxious, is restless, has poor concentration, may feel dazed, and sleeps badly. This response is often combined with depression (the normal response to loss) because many stressful events involve both threat and loss.

TABLE 5.1 Components of the psychological response to stressful circumstances
Emotional responses
◆ to threat: fear
◆ to loss: depression
Somatic responses
◆ to threat: autonomic arousal
◆ to loss: reduced physical activity
Difficulty in recall and numbing
Coping strategies

TABLE 5.2 Strategies for coping with stressful experiences
Potentially adaptive
◆ avoidance
◆ working through problems
◆ coming to terms with situations
Maladaptive
◆ excessive use of alcohol or drugs
◆ histrionic or aggressive behaviour
◆ deliberate self-harm

BOX 5.1 MECHANISMS OF DEFENCE

Repression (see text) is one of the mechanisms of defence proposed by Freud by which anxiety is kept from conscious awareness. Although the ideas have no strict scientific basis they are useful in making more understandable some of the behaviours of ill people and their families. Freud supposed that all the mechanisms are outside conscious awareness.

Repression is the exclusion from consciousness of impulses, emotions, or memories that would otherwise cause distress; for example, the memory of a traumatic event. Freud suggested that repression is a frequent response to severely stressful events.

Denial is a concept put forward to explain why people sometimes behave as if unaware of something of which they are, in fact, adequately informed. For example, someone who has been told that he is dying of cancer may behave as if unaware of the prognosis.

Regression is a concept to explain why people sometimes behave in a way more appropriate to an earlier stage of development; for example, child-like dependence on others. Regression occurs commonly among physically ill people. In the acute stage of illness regression is adaptive, enabling the person to accept a passive role while receiving intensive nursing care. If regression persists into the stage of recovery, it prevents self-help.

Displacement is the transfer of emotion from a person, object, or situation with which it is properly associated, to another which causes less distress. The concept is useful in understanding why, for example, a recently widowed man should blame a doctor for failing to provide adequate care for the wife, instead of blaming himself for putting his work before her needs in the last months of her life.

Projection is the attribution to another person of thoughts or feelings similar to one's own, thereby rendering one's own feelings more acceptable. For example, a person who dislikes a colleague may attribute reciprocal feelings of dislike to him. In this way the person can more easily justify his own feelings of dislike for the colleague.

Reaction formation is the unconscious adoption of behaviour opposite to that which would reflect true feelings and intentions. For example, excessively prudish attitudes to sex are sometimes (but certainly not always) a reaction to strong sexual urges that the person cannot accept.

Rationalization is the unconscious provision of a false but acceptable explanation for behaviour that has a less acceptable origin. For example, a husband may neglect his wife because he does not enjoy her company, but he may tell himself falsely that she is shy and does not enjoy going out.

Sublimation is the unconscious diversion of unacceptable impulses into more acceptable outlets. For example, turning the need to dominate others into the organization of good works for charity (in this, and the other examples given here, it needs to be understood that while the defence mechanism may be one reason for a particular behaviour, there are many other possible reasons).

Identification is the unconscious adoption of the characteristics or activities of another person, often to reduce the pain of separation or loss. For example, a widow may undertake the same voluntary work that her husband used to do.

2. *Physical symptoms of arousal* include palpitations and tremor. Fear responses are often described as 'fight or flight', and aggressive behaviour or running from the stressful situation are sometimes part of the stress response.

3. *Numbing and difficulty in recall* are common and sometimes experienced as a feeling that the events have not really happened.

4. *Coping strategies*: many people *avoid* the situation, and any direct reminders of it. As time passes difficulty in recall and avoidance lessen and are replaced by *working through* memories of the events, and *coming to terms* with the new situation.

Acute stress disorder

This term denotes an abnormal reaction to sudden stressful events. The basic response resembles the

TABLE 5.3 Acute stress disorder and post-traumatic stress disorder

Increased arousal
◆ anxiety and panic attacks
◆ restlessness and purposeless activity
◆ impaired concentration
◆ irritability
◆ insomnia
Depersonalization and derealization
'Dissociative' symptoms
◆ emotional numbness and 'being in a daze'
◆ difficulty in recall of the stressful events
Avoidance of reminders of the stressful events
Flashbacks (see text) and disturbing dreams
Maladaptive coping strategies (see text)

Acute stress disorder is diagnosed when symptoms last from 2 days up to 4 weeks

Post-traumatic stress disorder is diagnosed when symptoms last for 4 weeks or longer

normal response but it is more severe and there are some additional features (Table 5.3):

1. The **emotional response** includes intense anxiety, restlessness, purposeless activity, insomnia, and panic attacks. Some patients experience depersonalization and derealization.

2. **Somatic symptoms** include palpitations, sweating, and tremor.

3. **Dissociative symptoms**: this term is used to describe numbing and difficulty in recall, which are experienced as the feeling that the events have not really taken place, emotional numbing, being 'in a daze' (i.e. less aware of the surroundings), and the inability to remember important aspects of the stressful events. The term *flashbacks* is applied to sudden and repeated re-experiencing of visual images of traumatic experiences, which usually cannot be recalled easily at other times. There may also be recurrent frightening *dreams* of these events.

4. **Coping strategies** include *avoidance* of reminders of the stressful events, and of talking or thinking about them. Social contacts may also be avoided, thus depriving the person of potential sources of support. *Maladaptive coping* responses include 'flight' (e.g. running away from the scene of a road accident), the release of emotion through histrionic or aggressive behaviour, excessive use of alcohol, or deliberate self-harm.

By definition, acute stress disorder lasts no more than 4 weeks. Cases that last longer are called post-traumatic stress disorder (see below).

Aetiology

Many kinds of highly stressful event can provoke an acute stress disorder: for example, involvement in an accident or fire, physical assault, or rape. Since the stress response does not become abnormal in everyone exposed to the same events, there must be some kind of personal predisposition, but it is not known what it is. Acute stress disorder can occur among bystanders as well as those directly involved, and among those involved in rescuing or caring for others.

Immediate treatment

Most acute stress disorders can be managed by the family doctor or other clinician who is caring for the patient, and only the most severe need treatment by a specialist. There are four steps (see Table 5.4).

Reduce the emotional response Usually the person can be comforted effffectively by relatives or friends, and can talk to them about the stressful experience. If no close friend or relative is available, or if the response is severe, comfort may be supplied by a doctor, nurse, or social worker. Occasionally, when anxiety is severe, an anxiolytic drug is needed for a few days at most, or when insomnia is severe, a hypnotic drug for a few nights at most.

Encourage recall As anxiety is reduced, the person is usually able to recall and come to terms with the experience. When memories of the events remain fragmented, help may be needed to recall the events and integrate them into memory. Recall can be gradual—it used to be thought that acute emotional release should be encouraged but it now seems more important that the person fills in the gaps in memory and integrates the recall of the trauma with other memories (see cognitive therapy, below).

TABLE 5.4 Treatment of acute reactions to stressful experiences

◆ Reduce emotion by sympathetic listening and, in severe cases, short-term anxiolytics
◆ Encourage recall of, and coming to terms with, the events
◆ Help with more effective coping
◆ Help with residual problems

Develop more effective coping strategies Some people repeatedly react maladaptively to crises in personal relationships; for example, they drink to excess, behave in a histrionic or aggressive way, or take a drug overdose. Such people need to consider and try more adaptive ways of coping. Counselling to achieve this aim is called *crisis intervention* (see p. 258). (The management of patients who harm themselves is discussed further under deliberate self-harm, see pp. 180–2.)

Help with residual problems Sometimes an acutely stressful situation results in lasting adversity to which the person has to adjust. For example, a serious car accident may lead to permanent disability. When this happens the treatment of an acute reaction should be followed by help in readjustment (see p. 69).

Debriefing

After stressful events, a type of counselling known as debriefing is often made widely available. Subjects *talk* about the stressful events and are encouraged to express their thoughts and feelings at the time and since. They are *informed* about the nature of stress responses and how to manage them. Debriefing is usually offered to most of those involved, and is given soon after the events. In contrast, the measures recommended above are usually reserved for those most severely affected and those who lack other sources of support. Advocates of debriefing claim that its wider use reduces the incidence of subsequent post-traumatic stress disorder. Research does not support this claim and there is some evidence that debriefing may even worsen the long-term outcome.

Cognitive therapy

Cognitive therapy differs from debriefing crucially in its emphasis on *integrating recovered memories* with existing ones, and on *self-help*. It is described further under post-traumatice stress disorder (see below and p. 261).

Prolonged reactions to stress

Prolonged reactions typically follow exposure to extremely stressful events including *natural disasters* such as earthquakes; *man-made calamities* such as major fires, serious accidents, and the circumstances of *war*; and serious physical *assault* or *rape*. Of these, the most frequent are road traffic accidents, and physical and sexual assault. Not all of those involved even in the most severe events develop a prolonged reaction: many recover within the month that is the arbitrary limit for acute stress disorder. The most frequent *long-term consequences* of stressful events are:

◆ post-traumatic stress disorder;

◆ phobic disorder;

◆ depressive disorder.

Post-traumatic stress disorder

Clinical features

The symptoms of post-traumatic stress disorder are the same as those of acute stress disorder but they last for longer. The essential differences are: (i) that symptoms have *lasted for more than 4 weeks* (the arbitrary time limit for acute stress disorder); and (ii) *dissociative symptoms* are a required diagnostic criterion. The reason for this change of diagnosis after 4 weeks is that cases lasting for more than this period generally run a chronic course and require rather different treatment from that used for acute stress disorder. As explained above, there are a number of characterisic features (see Table 5.3):

1. *Symptoms of increased arousal*, such as severe anxiety, irritability, insomnia, and poor concentration. There may be panic attacks and, occasionally, episodes of aggression. Anxiety increases further during flashbacks or reminders of the traumatic event.

2. *Avoidance and 'dissociative' symptoms*, such as difficulty in recalling the events at will, detachment, an inability to feel emotion ('numbness'), and a diminished interest in activities. There is avoidance of reminders of the events and sometimes there is depersonalization and derealization.

3. *Intrusions* in which memories of the traumatic events appear suddenly as repeated intense imagery ('flashbacks') or distressing dreams.

4. *Depressive symptoms* are common and survivors of a major disaster often feel guilt.

5. *Maladaptive coping responses* include persistent anger (especially among those who believe they are innocent victims of others' misbehaviour); excessive use of alcohol or drugs; and episodes of deliberate self-harm, some of which end in suicide.

Post-traumatic stress disorder usually improves within months, but may persist for years.

Aetiology

The necessary cause of post-traumatic stress disorder is an *exceptionally stressful event* in which the person was involved directly or as a witness. However, only a minority of those involved in the same event develops the disorder. Reported rates vary from 4 per cent among earthquake victims to 45 per cent among battered

TABLE 5.5 Factors associated with developing post-traumatic stress disorder

◆ Age: children and old people are particularly vulnerable

◆ Family psychiatric disorder

◆ Childhood abuse

◆ Lack of social support

◆ Low intelligence

◆ Low self-esteem

women. Post-traumatic stress disorder is more common among those involved most directly in the stressful events, but the variation in response is not accounted for solely by the *degree of personal involvement*. Twin studies of Vietnam veterans suggest that, among young adults, part of the vulnerability is genetic. Other factors that increase vulnerability are shown in Table 5.5.

Physiological findings are consistent with the hyperarousal, except that cortisol levels are low. As cortisol levels are normally increased in response to stress, this finding may be a clue to aetiology, but its significance is not yet clear.

Psychological theories suggest that the disorder is caused by a failure to process emotionally charged information and that its persistence is explained by negative interpretations of the initial symptoms (e.g. 'I must be going mad'). This approach does not explain adequately why some people succeed in processing emotionally charged material while others develop negative interpretations and fail.

Assessment

Assessments are concerned with:

◆ the nature and severity of the stressful event;

◆ the nature and duration of the symptoms;

◆ patients' beliefs about the nature of their condition;

◆ disablement;

◆ personality;

◆ previous personal and family psychiatric history.

If the traumatic event has included *injury to the head* (e.g. from an assault or a road accident), a neurological examination should be carried out to exclude an injury to the brain.

Because patients who have prolonged reactions to stress may engage in litigation, it is important to record the assessment fully.

Treatment

Treatment is often difficult and specialist assessment and treatment are often required.

Psychological treatment

General measures include support, information about the condition, help to integrate memories of the events with the rest of the person's experience, and help with any associated grief, guilt, or anger.

Cognitive behaviour therapy is the most effective psychological method. It has three components:

1. **Recalling and sequencing** the fragmentary memories of the events, and relating them clearly to one another or to other memories.

2. **Correcting misinterpretations**, for example the idea that the person could have done more to help others, or that intrusive flashbacks are a sign of impending insanity.

3. **Confronting** any situations that trigger memories of the events.

Eye movement desensitization and reprocessing is a special treatment that comprises: (i) exposure (see p. 259) to imagined scenes of the traumatic events; (ii) the components of cognitive therapy set out above; and (iii) saccadic eye movements induced by following rapid movements of the therapist's finger (the procedure that is specific to the treatment). The treatment is more effective than placebo treatment but its success has not been shown to not depend on the specific eye movement component.

Medication

Anxiolytic drugs should be avoided because of the risk of dependency. Beneficial effects have been claimed for selective serotonin reuptake inhibitors (SSRIs), tricyclic antidepressants, and monoamine oxidase inhibitors (MAOIs). At the time of writing, the treatment of choice, taking into account side effects, appears to be SSRIs. Whatever medication is chosen, it should be accompanied by the general psychological measures described above.

Phobic disorder

Post-traumatic stress disorder is not the only lasting consequence of exposure to stressful events. Phobic reactions are common, especially fears of travel after road traffic accidents. Treatment involves gradual return to the situations that have been avoided (see p. 259).

Depressive disorder

Depressive disorder may follow traumatic experiences, and are often overlooked. The treatment of depressive disorder is described on pp. 108–14.

Reactions to special kinds of acute stress

Reactions to natural disasters and acts of terrorism

Disasters such as earthquakes, floods, and terrorist attacks may involve large numbers of people from the same community. Hence there may be few unaffected people who can comfort and support those affected. In these circumstances teams of counsellors can play a useful role along with those dealing with the physical consequences of the disaster.

Reactions to rape and physical assault

The response of victims of rape or physical assault is an acute stress disorder leading in some cases to a post-traumatic stress disorder. Along with some additional features, the person may:

◆ feel *humiliated, ashamed, and blame themselves* for having put themselves at risk;

◆ *lose confidence and self-esteem* and feel vulnerable to further attack;

◆ after rape, have *difficulty in trusting* others, especially in sexual relationships.

These problems should be talked over, and resolved as far as possible. *Counselling* can help to achieve these aims, as can help from a *victim support organization*. *Cognitive therapy* is also effective but it is less readily available.

Reactions to the stresses of war and torture, and among refugees

Some combatants develop acute reactions to stress, post-traumatic stress disorder, and other long-term consequences of exposure to stress. Similar reactions may develop among civilians in war zones, refugees, and victims of torture—any of whom may have additional problems of bereavement, remorse for the suffering of others, and the experience of rape. Some experience feelings of intense anger, shame, and humiliation. Treatment is similar to that for other post-traumatic disorders (see above) but with attention to the special circumstances of the case.

Long-term effects of sexual trauma in childhood

Sexually abused children experience anxiety, depression, and post-traumatic stress disorder. These respons-es eventually decline but some continue into adult life. As adults these people are prone to low self-esteem, psychosexual difficulties, and other problems.

Most adults who were sexually abused as children, retain some memory of the events, though these are often incomplete. Forgotten aspects are sometimes recalled again, for example after a chance encounter with some reminder of the events. Memories may also return during the history taking and discussion involved in psychological treatment. Occasionally, an adult who is receiving counselling or psychotherapy, suddenly recalls an episode of child abuse of which he was previously completely unaware. Sometimes such memories are confirmed by people who knew the patient at the time, but sometimes they are vigorously denied by others, including the alleged abuser. When this happens, it has to be decided whether the reports are true memories of actual events, or false memories induced by overzealous questioning, interpretation, or suggestion (the **false memory syndrome**). It is uncertain whether memories of sexual abuse can be completely forgotten for many years and then recalled—usually some fragment of memory is preserved. It is, however, generally agreed that:

◆ great care should be taken during history taking, counselling, and psychotherapy to avoid questions or comments that could suggest childhood sexual abuse;

◆ any apparent recall of events of which the person had no previous recollection should be considered most carefully and supporting evidence sought, before concluding that it is a true memory.

Normal and abnormal adjustment reactions

Normal adjustment

Adjustment refers to the psychological reactions involved in adapting to new circumstances. It may include short-lived *anxiety, depression, irritability* and *poor concentration*. Examples of life changes that may provoke normal or abnormal adjustment are: divorce and separation; a major change of work and abode such as the transition from school to university; and the birth of a handicapped child. Adjustment to bereavement and terminal illness have special features that are described later.

Adjustment disorder

Adjustment is judged to be abnormal—to be an adjustment disorder—if the distress involved is:

• greater than that which would be expected to the particular stressful events (this judgement is subjective and the diagnostic manuals offer no objective criteria); *or*

• accompanied by impairment of social functioning; *and*

• close in time to the life change (the diagnostic systems differ on how close—ICD specifies within 1 month and DSM allows up to 3 months); *and*

• not severe enough to meet the criteria for the diagnosis of another psychiatric disorder.

General practitioners and hospital doctors see many patients of this kind, often in relation to the life changes imposed by physical illness. These clinicians can usually judge better than a psychiatrist whether the patient's reaction is greater than that of most people with a similar illness.

Treatment

Treatment is designed to assist the natural processes of adjustment by reducing anxiety, encouraging problem solving, and discouraging maladaptive coping responses.

Anxiety reduction can usually be achieved by encouraging patients to talk about the problems and to express their feelings to a sympathetic listener. When anxiety is very severe, anxiolytic drugs may be needed but they should not be prescribed routinely or for long. Occasionally, a hypnotic drug is required for a few nights to restore sleep.

Problem solving Patients with adjustment disorder often feel overwhelmed by a series of life problems and are assisted by a problem-solving approach in which the patient is helped to:

• *list the problems* and think of ways of overcoming them;

• *consider* the advantages and disadvantages of various *solutions* to the problems;

• *select and implement actions* that seem most likely to succeed.

If the third step succeeds, the process is repeated with another problem; if it fails, the patient tries another approach to the first problem. Problem-solving counselling is discussed further on p. 257.

Crisis intervention This approach is used when a patient has responded to an acute life change—such as the sudden breaking up of an intimate relationship—

with a maladaptive coping mechanism such as deliberate self-harm. The approach (see p. 258) resembles problem solving but with additional help in examining the maladaptive coping responses, recognizing their disadvantages, and considering other ways of dealing with similar problems in the future.

Adjustment to special situations

Adjustment to physical illness

Illness behaviour Adjustment to physical illness involves a set of changes known as illness behaviour. This behaviour includes seeking medical advice, taking medication, accepting help, and giving up activities. Illness behaviours are at first adaptive, but if they persist too long they may become maladaptive. Occasionally, people adopt illness behaviours when they have no physical disorder. They are said to display *abnormal illness behaviour*, though it is not the behaviour that is abnormal but the circumstances in which it occurs—namely without a medical reason.

The sick role is a related concept. Society allows sick people to adopt a special role which comprises two privileges and two duties:

• *exemption* from some responsibilities;

• the *right* to help and care;

• the *obligation* to seek and cooperate in treatment;

• the *expectation* of a wish to recover and efforts to achieve this.

The sick role is usually adaptive. However, some people continue to adopt a sick role long after the illness is over, avoiding responsibilities and depending on others instead of becoming independent. Others adopt the sick role without ever having experienced any physical disorder.

Physical illness as a stressor The stress associated with physical illness may lead to *anxiety* and *depression*, and sometimes to *anger*. Most of these reactions are short lived, subsiding as the person adjusts to the new situation. The stressful effect of physical illness cannot be judged solely in terms of its objective severity; it depends also on the *patient's appraisal* of the illness and its likely consequences. This appraisal may be unrealistic and based on false assumptions. The latter may be shared by the relatives, thus reinforcing the patient's concerns, or contradicted by them, thus leading to family conflict.

Physical illness and its treatment as direct causes of psychiatric symptoms As well as acting as a psychological stressor, physical illness may induce psychiatric symptoms directly. Anxiety, depression, fatigue, weakness, weight loss, and certain abnormal behaviours can all be caused in this way. These associations are considered in Chapter 11 (see p. 151). Certain *medications* used in the treatment of physical illness may also affect mood, behaviour, and consciousness. These associations are considered on p. 152.

Denial As in adjustment to other situations, adjustment to physical illness often involves an initial stage of denial (see Box 5.1), which protects against overwhelming distress. If denial persists beyond the early stage of adjustment it prevents the working through of problems and interferes with full engagement with treatment. Denial can be reduced by helping patients to discuss their concerns, and by providing information to correct misunderstandings, for example about the likely amount of pain.

Treatment

When adjustment to physical illness is slow and incomplete, treatment can usually be provided effectively by the primary care or hospital team dealing with the physical illness. The clinician explains the nature of the physical illness and its treatment, and then discusses the patient's anxieties. The latter may include the effects of the illness on their family, or the threat of job loss. As anxiety diminishes, so should any maladaptive behaviours such as overdependence or poor adherence to treatment. To be effective, counselling must be based on a trusting relationship between the patient and physician or nurse. To achieve this relationship, sufficient time must be set aside—hurried consultations are unlikely to be effective. However, the necessary trusting relationship must not be allowed to become one of dependence.

Depressive and anxiety disorders as a response to physical illness Sometimes the stress of physical illness provokes an anxiety or depressive disorder. Such cases are treated in the same way as other anxiety or depressive disorders (see Chapters 6 and 8).

Adjustment to terminal illness

After terminal illness has been diagnosed, many people become anxious, depressed, guilty, or angry, and some adopt maladaptive ways of coping. Among patients dying in hospital about half have emotional symptoms. Understandably, these emotional reactions are more common in the young than in the old, and less common in the religious. The following symptoms are common among the dying.

1. **Anxiety** may be provoked by personal concerns about pain, disfigurement, or incontinence, and by concerns about others, especially the family.

2. **Depression** may be provoked by the loss of valued activities and the prospect of separation from loved ones. Depression and anxiety can also be the direct result of the physical disease or of the medication used to treat it (see Tables 11.3 and 11.4).

3. **Confusion** due to delirium is frequent among dying patients, caused, for example, by dehydration, drug side effects, and secondary infection (see p. 138).

4. **Guilt** may be caused by the belief that excessive demands are being placed on relatives or friends.

5. **Anger** may derive from ideas about the unjustness of impending death.

The response to the prospect of dying can be understood in terms of the concepts of denial and displacement (see Box 5.1), and of dependency and acceptance.

Denial is usually the first reaction to the news of fatal illness. It may be experienced as a feeling of disbelief and a consequent initial period of calm. Usually, denial diminishes as the patient gradually comes to terms with the situation. It may return with signs of the progress of the disease, when the patient may once more behave as if unaware of the nature of the condition.

Displacement Anger about the situation may be displaced onto doctors, nurses, and relatives. All may find this anger difficult to tolerate unless they understand its origins. Without this understanding they may be less inclined to spend time with patients, thereby increasing their feelings of isolation and anger.

Dependency is common among terminally ill people. It is adaptive at times when the patient is required to comply passively with treatment, but persisting or excessive dependency makes treatment more difficult, and increases the burden on the family.

Acceptance is the final stage of adjustment. The aim is to help the patient to reach this state before the final stage of the physical illness.

Treatment

Control of pain and confusion The first steps in treatment are to control pain and reduce confusion, as these symptoms distract patients from the psychological work needed to reach a satisfactory adjustment.

Explaining the illness and treatment Carers sometimes worry that explaining the terminal nature of the illness will increase the patient's distress. While excessive detail, given unsympathetically and at the wrong time, can have this effect, it is seldom difficult to decide how much to say provided that *patients are allowed to lead the discussion*. When patients ask about the prognosis they should be told the truth; evasive answers undermine trust. Patients notice when answers to their questions are evasive. When people avoid talking to them, they infer the truth from this avoidance although they are not told directly. Nevertheless, when patients do not at first indicate a desire to know the full extent of their problems, it is better to keep this information for a subsequent interview. The account should always be truthful, but the amount disclosed on a single occasion should be judged by the patient's reactions and by their questions. If necessary, the clinician should set aside time for further discussion when the patient seems ready for this. At an appropriate time, patients should be told what will be done to make their last days as comfortable as possible.

Sharing information Information given to patients should be known to all the staff concerned with their care and, provided the patient agrees, to involved relatives. Otherwise advice and opinions may conflict and those involved may draw back from patients, isolating them and increasing their difficulty in coming to terms with their situation.

Help for relatives Relatives may be anxious and depressed, and respond with denial, guilt, and anger. These reactions may make it difficult for them to communicate helpfully with the patient and with staff. Relatives need information about the disease and its treatment, and opportunities to talk about their feelings and to prepare for the impending bereavement.

Special nursing In many places terminal care nurses work with the patient and the family, liaising with the family doctor and with the hospital staff caring for the patient. These nurses are skilled in the psychological as well as the physical care of the dying.

Referral to a psychiatrist is indicated when:

- there is *doubt about the psychiatric diagnosis* (e.g. between adjustment disorder and depressive disorder);
- the patient has had a *previous psychiatric disorder*;
- the patient *refuses to discuss* the illness, or to make necessary decisions;
- the patient *refuses to cooperate* with treatment, in order to determine whether refusal is for rational reasons or has a psychiatric cause.

TABLE 5.6	The normal grief reaction
Stage I (hours to days)	
◆ Denial, disbelief	
◆ 'Numbness'	
Stage II (weeks to 6 months)	
◆ Sadness, weeping, waves of grief	
◆ Somatic symptoms of anxiety	
◆ Restlessness	
◆ Poor sleep	
◆ Diminished appetite	
◆ Guilt, blame of others	
◆ Experience of the presence of the deceased	
◆ Illusions, vivid imagery	
◆ Hallucinations of the dead person's voice	
◆ Preoccupation with memories of the deceased	
◆ Social withdrawal	
Stage III (weeks to months)	
◆ Symptoms resolve	
◆ Social activities resumed	
◆ Memories of good times	
◆ (Symptoms may recur at anniversaries)	

Grief: the response to bereavement

Normal grief

The normal response to bereavement goes through three stages (Table 5.6).

The **first stage** lasts from a few hours to several days. There is a lack of emotional response ('numbness'), often with a feeling of unreality, and incomplete acceptance that the death has taken place.

The **second stage** lasts from a few weeks to 6 months. There may be extreme sadness, weeping, and often overwhelming waves of grief. Somatic symptoms of anxiety are common. The bereaved person is restless, sleeps poorly, and lacks appetite. Many bereaved people feel guilty that they failed to do enough for the deceased; some project these feelings to clinical staff for failing to provide optimal care for the dead person. Some bereaved people have an intense experience of being in the presence of the dead person, and may experience vivid imagery, illusions, or sometimes hallucinations of that person's voice. The bereaved person is preoccupied with memories of the dead person, and often withdraws from social relationships.

In the **third stage** these symptoms subside, and everyday activities are resumed. The bereaved person gradually comes to terms with the loss, and recalls the good times shared with the deceased in the past. Often, there is a temporary return of symptoms on the anniversary of the death.

Abnormal grief

Grief is said to be abnormal when the symptoms are:

◆ *more intense* than usual and meet the criteria for (usually) a depressive disorder;

◆ *prolonged* beyond 6 months;

◆ *delayed* in onset.

Abnormal grief reactions are more likely in several circumstances:

◆ after a death that was sudden and unexpected;

◆ when the bereaved person was very close to, and dependent on, the deceased;

◆ when the survivor is insecure, or has difficulty in expressing feelings, or has suffered a previous psychiatric disorder;

◆ when the survivor cannot express grief easily, for example because she has to care for young children.

Helping the bereaved

Help for the bereaved resembles that for other kinds of adjustment reaction. The first step is to *listen* while the bereaved person talks about the loss and to enable him to express feelings of sadness or anger. When the person is seen soon after the loss, it is helpful to *explain* the normal course of grieving, and to forewarn about the possibility of feeling as if the dead person were present, or experiencing illusions or hallucinations. Without this warning, these experiences may be very alarming.

The bereaved person may need help to move from the early stage of denial of the loss to *acceptance* of reality by viewing the body and by later putting away the dead person's belongings. *Practical steps* should be discussed, for example, funeral arrangements and possible financial difficulties. A widow may need help in caring for young children. As time passes, the bereaved person should be encouraged to resume social contacts; to talk to other people about the loss; to remember happy and fulfilling experiences that were shared with the deceased; and to consider positive activities that the latter would have wanted survivors to undertake.

When *grief is prolonged* similar measures are used. When *grief is abnormally intense* and meets the criteria for depressive disorder, antidepressant drug treatment may be required. However, antidepressants do not relieve the distress of normal grief. An anxiolytic or hypnotic drug may be helpful in the first few days after bereavement if anxiety is severe or sleep greatly disrupted. However, medication should not be continued for more than a few days, and in most cases distress can be reduced by the opportunity to talk and weep.

Support groups are helpful, especially for young widows. The groups enable newly bereaved people to talk with others who have dealt successfully with the emotional and practical aspects of bereavement.

Further reading

Ehlers, A. (2000). Post-traumatic stress disorder. In *New Oxford Textbook of Psychiatry*. Ed. M. G. Gelder, J. J. Lopez-Ibor & N. C. Andreasen, pp. 758–71. Oxford University Press, Oxford.
A comprehensive overview of the syndrome and approaches to treatment.
Parkes, C. M. (1998). *Bereavement: Studies of Grief in Adult Life*, 3rd edn. Pelican, Harmondsworth.
Latest edition of classic description of bereavement reactions.

CHAPTER 6

Anxiety and obsessional disorders

Chapter contents

Normal and abnormal anxiety 73

Anxiety disorders 74

Generalized anxiety disorder 75
Phobic anxiety disorders 79
Panic disorder 83

Obsessive-compulsive disorder 85

Anxiety disorders are common in both primary care and general hospital practice. Many patients present with physical rather than psychological symptoms of anxiety. Also, anxiety disorders can be provoked by the stress associated with physical illness and its treatment. Thus anxiety disorders are encountered by clinicians working in all branches of medicine and they should be able to diagnose the conditions, arrange basic treatment, and know when to refer patients to a specialist.

Anxiety disorders are divided into generalized anxiety, phobic, and panic disorders each with a characteristic pattern of symptoms and disabilities, and each requiring somewhat different treatment. *Mixed states of anxiety and depression are common: these 'minor mood disorders' are described with depressive disorders to which they are more closely related* (see p. 103).

Obsessive-compulsive disorders are also considered in this chapter. Their relation to anxiety disorders is uncertain. They are classified with anxiety disorders in DSM-IV because there are many common features, but are classified separately in ICD-10 because there are some important differences.

Normal and abnormal anxiety

Normal anxiety is the response to threatening situations. Feelings of apprehension are accompanied by physiological changes that prepare for defence or escape ('fight or flight'), notably increases in heart rate, blood pressure, respiration, and muscle tension. Sympathetic nervous system activity is increased with, for example, tremor, polyuria, and diarrhoea. Attention is focused on the threatening situation.

Abnormal anxiety is a response that is similar but out of proportion to the threat and/or more prolonged, or occurs when there is no threat. With one exception, the symptoms of anxiety disorders are the same as those of a normal anxiety response. The exception is that the focus of attention is not the external threat (as in the normal response) but the physiological response itself. Thus in abnormal anxiety, attention is focused on a symptom such as increased heart rate. This focus of attention is accompanied by concern about the cause of the symptom. For example, a common concern is that rapid heart action is a sign of heart disease. Another common concern is that other people will become aware of the symptom and think it strange, for example, that they will notice trembling of the hands. Because these concerns are threatening, they activate a further anxiety response thus adding to the autonomic arousal, generating further concern, and setting up a vicious cycle of mounting anxiety.

Anxiety disorders

Classification

Anxiety disorders are states with marked and persistent mental and physical symptoms of anxiety that are not secondary to another disorder. Anxiety disorders are classified into those with continuous symptoms (**generalized anxiety disorder**) and those with episodic symptoms. The latter are divided into those in which episodes of anxiety occur in particular situations (**phobic anxiety disorders**) and those in which episodes can occur in any situations (**panic disorder**) (Fig. 6.1). Phobic anxiety disorders are classified further into **simple phobia**, **social phobia**, and **agoraphobia** (these terms are explained later). Some patients have both episodes of anxiety in particular situations, characteristic of agoraphobia, and random episodes, characteristic of panic disorder. These mixed disorders are called **panic with agoraphobia** in DSM (unfortunately the term in ICD10 is slightly different—agoraphobia with panic).

Prevalence

Anxiety disorders are common in the population with a 1-year prevalence of about 14 per cent, or about 10 per cent if simple phobias are excluded. They are encountered frequently in primary care and general hospital practice although many patients do not complain directly of anxiety, but instead ask for help with one or more of the physical symptoms of anxiety, such as

TABLE 6.1 Approximate prevalence of anxiety disorders	
	Approximate 1-year prevalence per 1000*
Generalized anxiety disorder	30
Phobic disorders	
Agoraphobia	20
Social phobia	30
Simple phobia**	45
Panic disorder	15
Obsessive-compulsive disorder***	10

*'Clinically significant' cases only, shown to the nearest 5 per thousand; ** if all cases are included (not just the clinically significant ones) the rate is approximately 85 per 1000; *** excluding cases co-morbid with another anxiety disorder.

From Narrow, W. E., Rae, D. S., Robins, L. N. *et al.* (2002). *Archives of General Psychiatry* **59**, 115–123.

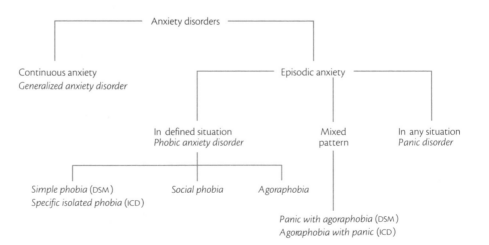

Fig. 6.1 Principles of classification of anxiety disorders.

palpitations. The approximate frequency of the various kinds of anxiety disorder is shown in Table 6.1. The figures are approximate and uncertain because different criteria have been used in the various surveys. They show, nevertheless, the relative frequency of the disorders.

Generalized anxiety disorder

Clinical features

Appearance The face looks strained and the brow furrowed; the posture is tense and the patient is restless and may tremble. The skin is pale, with increased sweating from the hands, feet, and axillae. Readiness to tears, which may erroneously suggest depression, reflects a generally apprehensive state.

Psychological symptoms are listed in Table 6.2. Patients with *poor concentration* sometimes complain of poor memory but true memory impairment does not occur in an anxiety disorder—if it is present a careful search should be made for an organic syndrome. Repetitive *worrying thoughts* are characteristic of generalized anxiety disorder. These thoughts may concern personal illness, fears about the health or safety of other people, or social anxieties.

Physical symptoms reflect overactivity in the sympathetic nervous system and increased tension in skeletal muscles. The list of possible symptoms is long, but they can be grouped conveniently by the systems of the body as shown in Table 6.2. A few items in the list require comment. Excessive wind results from the swallowing of air. Difficulty in inhaling caused by anxiety contrasts with the expiratory difficulty of asthma. Overbreathing causes further physical symptoms as explained below. Dizziness is not rotational but rather a feeling of unsteadiness. Some patients report blurring of vision although their visual acuity is normal. Headache is typically in the form of constriction or pressure, which is usually bilateral and frontal or occipital. Aching, especially in the back and shoulders, is common.

Some patients do not complain of anxiety but ask for help for one or more of the many physical symptoms of anxiety. Also, each of the physical symptoms of anxiety can also be caused by physical disease. Both points, which are important in diagnosis, are considered further under differential diagnosis (see below).

Sleep is disturbed in a characteristic way. On going to bed patients lie awake worrying; when at last they fall asleep, they wake intermittently. They often report unpleasant dreams, and occasionally 'night terrors' in which they wake suddenly feeling intensely fearful,

TABLE 6.2	Symptoms of generalized anxiety disorder
Psychological	Fearful anticipation
	Irritability
	Sensitivity to noise
	Restlessness
	Poor concentration
	Worrying thoughts
Physical	
◆ Gastrointestinal	Dry mouth
	Difficulty in swallowing
	Epigastric discomfort
	Excessive wind
	Frequent or loose motions
◆ Respiratory	Constriction in the chest
	Difficulty inhaling
	Overbreathing
◆ Cardiovascular	Palpitations
	Discomfort in chest
	Awareness of missed beats
◆ Genitourinary	Frequent or urgent micturition
	Failure of erection
	Menstrual discomfort
	Amenorrhoea
◆ Neuromuscular	Tremor
	Prickling sensations
	Tinnitus
	Dizziness
	Headache
	Aching muscles
Sleep disturbance	Insomnia
	Night terrors
Other symptoms	Depression
	Obsessions
	Depersonalization

sometimes remembering a nightmare, and sometimes uncertain why they are so frightened. Early waking with an inability to go back to sleep again is much less common among patients with a generalized anxiety disorder than among patients with a depressive disorder (see pp. 99–100). Therefore, early waking should always prompt a search for other symptoms of a depressive disorder.

Hyperventilation is breathing, usually in a rapid and shallow way, that is excessive in that it results in a fall in the concentration of carbon dioxide in the

TABLE 6.3	Symptoms and signs of hyperventilation
◆ Rapid shallow breathing	
◆ Dizziness	
◆ Tinnitus	
◆ Headache	
◆ Precordial discomfort	
◆ Weakness	
◆ Faintness	
◆ Numbness and tingling in the hands and feet	
◆ Carpopedal spasm	

blood. The resultant symptoms are listed in Table 6.3. Paradoxically, overbreathing produces a feeling of breathlessness that causes the patient to breathe even more vigorously. When a patient has unexplained bodily symptoms, the possibility of persistent overbreathing should be considered. The diagnosis should be made on the definite occurrence of this group of symptoms, and on observations of the patient's respiration pattern when the symptoms are present. The finding that symptoms produced by deliberate overbreathing resemble those experienced spontaneously does not prove that involuntary hyperventilation is the cause of the latter.

Panic attacks Some patients with generalized anxiety disorder experience occasional panic attacks, that is, sudden episodes of very severe anxiety. However, panic attacks are more characteristic of panic disorder (see p. 83).

Other symptoms are listed in Table 6.2. Although not major features of the disorder, they too may be the symptoms for which patients seek help.

Duration of symptoms By convention, generalized anxiety disorder is diagnosed only when symptoms of anxiety have been present for several months (6 months in DSM-IV). When symptoms have been present for a shorter time, the diagnosis is *stress* or *adjustment disorder* (see pp. 63 and 67).

Prevalence
Generalized anxiety disorder occurs in about 3 per cent of the population. It is slightly more common among women than men. The disorder is chronic and is therefore frequent among attenders in primary care.

Differential diagnosis
Generalized anxiety disorder has to be distinguished from other psychiatric disorders in which anxiety may be prominent and from physical illnesses that produce similar symptoms.

◆ **Depressive disorder** can present with symptoms of anxiety, and patients with chronic generalized anxiety disorder may ask for help when they feel depressed. *Diagnostic errors can be reduced by enquiring routinely about depressive symptoms* in patients presenting with anxiety. Usually the depressive symptoms are generally more severe than the anxiety symptoms, and other symptoms of depressive disorder will be present. The history, taken from an informant as well as from the patient, will usually reveal that the depressive symptoms appeared first. Sometimes *agitation* occurring in a severe depressive disorder (see p. 99) is mistaken for anxiety.

◆ **Schizophrenia.** Occasionally patients with schizophrenia complain of anxiety before they reveal other symptoms of schizophrenia. Errors in diagnosis can be reduced by asking anxious patients what they think is the cause of their symptoms. In reply, schizophrenic patients may reveal delusions (e.g. that they are anxious because they are being spied on).

◆ **Dementia** may first come to notice when the patient complains of anxiety. When this happens, the clinician may overlook the accompanying memory disorder or ascribe it to poor concentration. For this reason, memory should be assessed appropriately especially when older patients present with anxiety.

◆ **Withdrawal from drugs or alcohol or excessive use of caffeine** can cause anxiety, and the cause may be overlooked because patients wish to hide their drug or alcohol misuse. Reports that anxiety is particularly severe on waking in the morning suggests alcohol dependence (withdrawal symptoms are most likely at this time, see p. 188), though anxiety symptoms secondary to depressive disorder may also be worse on waking.

◆ Certain **physical illnesses** may present with symptoms similar to those of anxiety disorder. This possibility should be considered in every case, but particularly when no psychological explanation can be found for the anxiety.

  ◆ *Thyrotoxicosis* leads to irritability, restlessness, tremor, and tachycardia. Patients should be examined for an enlarged thyroid, atrial fibrillation, and exophthalmos; and thyroid function tests should be arranged in appropriate cases.

  ◆ *Phaeochromocytoma*, *hypoglycaemia*, *paroxysmal tachycardias*, and *Menière's disease* should be considered as occasional causes of episodic anxiety.

- *Other physical illness* may cause anxiety through psychological rather than physiological mechanisms (e.g. because the patient fears a fatal outcome). This sequence is particularly likely when the patient has a special reason to fear serious consequences (e.g. because a relative has died after developing similar symptoms). It is useful to ask anxious patients whether they know anyone who had similar symptoms.

- **Anxiety disorder mistaken for physical illness**. Any of the physical symptoms listed in Table 6.2 can be the presenting complaint of a patient with a generalized anxiety disorder. Special investigations carried out to exclude physical illness may be necessary, but if this error is made patients may be subjected to special investigations that increase anxiety because their negative results do not explain the symptoms.

Aetiology

Predisposing factors are of three kinds: genetic, childhood upbringing, and personality type.

1. **Genetic causes** are important in predisposing to anxiety disorders. The concordance for anxiety disorders of all kinds is greater among monozygotic than among dizygotic twins. However, most studies do not distinguish between the different kinds of anxiety disorder, so the size of the contribution of genetic factors to generalized anxiety disorder is uncertain.

2. **Childhood upbringing** has been thought to predispose to generalized anxiety disorder in adult life. However, despite much speculation, no specific causes have been identified. Anxiety is a common emotional disorder in childhood but most anxious children grow into healthy adults and not all anxious adults have been anxious children.

3. **Personality type**. Anxious and worry prone personalities (see p. 52) are linked to anxiety disorder but other personalities can predispose by making people less able to cope with stressful events.

Precipitating factors Generalized anxiety disorder usually begins in relation to stressful events, especially *threatening events* such as problems in relationships, with employment and with ill health.

Maintaining factors Generalized anxiety disorders are often maintained by *continuing stressful events*. They are also maintained by *ways of thinking* that make the symptoms of the disorder stressful; for example, fears that other people will notice that the patient is anxious, or that anxiety will impair performance at work. Such fears lead to a vicious circle that increases and prolongs anxiety.

Prognosis

By convention, the diagnosis of generalized anxiety disorder cannot be made until the symptoms have been present for several months (more than 6 months in DSM-IV). Without treatment, about 80 per cent of patients still have the disorder 3 years after the onset. *Prognosis is worse* when symptoms are severe, and when there is agitation, derealization, conversion symptoms, or suicidal ideas. Brief episodes of depression are frequent among patients with a chronic generalized anxiety disorder and it is often during one of these episodes that further treatment is sought. Hence the importance of a careful search for symptoms of a depressive disorder in all patients with generalized anxiety disorder.

Common features in the management of anxiety disorders

Although there are differences in the treatment of the various types of anxiety disorder, there are also many common features. Treatments are tested on patients who meet formal diagnostic criteria, but many patients seek help before their symptoms meet these criteria. For example, one criterion for generalized anxiety disorder is a duration of 6 months. Although it is clearly sensible to start treatment as soon as the patient asks for help, it has to be recognized that most of the procedures that are used have not been thoroughly evaluated with early cases. The usual approach to the treatment of anxiety disorders is as follows (Table 6.4).

TABLE 6.4 General treatment plan for anxiety disorders
Initial treatment
- Detect and treat any co-morbid depressive disorder
- Agree a clear plan
- Explain the nature and cause of symptoms, reassure about specific concerns
- Help in solving or coming to terms with stressful problems
- Advise about self-help methods
- If anxiety severe, use short-term benzodiazepine treatment
Further treatment
Continue the above and consider
- Relaxation training
- Respiratory control if hyperventilating
- Medication if anxiety still severe (see text)
- Referral for cognitive behaviour therapy (technique varies according to the type of disorder)

Initial treatment

Exclude depressive disorder Patients with chronic anxiety may ask for help when depressed; and depressive disorder may present with anxiety symptoms (see Differential diagnosis, above). If present, treatment for depression should be started (see p. 109).

Agree a clear plan Anxiety is prolonged by uncertainty and a clear management plan, agreed with the patient, helps to reduce it.

Provide and discuss information Anxiety disorders are maintained by fears about the nature and consequences of their symptoms. An explanation of the condition should be tailored to the particular concerns of the individual patient, but it is usually necessary to explain how fears that symptoms are caused by physical illness and concerns about other people's critical opinions, can cause vicious circles of anxiety. A simple diagram helps to explain this mechanism. Since anxious patients do not concentrate well on new information, it is useful to write down the essential points for the patient to study at home. Alternatively, a standard leaflet can be used, marked to indicate the points of most relevance to the patient, or a self-help book can be recommended (see below).

Identify and reduce or avoid any stressors Patients should be encouraged to deal with or come to terms with any social problems or other difficulties that appear to be maintaining the anxiety disorder. The general approach should be to help patients to: (i) identify stressors by keeping a *diary* of occasions when they felt anxious and the events at the time; (ii) think of ways of avoiding or dealing with the events; and (iii) try these out (see Problem-solving treatment, p. 257).

Advise about self-help methods Patients with anxiety disorders can help themselves in several ways, some of which apply generally while others are specific to the kind of disorder. The former include managing time, taking time off to relax, and reducing caffeine intake. The latter are described under the relevant disorders.

Limit the use of anxiolytics Anxiolytic drugs can bring rapid relief from anxiety at times of crisis. While it is easy to prescribe them, this should not be done routinely but kept for more severe disorders or cases in which immediate relief is essential (for example to fulfil an essential commitment). Anxiolytics should not be prescribed for more than about 3 weeks because of the risk of dependency (see p. 237).

Further treatment

Relaxation training can be provided within a primary care team. To be effective it must be practised regularly; some patients are better motivated by training in a group rather than individually. Some prefer to learn relaxation as part of yoga exercises.

Treatment for hyperventilation Although not applicable to every case, the treatment of hyperventilation is considered here because it may occur in several kinds of anxiety disorder:

♦ *To terminate an acute episode*, the patient should re-breathe expired air from a paper bag thereby increasing the alveolar concentration of carbon dioxide. Rebreathing during an episode is also an effective way of demonstrating that certain symptoms are caused by hyperventilation.

♦ *To prevent further episodes* of hyperventilation, patients should practise slow, controlled breathing, at first under supervision and then at home. A tape recording can be used to help the patient time his breathing appropriately. Such a tape can be made by the primary care team or obtained from a department of clinical psychology.

Consider antidepressants It may seem illogical to prescribe antidepressant medication for patients with anxiety disorders who do not have co-morbid depression. However, most antidepressants drugs have anxiolytic as well as antidepressant effects and, unlike other anxiolytics, they do not produce dependence. For this reason, they are suitable for long-term treatment of anxiety disorders. The anxiolytic effect of antidepressants is not immediate, instead the initial effect is sometimes to increase anxiety. For this reason the drugs should be started cautiously and sometimes with the addition of a benzodiazepine for a few days. Usually medication is continued for 6 months or more. Patients who relapse can resume their medication or be referred for cognitive behaviour therapy. The choice of drug, which varies a little with the type of disorder, is discussed later under the specific disorders.

Refer for cognitive behaviour therapy The treatments described so far can all be carried out by a primary care team. Cognitive behaviour therapy is provided by a clinical psychologist or a specially trained psychiatric nurse, though in some places there are waiting lists. Since techniques vary according to the type of disorder, they will be considered later in relation to the specific disorders.

Treatment of generalized anxiety disorder

In formal terms, generalized anxiety disorder cannot be diagnosed until symptoms have been present for 6 months. However, general practioners and other clinicians see many patients with similar symptoms before the 6-month period has passed, and they should be treated. *Depressive disorder* should be excluded in all cases.

General measures Treatment is based on the general measures described above. The following points apply particularly to generalized anxiety disorder.

Self-help methods As well as the general methods, patients should be encouraged to identify and deal with the worrying thoughts that are characteristic of generalized anxiety disorder. To do this, they should:

* write down the worrying thoughts so that they can be considered more objectively;

* consider for each problem whether anything can be done to resolve the worrying problem;

* if possible take the appropriate action; if no action is possible, set aside a brief 'worry time' each day, and for the rest of the day endeavour to use distraction to prevent worrying (this procedure is described more fully by Butler & Hope (1995), see further reading).

Anxiolytic medication As well as the occasional use of a benzodiazepine for short-term relief of anxiety, *buspirone*, a non-benzodiazepine anxiolytic (see p. 237) may be used. Buspirone is less likely than the benzodiazepines to cause dependence but its effects appear more slowly.

Antidepressant medication Several types of antidepressant can be used:

* *Tricyclics:* in this group, amitriptyline is an inexpensive and well-tried drug. Although anticholinergic side effects may be a problem, they are less frequent than in the treatment of depressive disorder because an anxiolytic effect can usually be achieved with a lower dose.

* *Specific serotonin reuptake inhibitors* (SSRIs) generally have fewer troublesome side effects than tricyclics and are less toxic in overdose (see p. 243). However, they may cause an increase in anxiety and agitation when first taken.

* *Monoamine oxidase inhibitors* (MAOIs) were the first antidepressants to be used to treat anxiety disorders but they are seldom used today because they interact with certain drugs and foodstuffs (see p. 245).

Cognitive behaviour therapy *Anxiety management* is described on p. 261. It combines relaxation with techniques to reduce worries about the physical symptoms of anxiety. Although research evidence is limited, clinical experience suggests that this is the psychological treatment of choice for generalized anxiety disorder.

Phobic anxiety disorders

The symptoms of phobic anxiety disorder are the same as those of generalized anxiety disorders, but there are three distinguishing features:

1. *Anxiety in particular circumstances only.* In some phobic disorders the relevant circumstances are so infrequent that the patient is free from anxiety for most of the time; in other cases the circumstances occur so frequently that the patient is seldom free from anxiety.

2. *Avoidance* of circumstances that provoke anxiety.

3. *Anticipatory anxiety* when there is the prospect of encountering such circumstances.

The circumstances that provoke anxiety include *situations*, such as crowded places, *living things*, such as spiders, and *natural phenomena*, such as thunder.

Phobic disorders are classified in three groups: simple phobia, social phobia, and agoraphobia. As explained above (p. 74) some patients have both agoraphobia and non-situational panic.

Simple phobia

A person with simple phobia is inappropriately anxious in the presence of a particular object or situation, or when anticipating this encounter, and has the urge to avoid the object or situation. The symptoms resemble those of generalized anxiety disorder (see p. 75). The urge to avoid the stimulus is strong, and in most cases there is actual avoidance. Anticipatory anxiety is often severe, for example a person who fears storms may become extremely anxious when there are only black clouds, which might precede a storm.

Simple phobias can be specified further by adding the name of the stimulus; for example, spider phobia. Sometimes terms such as arachnophobia (to denote spider phobia) or acrophobia (to denote phobia of heights) are used, but they have no advantage over the simpler terms. The following varieties of simple phobia require brief separate comments.

Phobias of blood, injection, and injury differ from other types of simple phobia in that there is a strong vasovagal response instead of the usual sympathetic reaction. Fainting is common.

Phobia of dental treatment About 5 per cent of adults have specific fears of this kind, which can become so severe that all dental treatment is avoided and serious caries develops.

Phobia of flying Anxiety during aeroplane travel is common. A few people have such intense fear that flying is impossible.

Phobias related to excretion Some people with this phobia become anxious when attempting to pass urine in public lavatories. Others have frequent urges to pass urine when away from home, fear being incontinent, and arrange their lives so as never to be far from a lavatory. A few patients have similar symptoms centred around defecation.

Phobia of vomiting People with this phobia fear that they may vomit in a public place, such as a bus or train, or fear that other people may do so.

Phobia of illness Some patients experience repeated fearful thoughts that they may have cancer, venereal disease, or some other serious illness. Such fears are a type of hypochondriacal symptom (see p. 91).

Prevalence

Simple phobias are common but very few patients seek medical help. The 1-year prevalence of clinically significant cases is about 45 per 1000 population (and nearly 100 per 1000 when all cases are counted).

Differential diagnosis

Some patients with longstanding simple phobias seek help when an unrelated **depressive disorder** makes them less able to tolerate the phobic symptoms. Apart from this association, simple phobia is seldom mistaken for another disorder.

Aetiology

Most of the simple phobias of adult life begin in childhood when simple phobias are extremely common (see p. 283). Why most childhood phobias disappear and a few persist into adult life is not known, except that the most severe phobias are more likely to do so. Simple phobias that begin in adult life often develop after a very frightening experience; for example, a phobia of horses following a dangerous encounter with a bolting horse. Sometimes, no cause can be identified.

Prognosis

There is little reliable information about the prognosis of simple phobias. Clinical experience indicates that simple phobias that began in childhood continue for many years, while those starting after a stressful experience in adult life may improve with time.

Treatment

Most of the general measures described on pp. 77–8 apply to simple phobia, except that it is usually inappropriate to prescribe antidepressants because anxiety in simple phobia is so intermittent. The following points apply particularly to simple phobia.

Self-help methods Patients should strive to enter repeatedly the situations that they have previously avoided, starting with those that provoke least fear and progressing to increasingly more difficult situations. They may be helped on the first few occasions by the reassuring presence of an understanding and trusted companion.

Medication Patients sometimes ask for immediate relief of symptoms when a longstanding phobia makes it difficult to fulfil a forthcoming important engagement (e.g. a claustrophobic person who requires an urgent MRI scan). In such circumstances, a benzodiazepine can be used, but in the short term only.

Cognitive behaviour therapy The treatment of choice for simple phobia is *exposure*, a more formal version of the procedure described above under self-help methods (see p. 259).

Social phobia

Social phobia is inappropriate anxiety in social situations. There are a number of principal features:

- *Specific concerns* (which they know to be irrational) about being observed critically by other people.

- *Situations that provoke anxiety* include: restaurants, canteens, and dinner parties; seminars, board meetings, and other places where it is necessary to speak in public; occasions when some action is open to scrutiny—for example, writing, eating, or drinking in front of another person (Table 6.5).

TABLE 6.5 Situations feared and avoided by patients with social phobia	
Common theme	Being observed and open to criticism
Examples	Committees, seminars
	Eating or drinking in public
	Social gatherings
	Writing or performing in front of others

- *Anticipatory anxiety.* People with social phobia also feel anxious when they anticipate entering such situations.

- *Avoidance* of these situations. Sometimes the avoidance is partial; for example, entering a social group but failing to make conversation, or sitting in an inconspicuous place in the group.

- *Symptoms* similar to those of other anxiety disorders (see p. 75), although **blushing** and **trembling** are particularly frequent.

- *Use of alcohol.* Some people take alcohol to relieve anxiety and alcohol abuse is more common among social phobics than among people with other phobias.

Onset and course

The condition usually *begins* with an acute attack of anxiety in some public place. Subsequently, anxiety occurs in similar places with episodes that become gradually more severe and with increasing avoidance.

Prevalence

The 1-year prevalence is about 30 per 1000. Social phobia is about equally common in men and women.

Differential diagnosis

- **Generalized anxiety disorder**. Social phobia is distinguished by the pattern of situations in which anxiety occurs.

- **Depressive disorder**. Social phobia is distinguished by the pattern of situations and the absence of the typical symptoms of depressive disorder (see p. 98). Sometimes people who have previously coped with social phobia seek help when they become depressed.

- **Schizophrenia**. Occasionally, patients with schizophrenia are anxious in, and avoid, social situations because of paranoid delusions.

- **Anxious/avoidant personality disorder**, characterized by lifelong shyness and lack of self-confidence, may closely resemble social phobia. However, personality disorder starts at a younger age and develops more gradually than social phobia.

- **Social inadequacy** is a primary lack of social skills with secondary anxiety. Speech is hesitant, dull, and inaudible, facial expression and gestures are awkward, and eye contact is avoided. People with social phobia possess these social skills but cannot use them when they are anxious.

Aetiology

The cause of social phobia is uncertain. Symptoms usually start in late adolescence, a time when many young people are concerned about the impression they are making on other people. It is possible that social phobias begin as exaggerated normal concerns, which are then increased and prolonged by thoughts that other people will be critical of any signs of anxiety.

Prognosis

There are no systematic data on the long-term course of social phobia. Clinical experience suggests that the phobias persist for many years, although most improve by mid life.

Treatment

The general measures are described on pp. 77–8, and the following specific points apply to social phobia.

Self-help methods Exposure to social situations is important but difficult to achieve in a graded way because social situations are not under the patient's control and do not always develop in predictable ways. Some patients can control anxious thoughts by distraction, with guidance from a self-help book. Exposure and distraction should be continued and extended during any drug treatment.

Antidepressant medication The usual choice is one of the SSRIs: paroxetine, fluvoxamine, and sertraline have been reported to be effective in social phobia in the short term although the long-term benefits are less certain. The MAOI moclobemide is also effective, at least by in the short term. Because its effect of inhibiting monoamine oxidase is reversible, precautions against dietary and drug interactions are less necessary than with other MAOIs. *While taking antidepressant medication, patients should practice exposure* to situations that they have previously avoided.

Anxiolytic medication provides immediate short-term relief, for example to help the patient deal with an important professional or social situation before more lasting treatment has taken effect. However, anxiolytics should not be used regularly because of the risk of dependence (see p. 237).

Beta-adrenergic antagonists are used occasionally to control tremor and palpitations unresponsive to anxiolytic treatment. Care should be taken to observe the contraindications for the use of these drugs and the precautions described in the manufacturer's literature.

Cognitive behaviour therapy combines exposure to feared situations with procedures to reduce the patient's anxiety-provoking thoughts (see p. 261). Though the evidence is limited, cognitive behaviour therapy is probably the treatment of choice for patients who do not respond to simple measures.

Dynamic psychotherapy Some clinicians consider that this treatment (see p. 262) benefits patients whose social phobia is associated with low self-esteem and longstanding problems in personal relationships. At the time of writing, there is insufficient evidence to decide the matter.

Agoraphobia
Clinical features

Agoraphobic patients are anxious when they are: away from home; in crowds; in situations they cannot leave easily; in social situations; and in open spaces (this last fear explains the name—'agoraphobia' contains the Greek word for 'market place'). Patients experience *anticipatory anxiety* and *avoid* situations that cause anxiety. *Anxious thoughts* are common with themes of fainting and loss of control. The anxiety symptoms are any of those shown in Table 6.2 together with *panic attacks*, *depression*, and *depersonalization*.

Situations that provoke anxiety and avoidance are listed in Table 6.6. The situations have in common the themes (noted above) of distance from home, crowding, and confinement. Examples include: buses and trains; shops and supermarkets; and places that cannot be left suddenly without attracting attention, such as a hairdresser's chair or a seat in the middle of a row at the cinema. Less common situations are open spaces such as parks and open country, and social situations such as parties or business meetings. As the condition progresses, patients avoid more and more of these situations until in severe cases they may be almost confined in their homes.

TABLE 6.6 Situations feared and avoided by patients with agoraphobia

Common themes	Distance from home
	Crowding
	Confinement
	Open spaces
	Social situations
Examples	Public transport
	Crowded shops
	Empty streets
	School visits
	Cinemas, theatres

The anxiety experienced in these situations is reduced by the reassuring presence of a trusted companion, or a reassuring object such as a few anxiolytic tablets, which are carried but never taken.

Anticipatory anxiety may be severe and appear several hours before the person has to enter a feared situation.

Course and outcome

Agoraphobia has two peak *times of onset*: in the early or mid twenties, and in the mid thirties. (Contrast the peak of onset of simple phobias in childhood and of social phobias in late teenage years.) The *first episode* of agoraphobia often occurs while the person is away from home, waiting for public transport, or shopping in a crowded store. Suddenly the person develops an unexplained panic attack, and either hurries home or seeks immediate medical help. This first episode subsides before long, but there is another when the same or similar situation is encountered again, and another hurried escape is made. This sequence recurs over and again and the person begins to avoid the situations. It is unusual to discover any immediate cause for the first panic attack, although some patients describe a background of problems at the time (e.g. worry about a sick child).

As the condition progresses, patients become increasingly *dependent on the spouse or other relatives* for help with activities, such as shopping, that provoke anxiety. These demands on the spouse sometimes lead to arguments, and serious marital problems are common.

Prevalence

The 1-year prevalence of agoraphobia is about 20 per 1000, with twice as many women as men being affected.

Differential diagnosis

- **Generalized anxiety disorder**, although this does not have the pattern of avoidance characteristic of agoraphobia.

- **Social phobia**. Although agoraphobic patients feel anxious in social situations and some social phobics avoid crowded buses and shops, the overall pattern of anxiety-provoking situations is different.

- **Depressive disorder**. Sometimes a person with longstanding agoraphobia seeks help when depressed. It is then important to identify and treat the depressive disorder.

- **Schizophrenia**. Rarely, patients with paranoid delusions avoid meeting people in a way that suggests agoraphobia. If they hide the delusions, diagnosis may be difficult but a thorough history and mental state usually shows the true diagnosis.

Aetiology

The development of anticipatory anxiety and avoidance after the first panic attack can be understood in terms of conditioning. The cause of the first panic attack is uncertain. It could be caused by panic disorder (see below) in which case agoraphobia is simply a variant of panic disorder. Alternatively, the first panic attack could have another cause such as an accumulation of stressful events, in which case agoraphobia and panic disorder are separate conditions. The matter is undecided and there may be different causes in separate cases. It is agreed, however, that agoraphobia is *maintained by avoidance*, which prevents deconditioning, and by *apprehensive thoughts*, such as fears of fainting or social embarrassment, which set up vicious circles of anxiety.

Prognosis

Agoraphobia that has been present continuously for a year is likely to persist for at least 5 years. Brief episodes of depressive symptoms often occur in the course of chronic agoraphobia.

Treatment

Treatment begins with the general measures described on pp. 77–8. The following points apply particularly to agoraphobia (Table 6.7). If the condition is severe, specialist assessment should be obtained at an early stage.

Self-help methods As soon as agoraphobia is diagnosed, patients should be strongly encouraged to return to situations that they have avoided (exposure). They should start with situations that provoke little anxiety and be helped to draw up a hierarchy of more difficult ones to approach later. They should use relaxation and distraction to control anxiety in the phobic situations. Most patients find exposure easier when accompanied by a trusted companion, at least on the first few occasions. It is essential that patients stay in the situation until anxiety has subsided, otherwise the phobic response will not decline and may even increase.

Antidepressants are of value not only for their general anxiolytic effect but also because some have antipanic effects (see p. 85). (Panic attacks are a common cause of relapse.) Their use should be combined with exposure, either as a self-help procedure or as part of cognitive behaviour therapy (see below). There is some evidence that the most effective treatment for agoraphobia is a combination of cognitive behaviour therapy and medication.

Cognitive behaviour therapy When the condition is even moderately severe, self-help is of limited value and cognitive behaviour therapy is required, either alone or combined with medication. The basic procedure, exposure, is the same as that used in self-help but it is supplemented by techniques for managing the anxiety experienced in the situation (see p. 261). The treatment has been shown to have long-term benefits. Cognitive behaviour therapy is a complex procedure requiring special training, and is usually provided by clinical psychologists or specially trained psychiatric nurses.

Panic disorder

Clinical features

The symptoms of a panic attack are listed in Table 6.8. Anxiety increases very quickly to a severe level and patients fear some kind of catastrophic outcome such as a heart attack. The diagnosis of panic disorder is made when the attacks occur unexpectedly (i.e. not in response to a known phobic stimulus), and when they are repeated. As the condition develops, situational panic may be added to the original spontaneous attacks. This progression blurs the distinction between agoraphobia and panic disorder.

Panic disorder patients often seek advice from general practitioners, cardiologists, and other physicians to

TABLE 6.7 Management plan for agoraphobia

- Adopt the general measures for anxiety disorders (see Table 6.4)
- Obtain specialist help for severe cases
- Prepare a hierarchy, arrange exposure with anxiety management
- Prescribe antidepressant if spontaneous panic attacks interfere with exposure (see text)
- Refer for cognitive behaviour therapy

TABLE 6.8 Symptoms of a panic attack

- Palpitations
- Dyspnoea
- Chest discomfort
- Sweating
- Trembling
- Dizziness or fainting
- Flushing
- Nausea
- Fears of an impending medical emergency
- Depersonalization

whom they complain not of anxiety, but of accompanying physical symptoms such as palpitations.

Prevalence

The prevalence of panic disorder is about 15 per 1000, and it is about twice as frequent among women as among men. Many other people have spontaneous panic attacks that are not sufficiently frequent to satisfy formal criteria for panic disorder—they number about 30 per 1000.

Differential diagnosis

Panic attacks occur in many conditions other than panic disorder, notably generalized anxiety disorder, phobic anxiety disorder (especially agoraphobia), hyperventilation (see pp. 75–6), depressive disorder, and during withdrawal from alcohol. Diagnosis is made by searching for symptoms of these other disorders and considering which symptoms developed first; for example, whether depression preceded or followed the onset of panic.

Aetiology

The causes of panic disorder are uncertain. It seems likely that is caused by a combination of excessive autonomic responsiveness to stressful events coupled with fears that the symptoms of autonomic arousal are evidence of an impending medical catastrophe (Box 6.1).

Prognosis

Systematic follow-up data have not been reported but clinical observation indicates that some patients who experience panic attacks recover within weeks of the onset. However, when panic attacks have persisted for 6 months or more the disorder usually runs a prolonged, although often fluctuating, course which may last for many years.

Treatment

The general measures described on pp. 77–8 form the basis of treatment. The following points apply particularly to panic disorder (Table 6.9).

TABLE 6.9 Management plan for panic disorder
◆ Adopt the general measures for anxiety disorders (see Table 6.4)
◆ Explain: the harmless nature of physical symptoms the vicious circle formed by concerns about symptoms and anxiety the effect of safety behaviours and avoidance
◆ Encourage self-help (see text)
◆ If panics are severe and/or frequent, consider medication (see text)
◆ Arrange cognitive therapy

BOX 6.1 THE AETIOLOGY OF PANIC DISORDER

The **biochemical hypothesis** is based on three sets of observations. First, certain *chemical agents can induce panic* attacks more readily in patients with panic disorder than in healthy people or patients with other kinds of anxiety disorder. These agents include yohimbine, an alpha-adrenergic antagonist that increases central sympathetic activity, carbon dioxide inhalation, and sodium lactate infusions, which act in unknown ways. Second, certain *drugs reduce panic attacks* (e.g. imipramine and SSRIs). Third, panic disorder is *more frequent among relatives* of panic disorder patients than among the general population, a finding consistent with a genetic cause but also with social transmission. So far there have been insufficient twin studies to be sure that the family aggregation is not due to the latter.

It has been proposed that regulation of the adrenergic and possibly also the 5-HT systems are abnormal in panic disorder. While there is no doubt that the noradrenergic system is highly active during panic attacks, it has not been shown that this activity is the cause of the disorder rather than the pathway through which another abnormality is expressed.

The **cognitive hypothesis** is based on the observation that, compared with other anxious patients, patients with panic disorder more often have fears concerning physical symptoms of anxiety. They fear, for example, that palpitations will be followed by a heart attack. It is proposed that these fears initiate a vicious circle in which anxiety leads to physical symptoms, which activate the fears, which in turn lead to more anxiety. There is experimental evidence in support of this hypothesis; for example, reducing fearful cognitions reduces panic.

Safety behaviours. Some patients carry out actions intended to avert the feared catastrophe, for example, breathing deeply or relaxing. Because they believe that these actions have prevented the feared events, for example a heart attack, patients do not find out that panic symptoms are not followed by the catastrophe that they fear, and their fear continues.

Information Clinicians who see patients soon after an initial panic attack should attempt to prevent progression to panic disorder by explaining that the physical symptoms are caused by anxiety and that, while frightening, they are harmless. They should explain also that anxiety is often accompanied by frightening thoughts about dying or losing control and that these thoughts cause a vicious circle of anxiety. When panic attacks are already established, it is often useful to compare them to a house alarm that is too sensitive so that it goes off when there is no real danger. Patients should be advised how safety behaviours prevent them from discovering that panic attacks are similarly a warning of non-existent danger (see above). They should be warned that if they avoid situations in which panic attacks have occurred they may develop agoraphobia.

Self-help methods The general measures described on pp. 77–8 help to reduce the general level of anxiety and may thereby reduce the panic attacks. Additional steps include: (i) writing down any thoughts during a panic attack, and considering them against the answer to the question 'What is the worst thing that could really have happened?'; and (ii) carrying a card on which is written the rational explanation for the panic attack, to be read as soon as the attack begins.

Antidepressant drugs As explained above (see p. 79), many antidepressants have long-term anxiolytic effects. Given in high doses, some also have antipanic effects that are useful when attacks are severe or frequent.

- *Imipramine* has been the most studied drug as a treatment for panic disorder. In high doses, its antipanic effect is as great as from high doses of benzodiazepines (see below) though its effect appears more slowly. Imipramine has anticholinergic and cardiac side effects (see p. 243), which limit its use in some patients. Treatment begins with very small doses because the first effect of imipramine in panic disorder is to increase apprehension, sleeplessness, and sympathetic overactivity. About a third of patients treated with imipramine relapse when the drug is stopped after 6 months, and need longer treatment. Clomipramine appears to be about as effective as imipramine.

- *SSRIs* also have an antipanic effect. Fluvoxamine, paroxetine, and sertraline have been shown to have therapeutic effects comparable to those of imipramine. SSRIs do not have the anticholinergic or cardiac side effects of imipramine but they have side effects of their own (see p. 244).

Anxiolytic drugs As explained above, the general rule in treating anxiety disorders is that anxiolytics should be used only for short periods, usually while other treatment is being initiated. This general rule has been broken in the use of alprazolam, a high potency benzodiazepine, as a treatment for panic disorder. High doses of up to 6 mg per day (equivalent to about 60 mg of diazepam) are used and continued for several months. The treatment is effective but up to a third of patients experience withdrawal symptoms when the drug is stopped, even when this is done slowly. The treatment was developed in the USA and has not been adopted widely in the United Kingdom. If it is used dosage should be increased slowly over 2–3 weeks, and withdrawn slowly over about 6 weeks. About a third of those who improve with alprazolam relapse if the drug is stopped after 6 months.

Cognitive therapy for panic disorder is a specialized treatment directed to changing the fearful cognitions that maintain the disorder (see p. 261). The short-term effects of cognitive therapy are as great as those of antidepressants or alprazolam and the relapse rate is lower. In practice, it is often used after a trial of drug treatment, but there is insufficient evidence of its effectiveness in patients who have been unresponsive to, or have relapsed after, such treatment.

Obsessive-compulsive disorder

Clinical features

Obsessive-compulsive disorders are characterized by obsessional thinking, compulsive behaviour, and varying degrees of anxiety, depression, and depersonalization (Table 6.10). Obsessional and compulsive symptoms were

TABLE 6.10 Symptoms of obsessional disorder
Obsessions
◆ thoughts
◆ images
◆ ruminations
◆ doubts
◆ impulse
Rituals
'Phobias' (see text)
Slowness
Other symptoms
◆ anxiety
◆ depression
◆ depersonalization

described on pp. 8–9, but the main features will be repeated here.

Obsessional thoughts are words, ideas, and beliefs recognized by the patient as his own. The thoughts intrude forcibly into the patient's mind and the patient attempts to exclude them. It is the combination of this sense of being compelled to think these thoughts and of resistance that characterizes obsessional symptoms. Obsessional thoughts may be single words, phrases, or rhymes; they are usually unpleasant or shocking to the patient, obscene, or blasphemous.

Obsessional images have the same characteristics of intrusion and resistance but appear as vividly imagined scenes, often of violence or of a kind that disgusts the patient, such as abnormal sexual practices.

Obsessional ruminations are internal debates in which continuous arguments are reviewed endlessly.

Obsessional doubts are thoughts about actions that may have been completed inadequately, such as failing to turn off a gas tap completely; or about actions that may have harmed other people, for example the idea that while driving his car past a cyclist the patient might have caused an accident which he did not notice at the time. Doubts may also be related to religious observances, such as the adequacy of confession.

Obsessional impulses are urges to perform acts, usually of a violent kind, for example leaping in front of a car or striking a child, or of an embarrassing kind, such as shouting blasphemies in church. The urges are resisted strongly, and are not carried out, but the internal struggle may be very distressing.

Obsessional rituals are repeated but senseless activities. They may be *mental activities*, such as counting repeatedly in a special way or repeating a certain form of words, or *behaviours*, such as washing the hands 20 or more times a day. Rituals are usually followed by temporary release of distress (although occasionally they increase it). Some rituals have an understandable connection with the obsessional thoughts that precede them, for example, repeated hand washing following thoughts about contamination. Other rituals have no such obvious connection; for example, routines concerned with laying out clothes in a complicated way before dressing may follow obsessional symptoms of an unconnected kind. The ritual may be followed by doubts whether it has been completed in the right way, and the sequence may be repeated over and again. Patients are aware that their rituals are illogical, and usually try to hide them.

Obsessional phobias Obsessional thoughts and compulsive rituals may worsen in certain situations; for example, obsessional thoughts about harming other people often increase in a kitchen or other place where knives are kept. When this happens, patients avoid the situations and this combination of fearful thoughts and avoidance is sometimes called obsessional phobia because it resembles the fear and avoidance of phobic patients (although the latter do not have fears that have the special features of obsessional thoughts).

Obsessional slowness Obsessional thoughts and rituals tend to slow the patient's performance of everyday activities. A minority of obsessional patients are afflicted also by extreme obsessional slowness that is out of proportion to other symptoms. The cause is not known.

Anxiety is an important symptom of obsessive-compulsive disorders. **Depressive symptoms** are often present. In some patients these are an understandable reaction to the obsessional symptoms, but in others there are recurring depressive moods that arise independently of the other symptoms. *Depersonalization* occurs sometimes, adding to the patient's disability.

Obsessional personality is described on p. 59. Although they share the same name, obsessional personality and obsessive-compulsive disorders do not have a simple one-to-one relationship. Obsessional personality is overrepresented among patients who develop obsessive-compulsive disorder, but about a third of obsessional patients have other types of personality. Moreover, although people with obsessional personality may develop obsessive-compulsive disorders, they are more likely to develop depressive disorders.

Prevalence

The 1-year prevalence is about 10 per 1000, with men and women affected about equally.

Differential diagnosis

Obsessive-compulsive disorders have to be distinguished from the following disorders in which obsessional symptoms can occur:

◆ **Anxiety disorders**. Obsessional symptoms are less severe than those of anxiety and develop later in the course of the disorder.

◆ **Depressive disorder**. Diagnosis can be difficult because the course of obsessive-compulsive disorder is often punctuated by periods of depression. Obsessional symptoms follow the depression in depressive disorders and precede it in obsessional disorder.

The correct diagnosis is important because obsessional symptoms in depressive disorders usually respond well to antidepressant treatment.

- **Schizophrenia**. When obsessional thoughts have a peculiar content, the clinical picture may suggest schizophrenia. Repeated mental state examinations will reveal other symptoms of schizophrenia and an informant may describe other behaviours that suggests this diagnosis.

- **Organic cerebral disorders**. Although obsessional symptoms may occur in dementia, they are seldom prominent and other features of dementia are present.

Aetiology
Predisposing causes

1. **Genetic**. Obsessive-compulsive disorder occurs more frequently among members of the families of obsessive-compulsive patients than among the general population. It is not certain whether this familial pattern indicates genetic causes rather than family environment because the necessary large-scale twin and adoption studies have not been carried out.

2. **Organic factors**. Parents with obsessive-compulsive disorder have an increased rate of minor, non-localizing neurological signs but no specific neurological lesion has been identified. Brain imaging has not shown any definite structural abnormality, but functional changes have been reported in the orbitofrontal cortex and caudate nucleus.

3. **Early experience**. Obsessional mothers might be expected to transmit a tendency to obsessional symptoms to their children through social learning. However, although children of such mothers are at increased risk for psychiatric problems, more of these problems are non-specific than obsessional.

Precipitating factors
Obsessive-compulsive disorders often begin when there are stressful events but no specific kind of stressful experience has been shown to be important.

Maintaining factors
Although checking behaviour and other rituals reduce anxiety for a short time their long-term effect is to reinforce and perpetuate the obsessional symptoms. Avoidance of cues that provoke symptoms has the same effect. (These findings are made use of in treatment, see below.)

Prognosis
About two-thirds of obsessional disorders improve within a year; the remaining third run a prolonged and usually fluctuating course with periods of partial or complete remission lasting a few months to several years. Prognosis is worse when the personality is obsessional, the symptoms are severe, and when there are continuing stressful circumstances.

Treatment
Treatment begins with the general measures to reduce anxiety, described on pp. 77–8. It is especially important to detect and treat any co-morbid depressive disorder. However, general measures are generally less effective for obsessive-compulsive disorder than for anxiety disorders, and specialist advice should usually be obtained at an early stage. The following additional measures apply (Table 6.11).

Information This is the important first step in treatment. Patients with an obsessive-compulsive disorder find their thoughts and actions so strange and irrational that they often fear that they are 'going mad' and could act on the impulses they are resisting. It is important to explain that obsessive-compulsive disorder does not progress in this way.

Reducing or avoiding stressors Obsessive-compulsive symptoms are often worse when there are stressful circumstances, especially those causing *anger* that the person finds hard to express. Alternative ways of dealing with these situations should be discussed or, if these cannot be found, ways of avoiding them.

Self-help methods It is important that patients resist rituals for although these produce short-term relief from distress, they maintain the disorder. Patients need a lot of support and encouragement to resist the very strong urge to carry out rituals. If the patient agrees, a relative or close friend can help but most patients are ashamed of the rituals and are therefore reluctant to accept such help.

TABLE 6.11 Management plan for obsessive-compulsive disorder

- Adopt the general measures for anxiety disorders (see Table 6.4)
- Refer to a specialist if disorder is severe
- Reassure about fears of loss of control or of 'going mad'
- Reduce or come to terms with stressors, especially those causing anger
- Help patient to resist rituals
- Prescribe a 5-HT uptake blocker (see text)
- Refer for cognitive behaviour therapy if there is no progress

Medication *5-HT uptake inhibitors* suppress obsessive-compulsive symptoms, and the action is independent of their antidepressant effect. Effective drugs include the SSRIs, fluvoxamine and fluoxetine, and the tricyclic drug clomipramine, which is a non-specific inhibitor of 5-HT uptake. The efficacy of SSRIs and clomipramine are similar with about half the patients improving substantially, although clomipramine may be slightly superior. All these drugs are slow to act, taking up to 6 weeks to reach their full effect. Medication is continued for 6 months, and for longer if the condition relapses when the drug is withdrawn. SSRIs are the usual first choice because clomipramine has to be given in high dosage, which is liable to produce anticholinergic and cardiac side effects. Clomipramine should be used only with physically healthy patients and treatment should usually be initiated by a specialist. Treatment with either type of drug should be maintained for up to 6 months and then reduced cautiously, watching for recurrence, and increased again for a further 2–3 months if symptoms reappear.

Anxiolytic drugs As with the anxiety disorders, anxiolytics should be used only for short-term relief of the distress.

Cognitive behaviour therapy *Exposure with response prevention* helps patients to suppress rituals while they return to any situations they have avoided (see p. 260). About two-thirds of patients with moderately severe rituals improve substantially, though far fewer recover completely. When rituals improve, associated obsessional thoughts usually improve as well. *Thought stop-*ping (see p. 260) is used occasionally for the minority of patients who have obsessional thoughts without rituals, but the results are seldom satisfactory. Recently, a novel form of cognitive therapy has been reported to give good results with these patients but at the time of writing this claim needs confirmation.

Psychosurgery was used, before modern treatments were developed, to treat severe and intractable cases of obsessive-compulsive disorder. Several kinds of operative lesion were used, mainly involving the frontal white matter. The immediate results of these procedures was a marked reduction in the obsessional symptoms but long-term benefits have not been proved. With improvements in other treatments, psychosurgery is now used very rarely.

Further reading

Butler, G. & Hope, T. (1995). *Manage your Mind: the Mental Fitness Guide*. Oxford University Press, Oxford.
A useful account of self-help methods for anxiety disorders and other conditions.
Kennerly, H. (1995). *Managing Anxiety: a Training Manual*. Oxford University Press, Oxford.
A practical guide to the psychological treatment of anxiety disorders.
Mavassakalian, M. R. & Prien, R. F. (eds) (1996). *Long-term Treatments of Anxiety Disorders*. American Psychiatric Press, Washington, DC.
A review of the evidence about the effectiveness of both pharmacological and psychological treatments.

CHAPTER 7

Physical symptoms not explained by organic pathology

Chapter contents

Classification of functional symptoms 89

Epidemiology 90

Aetiology 90

Management 92

Some common clinical problems 93

Self-inflicted and simulated illness 95

Concern about symptoms is a common reason for patients to seek medical help. Many of these symptoms, such as pain, weakness, and fatigue, remain unexplained by identifiable disease even after extensive medical assessment. Several general terms have been used to describe these types of symptom—somatization, somatoform, abnormal illness behaviour, medically unexplained symptoms, and functional symptoms. We prefer the term functional symptoms, which does not assume psychogenesis but only a disturbance in bodily functioning.

There are many kinds of symptoms (Table 7.1). They are considered in this textbook of psychiatry because psychological factors (including psychiatric disorder) are important in aetiology and because psychological and behavioural interventions have a fundamental role in treatment

A major obstacle to effective management of patients with functional symptoms is that they feel their doctors do not believe them. They are concerned that they may be thought to be 'putting it on'. However, the deliberate manufacture of symptoms or signs is very uncommon in ordinary practice and is considered on p. 95.

Classification of functional symptoms

Most functional symptoms are transient, but a sizeable minority persist and are often disabling. They are classified in two parallel ways:

1. **Medical syndromes** (such as fibromyalgia and chronic fatigue, chronic pain, and irritable bowel syndromes). Although the specific terms are useful in everyday medical practice, there is a substantial overlap in patterns of syndromes.

TABLE 7.1 Some common physical symptoms that may have psychological causes
Pain syndromes
◆ abdominal pain
◆ non-cardiac chest pain
◆ headache
◆ atypical facial pain
◆ muscular pain
◆ low back pain
◆ pelvic pain
Chronic fatigue
Non-ulcer dyspepsia
Irritable bowel
Palpitations
Dizziness
Tinnitus
Dysphonia
Premenstrual tension
Food intolerance

2. **Psychiatric disorders** (including anxiety, depression, and somatoform disorders). Well recognized psychiatric disorders such as depression and anxiety often present with somatic symptoms that may resolve with effective treatment of these disorders. In other cases psychological symptoms are not prominent and the appropriate psychiatric diagnostic category is a somatoform disorder as described below.

The existence of parallel classificatory systems is confusing. In practice functional symptoms are best classified in terms of the medical symptom (for example

chest pain) or syndrome (irritable bowel) with an additional second psychiatric diagnosis for the minority with an associated psychiatric disorder.

Epidemiology

Functional symptoms are common—about one-fifth of the population in all countries and communities. In primary care only a small proportion of people with functional symptoms ever receive a specific physical diagnosis (Fig. 7.1). Up to half will remain disabled by the symptoms at the 12 months' follow-up; outcome is poorest for patients with more intractable problems who are referred to specialist care.

Functional symptoms may occur alone, but also commonly accompany serious physical illness. For example following a heart attack or cardiac surgery, minor muscular chest aches and pains in the chest may be misinterpreted as evidence of angina, and lead to unnecessary worry and disability. Explanation and advice, sometimes in the context of a cardiac rehabilitation programme, may result in improvement in quality of life.

Aetiology

Functional symptoms are often put down to either physical *or* psychological causes. This simplistic separation of mind and body causes is unhelpful both in explaining aetiology or in planning treatment; it is also unacceptable to many patients. An alternative approach uses an interactive model in which physical, psychological, behavioural, and social factors all contribute to the formation of functional symptoms. This approach suggests that symptoms arise from minor physiological or pathological bodily sensations (Table 7.2) that are perceived by the patient as symptoms of illness and result in physical disability. From the patient's standpoint, illness fears that the

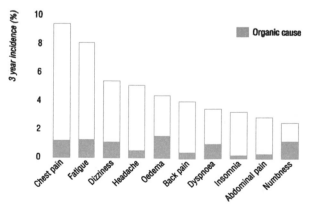

Fig. 7.1 Three year incidence of 10 common presenting symptoms and proportion of symptoms with a suspected organic cause in US primary care attendars. Reproduced with permission from Kroenke and Mangelsdorff (1989) Common symptoms in ambulatory care, American Journal of Medicine, 86, 262–8.

TABLE 7.2	Some causes of bodily sensations
Major physical pathology	
Minor physical pathology	
Physiological processes	
◆ autonomic effects of anxiety	
◆ lack of sleep	
◆ sinus tachycardia and minor arrhythmias	
◆ effects of prolonged inactivity	
◆ effects of fatigue	
◆ hangover	
◆ effects of overeating	

TABLE 7.3	Some factors affecting a patient's understanding of bodily sensations
Childhood and later experience of illness and its management	
◆ Knowledge of the illness	
◆ Press and television publicity	
◆ Experience of ill health of friends and family	
◆ Understanding of information given at previous consultations	

symptoms are due to disease are often reasonable. For example, a middle-aged man with a bad family history of heart disease may be understandably concerned about the implications of a chest pain which is, in fact, of musculoskeletal origin.

The extent to which these bodily sensations are noticed and the *interpretation* placed on them depend on the person's understanding, knowledge, and experience of illness (Table 7.3), on emotional arousal and personality (Fig. 7.2). It also depends upon social circumstances and upon the reactions of family, friends, and health care professionals.

Psychiatric disorder as a cause of functional symptoms

Psychiatric disorder is a common primary cause of functional symptoms. It may also be secondary to them (for example anxiety disorder), but may then exacerbate and maintain the physical symptoms. The psychiatric disorders associated with functional symptoms are divided into two broad groups:

1. **Psychiatric disorders causing functional symptoms**, most commonly *adjustment disorder*, *anxiety disorders of all kinds*, and *depressive disorder*.

BOX 7.1 SOMATOFORM DISORDERS

Somatization disorder Uncommon, multiple recurrent and changing physical symptoms not accounted for by physical pathology. Begins in early life, chronic and often fluctuating course.

Hypochondriasis Severe persistent anxiety about ill health and conviction of disease despite negative medical investigations and appropriate reassurance.

Body dysmorphic disorder Persistent, inappropriate concern about the appearance of the body (e.g. about the shape and size of the nose or breasts). Some patients demand cosmetic plastic surgery. Surgery only helpful in those with clear and reasonable expectations.

Pain disorder Poorly defined condition; chronic pain cannot be accounted for by any primary physical or mental disorder.

Undifferentiated somatoform disorder The commonest subcategory. A large, ill-defined, residual category of unexplained physical symptoms in spite of negative investigation and medical reassurance.

Conversion disorder See p. 94

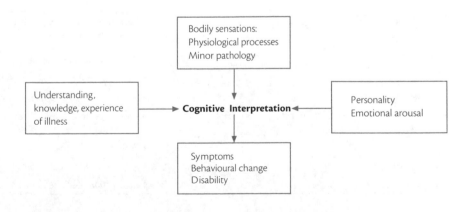

Fig. 7.2 Aetiology of medically unexplained symptoms.

2. **Somatoform disorders**, conditions characterized by *persistent abnormal concern* about physical health, and unexplained physical symptoms without an underlying psychiatric disorder or emotional arousal. The subclassification is summarized in Box 7.1 but is not particularly useful in everyday clinical practice.

Patients' understandable attempts to alleviate their symptoms may paradoxically exacerbate them. For example, excessive rest to reduce pain or fatigue may actually prolong it. Doctors may also unintentionally maintain symptoms by failing to address patients' concerns or by excessive investigation. Disability benefits can also be a disincentive for some patients to return to jobs they dislike, and litigation can maintain a focus on disability.

Management

Although it is always essential to consider physical disease as the cause of the patient's symptoms, an approach exclusively devoted to this can lead to difficulties if no disease is found. It is better to explain from the start that the symptoms may be either organic or functional, thus keeping open the option of a wider discussion of causes. In this way the problems have been framed from the outset in a way that allows psychological treatment to be presented as part of usual medical care rather than as an alternative that the patient may feel does not take his symptoms seriously. Table 7.4 summarizes the general principles of assessment.

Physical investigation

An appropriate physical examination and any medically indicated investigations are essential. Thereafter, any further test must be justified in terms of the likelihood and value of new information. Investigations that cannot be medically justified may increase the patient's anxiety.

TABLE 7.4 Principles of assessment of unexplained physical symptoms
◆ Organize any medically indicated physical investigation
◆ Identify the patient's concerns about the symptoms and belief of their cause
◆ Review any previous history of 'unexplained' symptoms
◆ Investigate how the patient reacts to and attempts to cope with the symptoms
◆ Use screening questions for depression and anxiety disorders
◆ Consider interviewing relatives

TABLE 7.5 Management of multiple somatic symptoms
◆ Explain that the symptoms are real and are familiar to you as a doctor
◆ Provide a positive explanation, including how behavioural, psychological, and emotional factors may exacerbate physiologically based somatic symptoms
◆ Identify and treat any depression or anxiety disorder
◆ Discuss the patient's and family's worries
◆ Give practical advice on coping with symptoms and encourage return to normal activity
◆ Discuss and agree the treatment plan
◆ Agree follow-up arrangements
◆ Follow-up review

Explanation and reassurance

Most patients are reassured by being told that the symptoms they have are common and rarely associated with disease and that their doctor is familiar with them, together with a promise of further review should the symptoms persist (Table 7.5).

Reassurance needs to be given carefully. It is essential to elicit all the patient's specific concerns before offering reassurance and to target this appropriately. Reassurance that fails to address patient's concerns is ineffective. When anxiety about disease is severe (hypochondriasis), repeated reassurance is not only ineffective but may even perpetuate the problem.

A positive explanation for symptoms is more helpful than a statement that no disease is present. Most patients accept explanations in terms of psychological and social factors as well as physiological ones provided they feel the symptoms are accepted as real. The explanation can usefully show the link between these factors—for example, how anxiety can lead to physiological changes that are experienced as somatic symptoms which, if regarded as evidence of disease, lead to increased anxiety.

TABLE 7.6 Non-specialist treatments of unexplained physical symptoms
◆ Discussion of, and help with, underlying problems
◆ Agreeing simple behavioural plans with the patient and family
◆ Advice about anxiety management
◆ Encouragement to use diaries as a basis for planning behavioural change
◆ Advice regarding a graded increase in activities
◆ Antidepressant medication if there is clear depressive disorder
◆ Explanation of self-help programmes

Further treatment

Most of those with unexplained symptoms respond to reassurance and explanation. Further treatment (Table 7.6) for the rest should aim to modify beliefs, reduce anxiety, and encourage a graded return to normal activity. Such treatment may include discus-sion of how anxiety can increase one's awareness of minor physical symptoms. Advice about simple ways of controlling negative thoughts (see p. 261) can be combined with encouragement to use physical relaxation techniques (see p. 259).

Antidepressant medication is indicated when there are definite symptoms of depressive illness, and is also valuable for atypical facial pain and some other pain syndromes whether or not there are prominent depressive symptoms. Other useful interventions include help in dealing with major personal family or social difficulties. Practical advice on coping with symptoms and advice about a graded return to normal activity is useful. Members of the primary care or hospital team other than doctors have important roles in treatment, follow-up, and practical help.

Referral

It is often tempting to refer difficult patients to another doctor but this can result in greater long-term difficulties without achieving a more effective treatment plan. When there is a clear reason for further medical or psychiatric referral, this should be discussed with the patient. The referral letter should clearly explain what is required of the specialist, for example confirmation of the diagnosis or advice on management.

Help from a psychiatrist might include more complex antidepressant drug regimens and specialist psychological interventions (Table 7.7). Among the latter, cognitive behavioural therapy has been shown to be effective in randomized controlled trials for a variety of functional syndromes, including non-cardiac chest pain and irritable bowel, and for hypochondriasis.

Some common clinical problems

Irritable bowel syndrome

In primary care about half of the patients seen with gut complaints have functional disorders, the most common type being irritable bowel syndrome. Most patients have relatively mild symptoms and can be managed effectively in primary care by a combination of improved diet, reassurance, and information. Antidepressant medication is indicated if there are also symptoms of depression.

One-third of patients seen in primary care with irritable bowel syndrome are referred to gastrointestinal specialists for futher assessment and treatment. Those that do not improve following the use of dietary measures, antimotility agents, and further information and reassurance may benefit from psychiatric or psychological referral. Cognitive behavioural treatment, antidepressant medication, and management of any associated psychiatric or social problems can be helpful.

Musculoskeletal pain and chronic pain

Musculoskeletal symptoms (for example neck pain, limb pain, low back pain, joint pain, and chronic widespread pain) are frequent reasons for consultation in primary care. Most patients can be effectively managed using the general measures summarized in Table 7.8. Early progressive mobilization and an early return to work should be encouraged.

The treatment of severe chronic pain is difficult, and patients are often referred to specialist pain clinics. Many have organic disease, but experience more pain than can be accounted for by the pathology. Analgesia should be made as effective as possible and patients should be encouraged to try other ways of coping with the pain. These procedures include distraction and reducing any

---

TABLE 7.7 Specialist treatments of unexplained physical symptoms

- Anxiety management
- Cognitive therapy to modify beliefs
- More complex antidepressant regimens
- Behavioural programmes to increase activity
- Illness-specific interventions (e.g. treating physical deconditioning in chronic fatigue)
- Management of complex associated social and psychiatric problems

---

TABLE 7.8 Simple management strategies for musculoskeletal pain

- Explain the difference between 'hurt' and 'harm'
- Reassure patients about the benign nature of their symptoms
- Help patients regain control over pain
- Encourage patients to 'pace' activities in small graded stages
- Advise that analgesic drugs should be taken on a regular rather than a pain contingent basis
- Set realistic goals
- Agree rewards for success, for example engaging in a favourite activity

behaviour that focuses attention on the pain (e.g. repeatedly rubbing or checking the area). Antidepressant medication is sometimes helpful even in patients who have no depressive disorder. Intensive specialist pain management programmes should be multidisciplinary and emphasize psychological techniques and the ways in which patients and their families can participate in planning treatment and monitoring progress.

Chronic fatigue syndrome

Depression, fatigue, and malaise are common following influenza, hepatitis, infectious mononucleosis, and other viral infections, but these usually improve over days and weeks.

Chronic fatigue syndrome is characterized by more persistent fatigue, and aching limbs with muscle and joint pains. Mild physical exertion is often followed by increased fatigue and pain so that patients alternate brief periods of activity with prolonged rest. Many patients are convinced that their symptoms are caused by a chronic virus infection or another, as yet, undetected medical condition. However, few cases are found to have a specific medical cause after thorough investigation.

In most cases, the causes of the syndrome are neither wholly psychological nor wholly organic, but a variable mixture of the two, with psychological factors becoming increasingly common over time. Inactivity and the resultant lack of physical fitness play a reinforcing role in chronic cases. Some patients have definite symptoms of depressive disorder, and they may improve with antidepressant treatment.

Treatment

The clinician explains that the syndrome is real, common, and familiar and that although there is no specific medical treatment, there are ways of achieving a good outcome. A graded programme of slowly increasing activity should be started with regular monitoring. Considerable effort is needed to ensure that patients practise progressively rather than alternating erratically between excessive activity and resting in bed. It is often appropriate to seek specialist advice for these patients; cognitive behavioural therapy and graded exercise therapy have both been shown to be helpful.

Multiple chronic functional symptoms

Patients who have multiple functional symptoms over long periods are said to have either somatization disorder or another subcategory of somatoform disorder. They are difficult to treat and the aim of management (Table 7.9) is often to limit distress and unnecessary investigation rather than to achieve a cure. The general

TABLE 7.9	Management of multiple chronic symptoms
◆ Take a full history and if possible interview relatives
◆ Review medical notes; discuss with doctors currently involved
◆ Negotiate with other doctors to simplify the medical care:
◆ limit the number of staff involved
◆ agree who has primary responsibility
◆ minimize the use of psychotropic drugs
◆ Arrange brief, regular appointments with the lead clinician
◆ Avoid repeated reassurance about the symptoms
◆ Focus on coping with disability and psychosocial problems
◆ Encourage graded return to normal activities

approach already described for the treatment of functional disorders is used, with an emphasis on avoiding inappropriate investigation and ensuring a consistent approach, if possible by a single doctor, usually the general practitioner. A psychiatric assessment may be useful in establishing a treatment plan although specialist psychiatric interventions are seldom of much value.

Dissociative and conversion disorders

In the past these disorders were called **hysteria**, but this term is not now used because it has acquired pejorative meanings. Conversion disorder refers to unexplained sensory and unclear symptoms; dissociative disorder refers to unexplained amnesia, fatigue, stupor, or identity disorder. The conditions are classified differently in DSM-IV and ICD-10. In the former, conversion disorder is listed among somatoform disorders and there is a separate category for dissociative disorder. In ICD-10, both conditions are grouped together in a single category dissociative disorder.

Conversion and dissociative *symptoms* also occur in many psychiatric disorders other than conversion and dissociative disorders, notably in anxiety, depressive, and organic mental disorders. A conversion (or dissociative) symptom is one that suggests physical illness but occurs in the absence of relevant physical pathology and is produced through unconscious psychological mechanisms. There are two obvious practical difficulties in applying this concept:

1. It is seldom possible to exclude physical pathology completely at the time when a patient is first seen.

2. It is difficult to be certain that the symptoms are produced by unconscious mechanisms rather than consciously and deliberately. (The deliberate feigning of symptoms is known as **malingering**.)

The *prevalence* of conversion and dissociative disorder varies between countries, being reported more often in less industrialized societies. In Western societies the prevalence is believed to be between 3 and 6 per 1000 for women, and substantially less for men. Most dissociative and conversion disorders of recent onset seen in general practice or hospital emergency departments recover quickly. Those that persist for longer than a year are likely to continue for many years more. Occasionally, organic disease may be present but undetectable when these patients are first seen, becoming obvious later. For this reason patients should be followed up most carefully.

Clinical features

Although conversion and dissociative symptoms are not produced deliberately, they are nevertheless shaped by the patient's concepts of illness. Sometimes, the symptoms resemble those of a relative or friend who has been ill. Sometimes they originate in the patient's previous experience of ill health; for example, dissociative memory loss may appear some years after head injury. Usually there are obvious *discrepancies between signs and symptoms* of conversion and dissociative disorder and those of organic disease; for example, a pattern of sensory loss that does not correspond to the anatomical innervation of the part. These discrepancies are important in diagnosis.

Motor symptoms include paralysis of voluntary muscles, tremor, tics, and abnormalities of gait. *Sensory symptoms* of conversion disorder include anaesthesiae, paraesthesiae, hyperaesthesiae, pain, deafness, and blindness. In general, the sensory changes are distinguished from those in organic disease by: (i) a distribution that does not conform to the known innervation of the part; (ii) their varying intensity; and (iii) their responsiveness to suggestion.

Dissociative symptoms are less common. Dissociative **amnesia** starts suddenly. Patients are unable to recall long periods of their lives and sometimes deny any knowledge of their previous life or personal identity. In a dissociative **fugue** the patient loses his memory and wanders away from his usual surroundings. In dissociative **stupor**, the patient is motionless and mute and does not respond to stimulation, but he is aware of his surroundings. **Multiple personality** is an exceedingly rare condition (of uncertain validity) in which there are sudden alterations between the patient's normal state and another complex pattern of behaviour (a second personality).

Management

Diagnosis depends partly on the exclusion of physical causes, but also on psychological assessment to identify psychological reasons for the onset and course of the symptoms. An important differential diagnosis is from

TABLE 7.10	Treatment of acute conversion disorder

- ◆ Medical and psychiatric history from patient and informants
- ◆ Full examination and appropriate investigation to excluded physical causes
- ◆ Sympathetic but positive reassurance that the patient is suffering from an acute temporary condition and does not have a disabling medical disorder
- ◆ Discussion of the expected rapid recovery
- ◆ Avoidance of reinforcement of disability or symptoms
- ◆ Offer continuing assessment and treatment of related psychiatric or social problems

physical disease. This depends on careful physical assessment highlighting any discrepancies in physical signs that are unlikely to have a physical basis. It is important to keep an open mind and to remember that conversion symptoms are common accompaniments to physical disorder.

Acute disorders seen in general practice or hospital emergency departments often respond to simple measures (Table 7.10). For *persistent cases* the general approach is similar, although the results are less satisfactory. Attention is directed away from the symptoms and towards problems that have provoked the disorder. Staff should show sympathetic concern for the patient, but at the same time encourage self-help and avoid reinforcing the disability. For example, a patient who complains of paralysis of the legs should be encouraged to return to walking, not offered a wheelchair. The main emphasis should be to try and concentrate the patient's attention on understanding problems and methods of solving them. More intense psychological exploration seldom produces results better than those of the simple measures described above.

Self-inflicted and simulated illness

Factitious disorder

The term factitious disorder refers to the intentional production of physical pathology or the feigning of physical or psychological symptoms, with the apparent aim of being diagnosed as ill. Factitious disorder differs from malingering in that it does not bring any external reward such as avoidance of duties or financial compensation.

Common symptoms include skin lesions ('dermatitis artefacta') and pyrexia of unknown origin. Sometimes the patient deliberately worsens an existing physical disorder; for example preventing the healing of varicose ulcers or neglecting the care of diabetes. At other times the whole condition is induced, for example by self-inflicted damage to the skin.

> **BOX 7.2 ETHICAL ISSUES OF FACTITIOUS DISORDERS**
>
> **Confidentiality**
>
> ◆ Disclosure to other parties (e.g. employers)
>
> ◆ Circulation of registers of 'blacklists'
>
> **Invasion of privacy**
>
> ◆ Searching patients' belongings
>
> ◆ Videotaping
>
> **Involuntary treatment**

There is no specific treatment. Supportive counselling is often offered, and helps some patients but many do not take up the treatment. If deliberate feigning of symptoms and signs is established, patients should be told sympathetically what has been discovered and offered help with whatever problems might have led to the behaviour. This should be part of a sympathetic plan that also offers psychological help. Box 7.2 summarizes the ethical issues.

Munchausen syndrome is an extreme and uncommon form of factitious disorder of poor prognosis, in which a patient gives a plausible and often dramatic history of an acute illness, with feigned symptoms and signs. Symptoms may be of any kind, including psychiatric symptoms. These patients often attend a series of hospitals, giving different names to each. Frequently, strong analgesics are demanded for pain. Patients often obstruct efforts to obtain additional information about them and may interfere with diagnostic investigations.

Munchausen syndrome by proxy refers to a form of child abuse in which a parent (or occasionally another adult, such as a nurse) gives a false account of symptoms in a child, and may fake physical signs (see p. 299).

Malingering

Malingering is the fraudulent simulation or exaggeration of symptoms with the intention of gaining financial or other rewards. It is the obvious external gain that distinguishes malingering from factitious disorder (see above). When malingering occurs it is most often among prisoners, the military, and people seeking compensation for accidents.

Malingering should be diagnosed only after a full investigation of the case. When the diagnosis is certain, the patient should be informed tactfully of this conclusion and encouraged to deal more appropriately with any problems that contributed to the behaviour.

Further reading

Mayou, R., Sharpe, M., and Carson, A. (2003). *ABC of psychological medicine*. BMJ Publishing group, London.
Includes general and more specific chapters on practical management.

CHAPTER 8

Mood disorders

Chapter contents

Depressive disorder 98

Mania 101

Mixed and alternating mood states 102

Classification of mood disorders 102

Minor mood disorders 103

Differential diagnoses 104

Epidemiology 105

Aetiology 105

Course and prognosis 107

Management of depressive disorders 108

Management of mood disorders following childbirth 114

Management of bipolar disorder 114

Changes of mood (depression/elation) are common in all psychiatric disorders and also frequently accompany physical illness. This chapter is about disorders in which mood change is the main psychopathological feature. The abnormality is more intense and persistent than normal variations in mood and often leads to problems in occupational and social functioning. There may be associated symptoms, such as disturbances of thinking and sleeping.

Depressive disorder is frequent in primary care and general hospital practice but is often undetected, especially when there are physical symptoms as well. Unrecognized depressive disorder may slow recovery and worsen prognosis in physical illness. It is important, therefore, that all doctors should be able to recognize the condition, treat the less severe cases, and identify those requiring specialist care because of suicidal risk or for other reasons. **Mania** is less common, but is important to recognize because it may lead to substantial impairment of functioning and may arise as a consequence of treatment of a depressive episode in a predisposed patient.

The central features of depressive disorder are low mood, pessimistic thinking, lack of enjoyment, reduced energy, slowness, poor concentration, and low self-esteem. The most readily available effective treatment for depressive disorder is antidepressant medicine, but all patients also require psychological and social support. Patients with recurrent disorders will often benefit from long-term drug treatment to prevent relapses.

The features of mania are elevated mood, over-activity, and poor judgement. Mania occurs as part of bipolar disorder, in which there may also be episodes of depression. Mania is considerably less common than depressive disorder; it is important that mania is recognized in its early stages because in the later stages the patient becomes increasingly unwilling to accept treatment. Long-term maintenance drug treatment to prevent relapse should be considered in the management of patients with recurrent **bipolar illnesses**.

Depressive disorder

General clinical features

Sadness is a normal emotion commonly experienced by healthy people in response to misfortunes, especially loss and including grief. It is often accompanied by some anxiety, lack of energy, general malaise, and poor sleep.

Depressive disorder More severe unhappiness is the central symptom of depressive disorder—a syndrome of symptoms associated with low mood, depressive thinking, and (in more severe cases) biological symptoms. Depressive symptoms also occur in many other psychiatric disorders, such as schizophrenia and dementia. Together with anxiety, depression is the commonest psychological complaint in patients seen in primary care and many cases are due to depressive psychiatric disorder.

Masked depression Sometimes the symptoms of depressive disorders are not immediately obvious because the patient smiles and denies feeling miserable, a condition described as masked depression. Diagnosing depressive disorder therefore requires a careful search for the whole range of symptoms described below, especially lack of pleasure in life, sleep disturbance, diurnal mood variation, and a pessimistic view of the future.

Mild depressive disorder

Mild depressive disorder occurs frequently and, despite its name, implies an unpleasant, disabling, and persistent syndrome. The wide range of mood, behaviour, and other symptoms (Table 8.1) are usually considered by the patient and by others to be distinctly different to their usual personality and behaviour.

The patient characteristically complains of low mood, lack of energy and enjoyment, and poor sleep. The pattern of the sleep disturbance is varied but it is often difficult to fall asleep, and sleep is restless with periods of waking during the night usually followed by sounder sleep a few hours before waking. Mood may vary during the day; usually it is worse in the evening than in the morning, in contrast to the more severe disorder.

TABLE 8.1 Features of mild depressive disorder
◆ Low mood
◆ Seen by others as different to normal character and behaviour
◆ Lack of energy or enjoyment
◆ Anxiety symptoms
◆ Poor sleep
◆ Mood often worse in the evenings
◆ Pessimism, but not suicidal ideation

Other symptoms include anxiety, phobias, and obsessional symptoms. Although anxiety may be a symptom in all degrees of depressive disorder, it can be just as severe in the mild as in the severe disorders.

TABLE 8.2 Symptoms and signs of moderately severe depressive disorder
Appearance
◆ Sad appearance
◆ Psychomotor retardation
Low mood
◆ Misery and unhappiness
◆ Diurnal variation—worse in morning
◆ Anxiety, irritability, agitation
Lack of interest and enjoyment
◆ Reduced energy
◆ Poor concentration
◆ Subjective poor memory
Depressive thinking
◆ Pessimistic and guilty thoughts
◆ Ideas of personal failure
◆ Hopelessness
◆ Suicidal ideas
◆ Self-blame
◆ Hypochondriacal ideas
Biological symptoms
◆ Early wakening and other sleep disturbance
◆ Weight loss
◆ Reduced appetite
◆ Reduced sexual drive
Other symptoms
◆ Obsessional symptoms
◆ Depersonalization, etc.

Moderate depressive disorder

In depressive disorders of moderate severity (Table 8.2), the central features are low mood, lack of enjoyment, reduced energy, and pessimistic thinking.

Appearance of patient

The patient's appearance is often characteristic. **Psychomotor retardation**, which is a slowing of mental and motor activity, is frequent. There may be **agitation** or a feeling of restlessness, which may manifest itself as an inability to relax, accompanied by restless activity. When agitation is severe the patient cannot sit for long and may pace up and down.

Mood

The patient is usually miserable. The low mood is usually experienced as having a different quality than ordinary sadness. There is *diurnal variation of mood*, which is characteristically worse in the morning than in the later part of the day (see Biological symptoms, below).

Anxiety and *irritability* are frequent.

Lack of interest and *loss of enjoyment* (**anhedonia**) are frequent and important symptoms, although not always complained of spontaneously. Patients show no enthusiasm for activities and hobbies that they would normally enjoy and describe a loss of zest for living and for the pleasure from everyday things. They often withdraw from social encounters.

Reduced energy is characteristic (although when accompanied by physical restlessness it can be overlooked). The patient feels lethargic, finds everything an effort, and leaves tasks unfinished. For example, a normally houseproud woman may leave beds unmade and dirty plates on the table. Understandably, many patients attribute this lack of energy to physical illness and seek help for this rather than for depression.

Poor concentration and complaints of *poor memory* are common. However, if the patient is encouraged to make a special effort, retention and recall can usually be shown to be normal. Sometimes, however, apparent impairment of memory is so severe that the clinical presentation resembles that of dementia. This presentation, which is particularly common in the elderly, is sometimes called **depressive pseudodementia** (see pp. 142–3).

Complaints about *physical symptoms* are common in depressive disorders. They take many forms but complaints of constipation and of aching discomfort in any part of the body are particularly common. Complaints about any pre-existing physical disorders usually increase, and *hypochondriacal* preoccupations are common.

Depressive thinking

Pessimistic thinking ('depressive cognitions') is when a low mood is associated with gloomy thoughts about the present, future, and past.

1. *Thoughts concerned with the present.* Patients see the unhappy side of every event, think that they are failing in everything they do, and that other people see them as a failure. They lose confidence and discount any success as a chance happening for which they can take no credit.

2. *Thoughts concerned with the future.* Patients expect the worst. They may foresee failure in their work, the ruin of their finances, misfortune for their families, and an inevitable deterioration in their physical health. These ideas of *hopelessness* are often accompanied by the thought that life is no longer worth living and that death would come as a welcome release. These gloomy preoccupations may progress to thoughts of, and plans for, suicide. *It is important to ask about suicide in every case of depressive disorder.* (The assessment of suicidal risk is considered further on pp. 172–5.)

3. *Thoughts concerned with the past.* These thoughts often take the form of unreasonable guilt and self-blame about minor matters; for example, patients may feel guilty about some trivial act of dishonesty in the past or about letting someone down. Usually, the patient has not thought about these events for years, but as the depression develops they flood back into memory accompanied by intense feelings of guilt. Gloomy preoccupations of this kind strongly suggest depressive disorder. Some patients have similar feelings of guilt but do not attach them to any particular event. Other memories are focused on unhappy events; patients remember occasions when they were sad, when they failed, or when their fortunes were at a low ebb. These gloomy memories become more frequent as the depression deepens.

Biological symptoms

This term is used to denote sleep disturbance, diurnal variation of mood, loss of appetite, loss of weight, constipation, loss of libido, and, in women, amenorrhoea. These symptoms are more common in severe depression than in cases of moderate severity (see below).

Sleep disturbance is of several kinds:

♦ *Early morning waking* is the most characteristic form of sleep disturbance. The patient wakes 2 or 3 hours before their usual time. Patients do not fall asleep again, but lie awake feeling unrefreshed and often restless and agitated. They think about the coming day with pessimism, brood about past failures, and ponder gloomily about the more distant future. This combination of early waking with depressive thinking is important in diagnosis.

• *Delay in falling asleep*, and waking during the night.

• *Excessive sleep*: the patient wakes late feeling unrefreshed.

Variation of appetite and weight The characteristic pattern is for loss of appetite and weight loss, which often seems greater than can be explained by the loss of appetite alone. Instead of eating too little and losing weight, some patients eat more and gain weight. Sometimes they do this because eating brings them temporary relief from their distressing feelings, in other cases it is a side effect of medication.

Loss of libido is usual.

Other psychiatric symptoms

Many other symptoms may occur as part of a depressive disorder, including **depersonalization**, **obsessional symptoms**, **phobias**, and **conversion symptoms**, such as fugue or loss of function of a limb (see Chapter 1). Occasionally one of these dominates the clinical picture.

Severe depressive disorder

As depressive disorders become more severe, all the features described under moderate depressive disorder occur with greater intensity. There may also be additional symptoms not seen in moderate depressive disorder, namely delusions and hallucinations ('psychotic' symptoms; a disorder with these symptoms is called **psychotic depression**) (Table 8.3).

TABLE 8.3 Symptoms of severe depressive disorder
Delusions of:
◆ worthlessness
◆ guilt
◆ ill-health
◆ poverty
◆ nihilism
◆ persecution
Hallucinations:
◆ auditory
◆ rarely visual

The **delusions** of severe depressive disorders are concerned with the same themes as the non-delusional thinking of moderate depressive disorders, namely, worthlessness, guilt, ill health and, more rarely, poverty. When delusions with this kind of content occur in depressive disorder, they are termed **mood congruent**. Such delusions have been described in Chapter 1, but a few examples may be helpful here. A patient with a **delusion of guilt** may believe that some dishonest act, such as a minor concealment in making a tax return, will be discovered and that he will be punished severely and humiliated. He is likely to believe that such punishment is deserved. A patient with **hypochondriacal delusions** may be convinced that he has cancer or a sexually transmitted disease. A patient with a **delusion of impoverishment** may wrongly believe that he has lost all his money in a business venture. A patient with **nihilistic delusions** may believe that he has no future, or that some part of him has ceased to exist or function (e.g. that his bowels are wholly blocked). A patient with **persecutory delusions** may believe that other people are discussing him in a derogatory way, or about to take revenge on him. When persecutory delusions are part of a depressive syndrome, typically the patient accepts the supposed persecution as something he deserves. **Mood-incongruent delusions** may also occur; when they do, the course of the illness may be more like schizophrenia.

Perceptual disturbances may also be found in severe depressive disorder. When **hallucinations** occur, these are usually auditory in the form of voices addressing repetitive words and phrases to the patient. The voices may seem to confirm their ideas of worthlessness (e.g. 'you are evil; you should die'), or to make derisive comments, or urge suicide. Visual hallucinations may also occur, sometimes in the form of scenes of death and destruction.

Suicidal ideas should be enquired about carefully in any patient with a severe depressive disorder. Rarely, there are **homicidal ideas** and when these occur they may concern family members, including children. Although rare, this possibility needs to be considered in puerperal depressive disorder (see pp. 103–4).

Variants of moderate and severe depressive disorder
The clinical picture of severe depressive disorder is varied and several terms are sometimes used to describe common patterns.

Agitated depression is a condition in which agitation is particularly severe. Agitated depression occurs more commonly among older patients.

Retarded depression is a condition in which psychomotor retardation is prominent.

Depressive stupor is a rare variant of severe depressive disorder in which retardation is so extreme that the patient is motionless, mute, and refuses to eat and drink. On recovering, patients can recall the events taking place at the time they were in stupor.

Atypical depression A minority of patients have prominent atypical features such as severe anxiety, severe fatigue, increased sleep, and increased appetite.

Mania

Mania, a syndrome which is in some ways the reverse of depression, occurs as part of **bipolar disorder**. The term bipolar disorder implies episodes of both mania and depressive disorder but the diagnostic category also includes those who, at the time of diagnosis, have suffered only manic illnesses (most patients with mania eventually develop a depressive disorder). When manic symptoms occur without significant psychosocial impairment, the syndrome is called **hypomania**.

Clinical features

The central features of the syndrome of mania are: elation or irritability, increased activity, and self-important ideas (Table 8.4).

TABLE 8.4   Clinical features of mania
Mood
◆ Euphoria
◆ Irritability
Appearance
Behaviour
◆ Overactivity
◆ Distractibility
◆ Socially inappropriate behaviour
◆ Reduced sleep
◆ Increased appetite
◆ Increased libido
Thinking and speech
◆ Flight of ideas
◆ Expansive ideas
◆ Grandiose delusions
◆ Hallucinations
Impaired insight

- **Elevated mood** may appear as elation, euphoria, cheerfulness, undue optimism, and as infectious gaiety. In other cases, it appears as irritability or a tendency to become angry. Mood often varies during the day, although usually not with the regular diurnal rhythm characteristic of severe depressive disorders (see p. 99). Sometimes elation is interrupted by sudden brief episodes of depression.

- **Appearance** often reflects the prevailing mood. Patients often select brightly coloured and ill-assorted clothes. When the condition is severe, they may appear untidy and dishevelled.

- **Behaviour**. Patients are *overactive*, often for long periods, leading to physical exhaustion. Manic patients are *distractible*, starting activities and leaving them unfinished as they turn repeatedly to new ones. Behaviour may be socially inappropriate due to a combination of increased activity, *disinhibition* and grandiosity. The patient may go on unrestrained buying sprees, dramatically increase their sexual activity. or increase their consumption of alcohol and/or drugs.

- **Libido**. Sexual activity is often increased.

- **Sleep** is often reduced but the patient wakes feeling lively and energetic and may often rise early and engage in noisy activity to the surprise and distress of other people.

- **Appetite** is increased, and food may be eaten greedily with little attention to conventional manners.

- **Speech** is often rapid and copious, reflecting thoughts that occur in quick succession ('pressure of speech'). When severe, the rapid succession of thoughts is difficult to follow; the term **flight of ideas** is used.

- **Thinking**. Expansive (grandiose) ideas are common. Patients believe that their ideas are original, their opinions important, and their work is of outstanding quality. Many patients become extravagant, spending more than they can afford, for example on expensive cars or jewellery. Others make reckless decisions to give up good jobs or embark on plans for risky business ventures. In severe cases there may be *grandiose delusions*. For example, the patient may believe that he is a religious prophet or an expert destined to advise statesmen about great issues. At times there are *delusions of persecution*, the patient believing that people are conspiring against him because of his special importance. *Delusions of reference* and *passivity feelings* may occur. The delusions often change in content over days.

◆ **Hallucinations** also occur in severe cases. They are usually consistent with the mood and fluctuate in content, taking the form of voices speaking to the patient about his special powers or, occasionally, of visions with a religious content.

◆ **Insight** is invariably impaired. Patients may see no reason why their grandiose plans should be restrained or their extravagant expenditure curtailed. They seldom think of themselves as ill or in need of treatment.

Most manic patients can exert some control over their symptoms for a short time. Many do so when the interviewer is assessing the need for treatment, with the result that the severity of the disorder may be underestimated. For this reason it is important, whenever possible, to interview an informant as well as the patient.

Clinical patterns

Mild mania Physical activity and speech are increased; mood is labile, mainly euphoric but at times irritable; ideas are expansive; and the patient often spends more than he can afford. By definition, there is some social impairment in this and other patterns of mania (without it, the diagnosis is hypomania).

Moderate mania There is marked overactivity with pressure and disorganization of speech; the euphoric mood is increasingly interrupted by periods of irritability, hostility, and depression; and grandiose and other preoccupations may become delusional.

Severe mania There is frenzied overactivity; thinking is incoherent and delusions become increasingly bizarre; and hallucinations are experienced. Very rarely, however, the patient becomes immobile and mute instead of overactive and talkative (*manic stupor*).

Mixed and alternating mood states

Occasionally, manic and depressive symptoms occur together, as a mixed mood state. For example, an overactive and overtalkative patient may have profound depressive thoughts, including suicidal ideas.

In alternating mood states, mania and depression follow one another in a sequence of rapid changes. Thus, a manic patient may be intensely depressed for a few hours and then quickly become manic again. Occasionally, states of mania and depression follow one another regularly with intervals of a few weeks or months between them. The disorder is called **rapid cycling** when four or more episodes of mood disorder (depressive, manic, or mixed) occur within a 12-month period.

Classification of mood disorders

The classification of mood disorders is descriptive and based on clinical characteristics. There are three broad approaches:

1. **Aetiology**: the extent to which symptoms are caused by factors within the individual person (*endogenous*) or by external stressors (*reactive*). Both types of cause are present in every case and this is not a useful basis for classification.

2. **Symptoms**: the nature and intensity of depressive symptoms (*neurotic* and *psychotic*). This approach is also unsatisfactory because there appears to be a gradation of severity of the disorder rather than distinct patterns.

3. **Course**: apart from classifying depression as a single episode, recurrent, or persistent, there is an important distinction between those who only have depressive disorders (*unipolar*) and those who also have manic episodes (*bipolar*). All manic patients are classified as bipolar, even if there has been no episode of depressive disorder. This distinction has a genetic basis and has implications for treatment.

The categories used for classification in ICD-10 and DSM-IV are broadly similar, although the terms are not quite the same (Table 8.5). For most clinical purposes it is useful to *describe* mood disorders systematically as shown in Table 8.6. Depressive episodes can be divided into mild, moderate, or severe, using standard criteria. Within these main diagnostic categories it is possible to specify disorders that have a seasonal pattern and those in which general medical conditions or substance dependence appear to be aetiological factors.

TABLE 8.5 Classification of affective disorders

ICD-10	DSM-IV
Manic episode	Manic episode
Depressive episode	Major depressive episode
◆ Mild	
◆ Moderate	
◆ Severe	
Bipolar affective disorder	Bipolar disorders
Persistent mood (affective) states	
◆ Cyclothymia	Cyclothymia
◆ Dysthymia	Dysthymia

TABLE 8.6	Systematic scheme for the description of affective disorders
The episode	
◆ Severity	Mild, moderate, or severe
◆ Type	Depressive, manic, mixed
◆ Special features	With neurotic symptoms
	With psychotic symptoms
	With agitation
	With retardation or stupor
Course	Unipolar or bipolar
Aetiology	Predominantly reactive
	Predominantly endogenous

The classification includes two categories for less severe and more chronic illnesses:

1. **Dysthymia**, with chronic, constant, or fluctuating mild depressive symptoms.

2. **Cyclothymia**, with chronic instability of mood with mild depressive and manic symptoms.

Minor mood disorders

In primary care, the most frequent presentation of mild depressive disorder is a mixture of anxiety and depression; often referred to as **minor mood (or affective) disorder**. This term, which does not appear in either ICD-10 or DSM-IV, covers a range of disorders in which the symptoms are not sufficiently severe to meet diagnostic criteria for depressive disorder, but may still be disabling for the patient. Such conditions are common in general practice. Estimates of prevalence vary from 18 to 79 per 1000 for men, and from 27 to 165 per 1000 for women. Looked at in another way, minor mood disorders probably make up about two-thirds of the psychiatric disorders seen in general practice. The most frequent symptoms are:

◆ anxiety and worrying thoughts;

◆ sadness and depressive thoughts;

◆ irritability;

◆ poor concentration;

◆ insomnia;

◆ fatigue;

◆ somatic symptoms, including abdominal discomfort, indigestion, flatulence, and poor appetite; palpitations, praecordial discomfort, and concerns about

heart disease; headache and pain in the neck, back, and shoulders;

◆ excessive concern about bodily function.

About half of patients with minor mood disorders improve within 3 months and a further quarter within 6 months. The rest continue to suffer from minor mood disorder, or become more severe so that they are diagnosed as having anxiety disorders, depressive disorders, or somatoform syndromes.

Mood disorder following childbirth

Following childbirth, women may experience several forms of mood disturbance (see Chapter 11).

Mild depression (baby blues) This occurs in the first few days following childbirth. It is a normal phenomenon, occurring in about 70 per cent of mothers and is self-limiting, usually disappearing within a few days. The main symptoms are irritability, lability of mood, muddled thinking, and tearfulness. Of these symptoms, lability of mood is particularly characteristic. All these symptoms reach their peak on the third or fourth postpartum day. Both the frequency of the emotional changes and their timing suggests that maternity 'blues' may be related to a readjustment in hormones after delivery, but there is no direct evidence to support this idea.

Postnatal depressive disorder A depressive disorder occurring in the first 3 months after childbirth occurs in about 10 per cent of mothers and the symptoms of are similar to a depressive disorder occurring at any other time, although tiredness, irritability, and anxiety may be more prominent than depressive mood and there may be prominent phobic symptoms. There are several factors that are thought to be involved in the aetiology of postnatal depressive disorder and these are probably exacerbated by the psychological adjustments required after childbirth, by loss of sleep, and by the hard work involved in the care of a baby. Some of these women have a history of psychiatric illness and some have experienced stressful events near the time of onset of the disorder. Depressive disorder can have a negative effect on bonding between mother and baby and this can delay the infant's development. Efforts should be made, therefore, to identify mothers who are developing a depressive disorder following childbirth and, increasingly, simple screening tests such as the Edinburgh Postnatal Depression Scale are being used.

Puerperal psychosis usually begins in the first or second week after delivery and occurs in about 1 in 500 births (see Chapter 11). It is more frequent among primiparous women, those who have suffered previous serious major psychiatric disorder, and those with a family history of psychiatric disorder. Delirium used to be common before antibiotics were introduced to treat puerperal sepsis. Nowadays, the usual clinical picture is of a severe psychotic mood disorder or schizoaffective disorder, although varying levels of confusion and disorientation lend an organic 'flavour' to the clinical picture.

Seasonal affective disorder (SAD)

Some people repeatedly develop a depressive disorder at the same time of year. In some cases this timing reflects extra demands on the person at a particular time of year; in other cases there is no such extra demand, and it has been suggested that the cause is related to changes in the season, for example, in the length of daylight. Although these affective disorders are characterized mainly by the season at which they occur, they are also said to be characterized by some symptoms that are less common in other affective disorders, for example hypersomnia and increased appetite with cravings for carbohydrates.

The most common pattern is of onset in the autumn or winter, and recovery in the spring or summer. This pattern has led to the suggestion that shortening of daylight is important. Some patients improve after exposure to artificial light, usually given in the early morning (see p. 253). It is uncertain for which patients the treatment is effective, or how lasting are its effects.

Differential diagnoses

Depressive disorders

These disorders have to be distinguished from the following conditions.

- **Normal sadness**. The distinction from normal sadness depends on the presence of other symptoms of the syndrome of depressive disorder.

- **Grief**. Although depressive disorder resembles uncomplicated grief in many ways, severe pessimism, suicidal thoughts, profound guilt, and psychotic symptoms are all rare in grief. Severe symptoms persisting for more than 2 months after bereavement suggest a depressive disorder.

- **Anxiety disorder**. Mild depressive disorders are sometimes difficult to distinguish from anxiety disorders. Accurate diagnosis depends on assessment of the relative severity of anxiety and depressive symptoms, and on the order in which they appeared. Similar problems arise when there are prominent *phobic* or *obsessional* symptoms. (These points are discussed further in Chapter 6.)

- **Functional physical symptoms** (see Chapter 7). It is not uncommon for depressive disorder to present with concern about non-specific and medically unexplained physical symptoms, without a direct complaint of psychological symptoms. Careful enquiry will elicit these additional symptoms.

- **Schizophrenia**. The differential diagnosis of depressive disorder from schizophrenia depends on a careful search for the characteristic features of schizophrenia (see Chapter 9). Diagnosis may be difficult when a patient has both depressive symptoms and persecutory delusions, but the distinction can usually be made by examining the mental state carefully and by establishing whether the delusions followed, and are consistent with, the depressive symptoms (mood-congruent depressive disorder) or whether the delusions came first or are not congruent with the mood disorder (schizophrenia). For example, in depressive disorder, persecution is usually accepted as the deserved consequence of the patient's own failings; in schizophrenia it is strongly rejected. Some patients have symptoms of both depressive disorder and schizophrenia; these *schizoaffective disorders* are discussed in Chapter 9. A depressive syndrome may also occur following treatment of the psychotic symptoms of schizophrenia; it is called *post-psychotic depression*.

- **Dementia**. In middle and late life, depressive disorders may be difficult to distinguish from dementia because some patients with depressive disorder complain of considerable difficulty in remembering and some demented patients are depressed. In depressive disorders, difficulty in remembering occurs because poor concentration leads to inadequate registration. The distinction between the two conditions can often be made by careful memory testing. Standard psychological tests are required in doubtful cases, but even these may not decide the issue. If memory disorder does not improve with recovery of normal mood, dementia is probable (see pp. 142–3).

- **Substance abuse**. Depressive symptoms are common in substance abuse and some patients with depressive disorder abuse alcohol or non-prescribed drugs to relieve their distress. The sequence of the depressive symptoms and substance abuse should be determined, as well as the presence of the features of depressive disorder other than low mood.

Manic disorders

Manic disorders have to be distinguished from: schizophrenia, organic brain disease involving the frontal lobes (including brain tumour and general paralysis of the insane), endocrine disorders, and states of excitement induced by amphetamines and related drugs.

- **Schizophrenia.** Diagnosing manic disorders from schizophrenia can be most difficult. In manic disorders, auditory hallucinations and delusions can occur, including some delusions that are characteristic of schizophrenia—such as delusions of reference. In mania these symptoms usually change quickly in content, and seldom outlast the overactivity. When there is a more or less equal mixture of features of the two syndromes, the term *schizoaffective* (or 'schizomanic') is used. These conditions are discussed further in Chapter 9.

- **Dementia** should always be considered, especially in middle-aged or older patients with expansive behaviour and no past history of affective disorder. In the absence of gross mood disorder, extreme social disinhibition (e.g. urinating in public) strongly suggests frontal lobe pathology. In such cases appropriate neurological investigation is essential.

- **Endocrine disorders.** Hyperthyroid states may cause symptoms suggestive of mania. Physical signs of elevated thyroid should be sought and blood levels of thryoid hormones estimated.

- **Abuse of stimulant drugs.** The distinction between mania and excited behaviour due to the abuse of amphetamines depends on the history, together with examination of the urine for drugs before treatment with psychotropic drugs is started. Drug-induced states usually subside quickly once the patient is in hospital and free from the drugs (see Chapter 13).

Epidemiology

Major depressive disorders are frequent with a prevalence in Western countries of 20–30 per 1000 for men and 40–90 per 1000 for women. The lifetime risk is about 1 in 10 for men and 1 in 4 for women. It is not certain why consistently higher figures are reported for women. Depressive disorders are more common in urban than rural populations and, in general, the prevalence is higher in groups with adverse socioeconomic factors (e.g. in homeless people). The high prevalence means that depressive disorders are one of the most important causes of disability in all countries. Depressive disorders cause both direct costs to health services and much greater indirect costs due to inability to work.

Bipolar disorder is less common. The prevalence is between 1 and 6 per 1000 and the lifetime risk is rather less than 1 in 100. First-degree relatives are at much higher risk—with a 12 per cent lifetime risk of bipolar disorder, a 12 per cent lifetime risk of recurrent depressive disorder, and a 12 per cent risk of dysthymic or other mood disorders.

A primary care doctor responsible for 2000 patients of all ages may expect to see 20–30 patients a year presenting with major depression and perhaps one or two patients presenting with an episode of mania.

Aetiology

In broad terms, mood disorders are caused by an interaction between: (i) **stressful events**; and (ii) **constitutional factors** resulting from genetic endowment and childhood experience. These aetiological factors act through biochemical and psychological processes, which have been partly identified by research. More is known about the aetiology of depressive than of manic disorders. For this reason, and because it illustrates the multifactorial approach to aetiology in psychiatry, we focus here on depressive disorders.

Genetic causes

Genetic factors have been studied mainly in moderate to severe cases of mood disorder, rather than in milder cases. Parents, siblings, and children of severely depressed patients have a higher lifetime risk for mood disorder (10–15 per cent), than the general population (1–2 per cent). **Twin studies** indicate that these high rates among families are due to genetic factors. Thus the concordance of bipolar disorder is the same (about 70 per cent) among monozygotic twins reared together and monozygotic twins reared apart, and higher than the concordance between dizygotic twins (23 per cent). Studies of **adopted children** confirm the importance of genetic causes of depressive disorder because the risk of developing the disorder is higher in a child who was born to a parent with a history of serious depressive disorder, but raised by adoptive parents with no such history, than in a child who was born to parents with no history of serious depressive disorder. Bipolar disorders are more frequent in the families of bipolar probands than in the families of unipolar probands. However, unipolar cases are frequent in the families of bipolar as well as unipolar probands. Thus unipolar cases may be of more than one genetic type. Although the circumstantial evidence for genetic factors is therefore strong, no single gene, or combination of genes, causing depression have yet been consistently identified.

Personality

It has been suggested that genetic factors might predispose to affective disorder through an effect on personality, or alternatively that variations in personality (e.g. cyclothymic personality, see p. 52) reflect the same genetic factors that cause illness. Unipolar depressive disorders have not been found to be associated with a single personality type.

Predisposing environmental factors

Depressive disorders often seem to begin after prolonged adversity, such as difficulties in marriage or at work. These adverse circumstances seem to prepare the ground for a final acute stressor, which precipitates the disorder. For example, there is evidence that having the care of several young children, poor economic circumstances, and an unsupportive marriage increase vulnerability to depression.

Looked at another way, certain factors *protect* against the action of stressors and people who lack them are more vulnerable. Thus, some women appear to be more vulnerable to depressive disorder when they have nobody with whom they can confide. Clearly, there is some overlap between the concepts of vulnerability and protective factors.

Precipitating environmental factors

Clinically, depressive disorders often seem to follow stressful *life events*. This association is not necessarily causal: instead it might be coincidental or the stressful event itself might be a consequence of the early, but unrecognized, stages of the illness (e.g. losing a job because of deteriorating performance) rather than a cause in its own right (e.g. losing a job when a whole factory closes). Epidemiological research has shown that there is an excess of life events *independent* of the illness in the week preceding a depressive disorder, but this association is *non-specific* since life events also occur in excess in the weeks before the onset of schizophrenia, and before acts of deliberate self-harm. The effect is substantial: the risk of developing a depressive disorder is increased about six-fold in the 6 months after experiencing moderately severe life events (the corresponding figure for schizophrenia is about three-fold). Loss events, such as bereavement, are particularly likely to lead to depressive disorder.

Life events also provoke mania, but less often than depressive disorder. Surprisingly, mania can follow an event that would be expected to produce a depressive response (e.g. a bereavement) as well as an event that would be expected to produce elation (e.g. success and excitement).

Physical conditions as predisposing or precipitating factors

Most physical conditions are non-specific stressors but a few appear to precipitate depressive disorder by direct biological mechanisms. They include influenza and some other viral infections, childbirth (see pp. 158–9), and Parkinson's disease.

A number of psychoactive substances, brain injury, some neurological endocrine disorders, and several other physical illnesses can produce secondary manic illnesses. In addition, in some people with a family history of bipolar disorder, antidepressant medication can precipitate a manic episode.

Mediating processes

Two kinds of complementary mediating processes have been studied: psychological and biochemical.

Psychological mediating processes

Depressed patients think in a gloomy, self-deprecating way that worsens and prolongs the initial change of mood. Their abnormal thinking can be divided into three components:

1. They *remember unhappy events* more easily than happy ones.

2. They have *intrusive gloomy thoughts* ('negative thoughts'), for example, 'I am a failure as a mother'.

3. They have *unrealistic beliefs*, for example, 'I cannot be happy unless I am liked by everyone I know'.

Depressed patients also think in illogical ways ('**cognitive distortions**'), such as drawing a general conclusion from a single event; for example 'I have failed in this relationship, so I will never be loved by anyone'. These illogical ways of thinking allow the intrusive gloomy thoughts and the unrealistic expectations to persist despite evidence to the contrary.

Repeated negative thoughts deepen the depressive mood, while unrealistic beliefs convert everyday experiences into stressful problems. These ways of thinking may also explain why some disorders persist after the original causes have passed, since they set up a vicious circle in which depressive thinking generates low mood, which then perpetuates the depressive thinking.

It is not known whether these modes of thought precede the depressive disorder and play a part in its onset.

Biochemical mediating processes

There is increasing evidence of biochemical abnormalities, at least in the more severe depressive disorders, but their nature is uncertain. Also, it is not known whether there is a single abnormality present in every patient with depressive disorder, or whether different abnormalities lead to the same clinical picture.

The strongest evidence is for an abnormality of **5-HT (serotonin) function**. There are three main strands of evidence:

1. *Concentrations of the main 5-HT metabolite (5-HIAA) are reduced* in the cerebrospinal fluid (CSF) of patients with severe depressive disorders. This is very indirect evidence since concentrations of 5-HT in the brain could be very different from those in CSF.

2. *5-HT concentrations are reduced* in the brains of depressed patients who have died by suicide. This reduction could, however, be caused by drugs used to commit suicide or by post-mortem changes.

3. *Neuroendocrine functions that involve 5-HT transmission are reduced* in depressed patients. However, the findings of an abnormality in neurons controlling endocrine function is not necessarily evidence for the same abnormality in neurons controlling mood.

If low 5-HT function is important in causing depressive disorder, then increasing this function should be therapeutic. All antidepressant drugs increase 5-HT function but until recently most have also had effects on other neurotransmitter systems. Recently, drugs have been developed that have specific 5-HT effects (the SSRIs, see Chapter 16) and these have antidepressant effects. The action of transmitter systems in the brain, however, is through checks and balances. Hence it cannot be argued that, because increasing 5-HT function improves depressive disorder, reduced 5-HT function causes the disorder. The point becomes more obvious when parkinsonism is considered: in this disorder, anticholinergic drugs have therapeutic effects but the abnormality is of a loss of dopaminergic function. Recently, the picture has become more complex with the discovery that there are several kinds of 5-HT receptor, each with different functions. It seems possible that antidepressant drugs exert their effects mainly on $5-HT_2$ receptor function.

Noradrenergic function also seems to be reduced in depressive disorders. Most antidepressant drugs affect this transmitter system; they affect both pre- and post-synaptic noradrenergic neurons in a complicated way, but the overall action is a brief initial increase of function followed by a decrease. It seems unlikely, therefore, that the beneficial effect of antidepressant drugs can be due to a direct effect on noradrenergic receptors since, as just mentioned, noradrenergic function appears to be decreased in depressive disorders.

Endocrine abnormalities

A causal role for endocrine abnormalities is suggested by the association of mood disorder with Cushing's syndrome, Addison's disease, and hyperparathyroidism (Cushing's syndrome is sometimes associated with elation rather than depression of mood). It has also been suggested that depressive disorders occurring after childbirth or at the menopause are related to endocrine changes at these times but there is no strong evidence for this.

Among endocrine causes, interest has centred on **cortisol**. Plasma cortisol is increased in about half of patients with depressive disorder. However, this increase in cortisol is not specific to depressive disorder; it occurs also in mania and schizophrenia. The change does not seem to be just a reaction to the stress of being ill, for it involves a change in the diurnal pattern of secretion of cortisol (being high in the afternoon and early evening after which time it normally decreases), a change not seen after exposure to stressors. It has been suggested that the elevation of cortisol may arise after a *prolonged* life stress and may predispose to depression by interfering with brain 5-HT function.

Conclusion

Genes *predispose* to depressive disorder and mania, although the precise mode of inheritance is unknown. Recent adverse social circumstances also predispose to depression. People who lack confiding relationships seem to be more vulnerable than others to stressful circumstances. An accumulation of long-term problems may increase vulnerability to acute stressors. Depressive disorder is *precipitated* by stressful life events (especially loss), and by certain kinds of physical illness. Depressive disorders are *maintained* by continuing stressors and in some cases by depressive thinking.

Course and prognosis

Unipolar depressive disorders may start at any time from childhood to late life, the most common age of onset being in the late twenties. Untreated illnesses can last 6 months or more, with a significant minority lasting for years. With treatment, each episode lasts 2–3 months on average. Most patients eventually recover from the episode, although recurrences are common. At least half of those who have a single episode followed by complete recovery will eventually have another episode.

Bipolar disorders usually begin in the first half of life, 90 per cent starting before the age of 50. They run a recurring course with recovery between episodes of illness. Each episode generally lasts several months—on average about three. Most patients experience depressive as well as manic episodes, but a few have only manic episodes.

Suicide is substantially more frequent among patients with affective disorder than among the general population. Among patients with severe depressive disorder about 1 in 10 eventually commits suicide.

Puerperal psychosis Most patients recover fully from puerperal psychosis but a few (mostly those with a schizophrenic psychosis) remain chronically ill. At a subsequent birth, the recurrence rate for puerperal depressive illness is between 1 in 2 or 3 (compared with 1 in 500 for those without a previous puerperal psychosis). At least half the women with a puerperal depressive illness go on to develop a depressive illness unrelated to childbirth.

Management of depressive disorders

Most patients with depressive disorders are treated in primary care. However, not all those needing treatment are recognized. This is partly due to a lack of understanding of the recognition and treatment of the condition.

Detection of depressive disorders

It is important that all doctors remain aware of the high prevalence of depression in all settings. The detection of depression can be improved if the doctor always remembers to ask two simple screening questions:

1. During the last month, have you often been bothered by feeling down, depressed, or hopeless?

2. During the last month, have you often been bothered by little interest or pleasure in doing things?

Doctors with good interviewing skills are also more likely to detect depression and to produce better outcomes, possibly because good interviewing provides non-specific benefits as well as leading to improved diagnosis and the provision of effective treatment.

Assessment

A patient who is suspected of having a depressive disorder needs a comprehensive assessment that includes a consideration of medical, psychological, and social needs and an assessment of the risks (Table 8.7).

Diagnosis depends on thorough history taking and examination of the physical and mental state of the patient. Differential diagnosis has been discussed earlier in this chapter (see p. 104). Particular care should be taken:

- not to overlook a depressive disorder in a patient who complains of the physical symptoms of depression such as fatigue or poor sleep rather than depressed mood ('masked depression');

- not to diagnose a depressive disorder simply on the grounds of prominent depressive symptoms; the latter could be part of another disorder, for example an organic psychiatric syndrome caused by cerebral neoplasm;

- to remember that certain drugs can induce depression (see p. 152);

- to determine if the patient has suffered from a previous episode of mania, in which case the diagnosis

TABLE 8.7	Assessment of depressive disorder
Diagnosis	History
	Mental state
	Relevant physical examination
	Relevant physical investigation
	Informants' accounts
Severity	Biological symptoms
	Psychotic symptoms
	Suicide risk, risk to others
	Effect on social functioning
Aetiology	Psychological
	Social
	Physical illness
	Drug therapy
	Constitutional
Social consequences	Patient's everyday life
	Partner and family
	Dangers at work
Social resources	Family support
	Housing
	Work

would be bipolar depression and the treatment would be as described below (see p. 117).

Severity The severity of the disorder is judged from the symptoms and behaviour. Whenever possible, an informant should be interviewed as well as the patient. More severe illnesses are accompanied by 'biological' symptoms, and by the presence of 'psychotic' symptoms (e.g. hallucinations and delusions). The risk of *suicide* must be judged in every case (the methods of assessment are described in Chapter 12). It is also important to assess how far the depressive disorder has reduced the patient's capacity to work or to engage in family life and social activities. In this assessment, the duration and course of the condition should be taken into account as well as the severity of the present symptoms and disability. The length of history not only affects prognosis, it also gives an indication of the patient's capacity to tolerate further distress. A long continued disorder, even if not severe, can bring the patient to the point of desperation.

Aetiological factors Possible aetiological factors may include both known medical and psychiatric causes and precipitating, predisposing, maintaining, and pathoplastic factors. Precipitating causes may be psychological and social (the life events discussed earlier in the chapter) or they may be physical illness or its treatment. In assessing such causes enquiries should be made into the patient's work, finances, family life, social activities, general living conditions, and physical health. Problems in these areas may be recent and acute, or chronic background difficulties may exist such as prolonged marital tension, problems with children, and financial hardship. In planning treatment, maintaining factors are usually of the most relevance.

Social consequences The impact on the patient's everyday life should be considered by asking about ability to work, effects on leisure interests, and, particularly, consequences for family life. Such information is not only an indication of the severity of the disorder, but may bring up issues that require advice and discussion with the patient and family. The effect of the disorder on other people should also be considered. It is important to consider whether the patient could *endanger other people* by remaining at work (e.g. as a bus driver). Effects in the family are important, especially the effects on young children; a severely depressed mother may neglect her children. Danger may also arise when there are depressive delusions that could lead to action. Severely depressed mothers may sometimes kill their children because of the belief that they are doomed to suffer if they remain alive. Severely depressed patients occasionally kill their spouses. In the longer term, depressive disorder in either parent is associated with the development of emotional disorder in the children.

Social resources The patient's social resources should be considered next. Enquiries should cover family, friends, and work. Supportive families and friends can help patients through periods of depressive disorder by providing company, encouraging them when confidence is lost, and guiding them into suitable activities. For some patients, work is a valuable social resource, providing distraction and comradeship. For others it is a source of stress. A careful assessment is needed in each case.

Treatment of the acute phase of depression

Treatment of depressive disorder can be divided into three main stages (Fig. 8.1):

1. An **acute phase** to relieve symptoms of depression and achieve recovery.

2. **Continuation** therapy to preserve the improvement.

3. A **maintenance phase** to protect vulnerable patients from further episodes.

There are several effective treatments for depressive disorders and the choice of treatment for each individual patient will depend on several factors, including the severity of the disorder, the patient's own preferences, and the availability of the treatments.

General aspects of acute phase treatment

As well as the specific treatments outlined above, non-specific and supportive measures are very important. The patient may have an unclear view of the nature of depressive disorder and its treatment. The doctor should therefore provide a clear outline of the nature of the disorder and the available treatments, including both likely benefits and possible adverse effects, and should discuss the patient's preferences and agree a treatment plan. Active follow-up with early identification of any problems leads to better adherence to the prescribed therapy and improved outcomes. During the initial weeks of treatment, patients should be seen and supported—those with severe disorders may need to be seen every 2 or 3 days, while others are usually seen weekly. The possibility of the emergence of a manic episode should be kept in mind when depression is being treated because the first manic episode follows treatment for a depressive disorder in some patients with bipolar disorder.

It is important to advise the patient that there are a number of things that they can do themselves to promote recovery from depression.

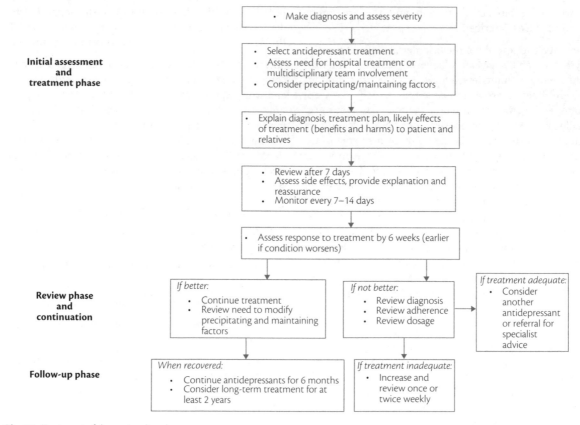

Fig. 8.1 Treatment of depressive disorders.

◆ **Activity**. The level of activity should be considered for every patient. Depressed patients give up activities and withdraw from other people. In this way, they become deprived of social stimulation and rewarding experiences, and their original feelings of depression increase. It is important to make sure that patients are occupied adequately, but also that they are not pushed into activities in which they may fail because of slowness or poor concentration. Hence, the range of activity appropriate for a depressed patient is narrow and changes as the illness runs its course. If the patient is treated at home, it may be helpful to discuss with relatives how much the patient should do each day.

◆ **Diet**. Appetite may be diminished in depression and the patient should be encouraged to eat regularly and healthily.

◆ **Sleep**. Simple advice should be given on how to deal with any insomnia that accompanies the depression (see p. 167).

In can be helpful to involve the patient's relatives in the treatment plan. In particular, they should be helped to understand the disorder as an illness, to avoid criticizing the patient, and to encourage appropriate activity.

Even when not being treated with a specific psychological treatment, all depressed patients require support, encouragement, and repeated explanation that they are suffering from illness not moral failure. When the depressive disorder appears to have been precipitated by life problems, discussion and problem-solving counselling may be required. However, when the depressive disorder is severe, discussion of problems may increase hopelessness. The more depressed the patient, the more the doctor and others should take over problems in the early days of treatment. When mood improves, the problems can be reconsidered.

Specific treatments for depressive disorder
Antidepressant drug treatment

Antidepressant drugs are the most widely available effective treatment for depressive disorder and are prescribed widely in both primary and secondary care. As with most effective treatments, they are not without adverse effects so their use should generally be restricted to patients with at least a moderate level of symptom severity in whom depressive symptoms are causing impaired functioning.

There are several groups of antidepressant drugs which are fully described on pp. 242–8. The usual first choice is a selective serotonin reuptake inhibitor or a tricyclic drug.

Combined drug regimens

Combined treatment may be useful when patients have not responded to monotherapy, although there is limited evidence on its efficacy. Combinations of drugs are more likely to lead to interactions and adverse effects and should generally be initiated by a specialist, used cautiously, and monitored carefully.

The most commonly recommended combination treatment is lithium plus an antidepressant, which is effective in some patients who have not responded to the antidepressant alone. Combinations of tricyclics and MAOIs and tricyclics and a SSRI may be effective in some patients unresponsive to either drug given separately.

Electroconvulsive therapy (ECT)

ECT is described more comprehensively on pp. 252–3. The antidepressant action of ECT is quicker than that of antidepressant drugs, but it causes more adverse effects, especially impairment of short-term memory. For these reasons, ECT is mainly used to treat severe depressive illness in only a couple of situations:

1. The depressive disorder has not responded to adequate antidepressant drug treatment.

2. A rapid response is necessary because of high suicidal risk or severe psychomotor retardation.

ECT is probably most effective in severe depressive disorder with delusions and/or psychomotor retardation.

Psychological treatment

Supportive and problem-solving treatments All depressed patients and their families need supportive care to sustain them until improvement takes place. Persistent interpersonal problems maintain depression and problem solving can resolve the difficulties. The least severe illnesses can usually be treated by problem solving and psychological and social support; more severe depressive disorders are usually treated with drug treatment with psychological and social support (though a few receive cognitive therapy, see below).

Dynamic psychotherapy Although depressed patients often express guilt and regrets about experiences in their recent or remote past, these feelings generally resolve as mood improves and there is no evidence that dynamic psychotherapy speeds this process. Indeed, it is generally better not to dwell on past events in the early stages of treatment for this may only increase the patient's guilty introspection.

Cognitive therapy (see p. 258) is as effective as antidepressant drugs in the treatment of moderate depressive disorders and may also prevent relapse. In practice, cognitive therapy is seldom used for these purposes, because antidepressant drug treatment is simple, generally effective, less time consuming, and hence more available. Cognitive therapy may be useful for helping residual depressive symptoms that remain after antidepressant treatment. Cognitive therapy is sometimes used for recurrent or chronic depressive disorders in which depressive thinking seems to make the patient more vulnerable to life events or to perpetuate the disorder. However, this use has not been thoroughly evaluated by clinical trials.

Interpersonal psychotherapy is a standardized form of brief psychotherapy that focuses on improving the patient's interpersonal functioning and identifying the problems associated with the onset of the depressive episode. Interpersonal therapy has been shown to be effective for outpatients with unipolar non-psychotic depressive disorders but in practice antidepressant drugs and problem solving are used more often.

Tailoring the treatment according to the severity of the disorder

The appropriate treatment for a person with depressive disorder depends on the severity of the disorder. All treatments have adverse effects and financial costs as well as benefits, and so it is important to make sure that the likely benefits are worth the costs. There is little point in providing an intensive and expensive psychotherapy to a patient with a mild disorder that is likely to resolve spontaneously and quickly. On the other hand, a patient with a severe disorder may need early intensive drug treatment, or inpatient care (such a patient is also likely to need urgent referral to the specialist mental health services).

Mild depressive disorders

Mild depressive disorders seldom require treatment with antidepressant drugs or an intensive psychological treatment, especially when they are clearly reactions to stressful life events that have resolved. Patients should receive a clear explanation of the problem and their part in overcoming it, and should be encouraged to talk about their feelings and discuss their problems. The patient should be encouraged to eat well, take exercise, and try to get sufficient sleep. Such help is particularly important after bereavement or other kinds of loss. Self-help reading materials may also be helpful.

Many patients with mild depressive disorders have slept badly for weeks. A hypnotic drug may be given for a few days to restore sleep, but such treatment should not be prolonged. If the depressive symptoms do not respond quickly to social and psychological measures and if sleep problems persist, sedative antidepressants should be prescribed to be taken at night.

Should the patient remain at work? When the disorder is mild, work can be a valuable distraction from depressive thoughts, and can provide companionship.

Moderately severe and severe depressive disorder

All except mild depressive disorders should be treated with antidepressant drugs or with specific psychological treatments. The decision about which treatment to try first should be made jointly by the doctor and patient and will depend on the severity of the symptoms, the patient's preferences, and the availability of the treatments.

Is antidepressant drug treatment required? Antidepressant drugs are effective for most patients with a depressive disorder of at least moderate severity, and particularly those with biological symptoms. A history of previous response to medication and severe symptoms both suggest a good response to treatment. No single antidepressant is clearly more effective than another and the choice for a particular patient depends on:

* the response of the patient to any previous antidepressant medication;

* adverse effects;

* concurrent medical illnesses;

* concurrent mediaction;

* toxicity in overdose;

* cost.

Doctors should become familiar with the use of one or two drugs from each group.

Is psychiatric referral appropriate? Moderately severe depression is usually treated by non-specialists, for example, general practitioners. However, it is essential to consider in every case whether psychiatric referral is

TABLE 8.8 Situations when a patient should be referred for specialist advice
◆ In all severe and some moderately severe cases, especially when there is a substantial risk of suicide or harm to the welfare or life of another person (particularly dependent children)
◆ When the diagnosis is in doubt
◆ When a patient has failed to respond to antidepressant treatment
◆ When day or inpatient care is required
◆ When cognitive behaviour treatment may be required

required (Table 8.8) and, if so, whether the referral should be for outpatient treatment or whether immediate inpatient or day patient care is required (see below).

Is hospital care needed? In deciding the need for inpatient or day patient care, consideration is given to:

* severity and risk to the patient and to others, especially to any dependent children;

* the patient's ability to look after himself;

* the availability of social support (a patient living alone may need hospital care for a disorder that could be treated at home if there was a supportive family member who could be present day and night).

Should the patient remain at work? When the disorder is more severe, retardation, poor concentration, and lack of drive are likely to impair performance, and this failure may add to feelings of hopelessness. Sometimes, poor performance at work may endanger other people, and when the potential for such danger is great (as in the case of driving a heavy goods vehicle) the patient should not work even if the risk of failure is small.

What information do the patient and family need about medication?

It is essential that the drugs are taken in the full prescribed dose. A depressed patient's adherence to antidepressant treatment can be improved by informing the patient and the family about the nature of the medication, its potential benefits and side effects, any possible toxic effects, and the importance of continuing a full dosage for an adequate period of time. It is important to explain that, although side effects will appear quickly, the therapeutic effect is likely to be delayed for 2–3 weeks. Patients should be warned about the effects of taking alcohol because of its sedative effects. They should be advised about driving, particularly that they

TABLE 8.9	Steps to follow if there is a lack of response to antidepressant treatment

- Review diagnosis
- Check compliance with present treatment
- Review psychological and social causes
- Increase dose to maximum
- Consider change to antidepressant of a different group*
- Obtain specialist opinion concerning need for hospital admission and further treatment*
- Combined drug treatment*
- Consider ECT*

*These steps usually require a specialist opinion (see text).

should not drive while experiencing sedative or any other side effects that might impair their performance.

Failure to respond to treatment

Around 30 per cent of patients with a depressive disorder do not respond within 6 weeks to a combination of antidepressant drugs, graded activity, and psychological treatment. In these cases the *treatment plan should be reviewed* at 6 weeks and earlier in severe cases (Table 8.9).

- *Is the diagnosis correct?* The diagnosis should be reviewed carefully.

- *Have stressors been overlooked?* A check should be made for stressful life events or continuing difficulties that may have been overlooked.

- *Is the patient taking the full prescribed dose of medicine?* Check again that the patient has been taking the medication in the full amount. If not, the reasons should be sought. Some patients are convinced that no treatment can help, others are unable to tolerate drug side effects.

- *Should the dose be increased?* If the preceding enquiries reveal nothing, the dose of antidepressant may be increased if it is not already maximal.

- *Should the medication be changed?* If the patient cannot tolerate the drug, or there has been no response to the maximum tolerated dosage, an antidepressant drug from another group may be tried.

- *Frequent supportive interviews should be continued* with monitoring of severity, and the patient reassured that depressive disorders almost invariably eventually get better. Meanwhile, provided that the patient is not too depressed, any problems contributing to the depressed state should be discussed further.

- *Is a specialist opinion required?* If serious depression persists, specialist advice should be obtained concerning the need for combined antidepressant drug treatment, day care, admission to hospital, or, in the most severe cases, electroconvulsive therapy.

Continuing failure to respond

Disorders that do not fully respond to at least two adequate courses of antidepressant medicine are called **treatment resistant**. In these cases, it is usually worth trying alternative treatments, for example, cognitive therapy may be effective in patients with residual symptoms of depression following antidepressant treatment. For most patients however, the next step is combination therapy. The best established combinations are:

- lithium augmentation of an antidepressant drug.; particular care is required if lithium is added to a 5-HT uptake blocker since this produces neurotoxic side effects in a few cases;

- thyroid hormone augmentation of antidepressant drug, usually with triiodothyronine, although the evidence on this is limited;

- MAOI augmentation of a tricyclic drug. The reverse procedure of adding a tricyclic drug to a MAOI should *not* be used because it is more likely to cause serious toxic effects.

Specialist advice should be sought before using any of these drug combinations.

ECT should also be considered in the treatment of patients with depressive disorders that do not respond to drugs.

Continuation therapy

The continuation phase of treatment focuses on maintaining improvements made during treatment of the acute phase for the next 6 months or so. After recovery from a depressive disorder the patient should be followed up for several months either by the family doctor or by a psychiatrist. At this stage it is often valuable to discuss possible precipitants of the illness with the patient and in joint interviews with close relatives. This discussion is particularly important when there have been repeated depressive disorders provoked by life events.

Some residual symptoms may take several months to disappear and many patients are particularly vulnerable to relapse during this period. With antidepressant medicines, the same dose of the successful treatment should be continued during the continuation phase. Patients will need encouragement to continue with treatment, deal with any adverse effects, and advice about the appropriate level of activity and about returning to work.

Prevention of relapse

Maintenance medication Patients who responded to acute phase treatment, remained well during the continuation phase, and are at moderate or high risk of relapse (e.g. those with a history of relapse relatively soon after successful treatment of depression, or on the ending of continuation therapy) will benefit from long-term therapy for at least 2 years with antidepressants at the same dose that was effective in the acute phase. On average long-term drug treatment halves the risk of relapse.

Cognitive therapy may also reduce the relapse rate after a moderately severe depressive disorder but there is less evidence than for maintenance for antidepressant drugs. Cognitive therapy is sometimes tried for patients who have *repeated* episodes of depression, despite maintenance medication, that are apparently related to depressive forms of thinking.

Life changes If the depressive disorder was clearly related to stressors such as overwork or complicated social relationships, the patient should be helped to change to his lifestyle in the hope that this will reduce recurrence.

Recognizing early signs of relapse It can also be helpful to have a written, agreed care plan should depressive symptoms recur. The patient should be fully involved in this process by being helped to understand the risk of relapse, taught to recognize warning signs, and by agreeing on an appropriate action plan. When appropriate, the patient's relatives should be involved.

Management of mood disorders following childbirth

Baby blues

The patient and her partner should be reassured that the condition is common and short lived. No other treatment is needed.

Postnatal depressive disorder

Postnatal depression is assessed in the same way as other depressive disorders, with attention to any ideas that suggest a risk to the child (see p. 149). The Edinburgh Scale (see Box 8.1) can aid assessment and suggests topics to be explored further in the interview. If there is doubt about the risk to the child, or when risk is judged to exist, a specialist opinion should be obtained. Patients need a clear explanation of the nature of the condition and the plan of treatment, together with support from the medical team and, if possible, from the extended family. The general practitioner should liaise with the midwife, health visitor, and any specialist mental health services involved in the case to ensure necessary support and frequent monitoring. Additional help with child care may be needed. If the severity of the disorder is more than mild, or if a mild disorder persists for longer than a few weeks, treatment with antidepressant drugs may be indicated. The psychological components of the treatment plan resemble those for other depressive disorders (see above). Most cases can be treated in the community. However, when the disorder is severe or if there is a risk of self-harm or harm to the baby, hospital treatment may be required. If admission is necessary—especially if it is likely to be prolonged—then there are advantages to treatment in a specialist mother and baby unit if one is available.

Puerperal psychosis

The treatment of puerperal psychosis is the same as that for psychotic disorders occurring outside pregnancy (see pp. 116 and 117). When the disorder is not severe and the mother has no ideas of harming herself or the baby, treatment can be at home along the lines described above for non-psychotic postnatal depressive disorder. When the disorder is severe, or there are ideas of harm to the self or the baby, the mother should usually be admitted to hospital, if possible to a special mother and baby unit. If antidepressant or antipsychotic drugs or lithium have to be prescribed, then breast-feeding will have to be stopped. ECT is often used because it has a rapid effect, which if successful enables the mother to resume the feeding and care of her baby.

Women who have had a puerperal psychosis should be referred to a psychiatrist if they become pregnant again and monitored closely during subsequent deliveries. Patients who have a history of bipolar disorder and who are taking long-term lithium therapy will need specialist assessment. In some cases the lithium can be gradually stopped before the first trimester to minimize the risk of fetal abnormality, or before the delivery and restarted soon after but with no breast-feeding. Patients with schizoaffective disorders may need continued antipsychotic therapy—conventional antipsychotics are usually favoured.

Management of bipolar disorder

Assessment

The assessment of a depressive episode in a patient with bipolar disorder is essentially the same as the assessment of a unipolar depressive episode (see above), although the treatment is different, as described below.

BOX 8.1 EDINBURGH POSTNATAL DEPRESSION SCALE (EPDS)

The EPDS was developed for screening postpartum women in outpatient, home visiting settings, or at the 6-8 week postpartum examination. It has been utilized among numerous populations including US women and Spanish speaking women in other countries. The EPDS consists of 10 questions, and can usually be completed in less than 5 minutes. Resposes are scored 0, 1, 2, or 3 according to increased severity of the symptom. Items marked with an asterisk (*) are reverse scored (i.e. 3, 2, 1, and 0). The total score is the sum of the scores for each of the 10 items. Validation studies have utilized various threshold scores to determine which women were positive and in need of referral. Cut-off scores ranged from 9 to 13 points. Therefore, to err on the safe side, a woman scoring 9 or more points or indicating any suicidal ideation – scoring 1 or higher on question 10 – should be referred immediately for follow-up. Even if a woman scores less than 9, if the clinician feels the client is suffering from depression, an appropriate referral should be made. The EPDS is only a screening tool. It does not diagnose depression – that is done by appropriately licensed health care personnel. Users may reproduce the scale without permission providing the copyright is respected by quoting the author names, title, and source of the paper in all reproduced copies.

Instructions for users
1. The mother is asked to underline 1 of 4 possible responses that comes the closest to how she has been feeling the previous 7 days.
2. All 10 questions must be completed.
3. Care should be taken to avoid the possibility of the mother discussing her answers with others.
4. The mother should complete the scale herself, unless she has limited English or difficulty reading.

Name: **Date:**
Address: **Baby's age:**

As you have recently had a baby, we would like to know how you are feeling. Please **underline** the answer which comes closest to how you have felt **in the past 7 days**, not just how you feel today.

Here is an example, already completed:
       I have felt happy
            Yes, all the time
            Yes, most of the time
            No, not very often
            No, not at all
This would mean: "I have felt happy most of the time during the past week". Please answer the following 10 questions in the same way.

In the past 7 days:

1. I have been able to laugh and see the funny side of things
   As much as I always could
   Not quite so much now
   Definitely not so much now
   Not at all

2. I have looked forward with enjoyment to things
   As much as I ever did
   Rather less than I used to
   Definitely less than I used to
   Hardly at all

*3. I have blamed myself unnecessarily when things went wrong
   Yes, most of the time
   Yes, some of the time
   Not very often
   No, never

4. I have been anxious or worried for no good reason
   No, not at all
   Hardly ever
   Yes, sometimes
   Yes, very often

*5. I have felt scared or panicky for no good reason
   Yes, quite a lot
   Yes, sometimes
   No, not much
   No, not at all

*6. Things have been getting on top of me
   Yes, most of the time I haven't been able to cope at all
   Yes, sometimes I haven't been coping as well as usual
   No, most of the time I have coped quite well
   No, I have been coping as well as ever

*7. I have been so unhappy that I have had difficulty sleeping
   Yes, most of the time
   Yes, sometimes
   Not very often
   No, not at all

*8. I have felt sad or miserable
   Yes, most of the time
   Yes, quite often
   Not very often
   No, not at all

*9. I have been so unhappy that I have been crying
   Yes, most of the time
   Yes, quite often
   Only occasionally
   No, never

*10. The thought of harming myself has occurred to me
   Yes, quite often
   Sometimes
   Hardly ever
   Never

EDINBURGH POSTNATAL DEPRESSION SCALE (EPDS)
J.L. Cox, J.M. Holden, R. Sagovsky
From: *British Journal of Psychiatry* (1987), 150, 782–786.

The assessment of a manic patient is difficult, and the help of a *specialist will usually be required*. In the assessment of mania, the steps are those already outlined for depressive disorders. They are: (i) decide the diagnosis; (ii) assess the severity of the disorder; (iii) form an opinion about the causes; (iv) assess the patient's social resources; and (v) judge the effect on other people.

Diagnosis depends on a careful history and examination. Whenever possible, the history should be taken from relatives as well as from the patient because the patient seldom recognizes the full extent of the abnormal behaviour. Differential diagnosis has been discussed earlier in this chapter; it is important to remember that mildly disinhibited behaviour can result from intoxication with drugs or alcohol or, rarely, from frontal lobe lesions (e.g. by a cerebral neoplasm).

Severity and the degree of psychosocial dysfunction should be carefully considered because this has important implications for diagnosis (e.g. for discriminating between hypomania and mania, see p. 101) and management. For this purpose it is essential to interview another informant. Manic patients are able to exert a degree of self-control during an interview with a doctor, and then behave in a more disinhibited and grandiose way immediately afterwards. At an early stage of the disorder it is easy to be misled by patients in this way and to miss the opportunity to persuade them to enter hospital before causing difficulties for themselves, for example, through ill-judged decisions at work or unaffordable extravagance.

Usually, the *causes* of a manic disorder are largely endogenous; some cases follow physical illness, treatment by drugs (especially steroids), or operations. It is important to identify any life events that may have provoked the onset and also to identify maintaining factors.

The patient's *resources* and the *effects of the illness* on other people should be assessed along the lines already described for depressive disorders. Even for the most supportive family, it is extremely difficult to care for a manic patient at home for more than a few days unless the disorder is exceptionally mild. The patient's responsibilities in the care of dependent children or at work should always be considered carefully.

Treatment of mania

General aspects of treatment

It is important to commence treatment for a manic episode as quickly as possible because of the high likelihood of serious personal and social consequences that might follow from the errors of judgement that are characteristic of the disorder. The general practitioner will need to contact the specialist services urgently, and should commence effective drug treatment if the diagnosis is clear and the patient is agreeable. Milder manic episodes may be treated on an outpatient basis, but more severe disorders with associated loss of judgement will almost always need initial treatment as an inpatient. When the disorder is more severe, compulsory admission is likely to be needed.

Almost all patients with a manic episode will need drug treatment and, because it is important to commence this as soon as possible, many patients with a previous bipolar disorder keep a small supply of antipsychotic medication to take if they experience prodromal symptoms of mania (see below).

The clinical status should be monitored frequently. Progress is judged not only by the mental state and general behaviour, but also by the pattern of sleep and by the regaining of any weight lost during the illness. As progress continues, antipsychotic drug treatment is reduced gradually. It is important, however, not to discontinue the drug too soon, otherwise relapse may occur.

During treatment a careful watch should be kept for the appearance of depressive symptoms because transient but profound depressive mood change and depressive ideas are common among manic patients. Also, the clinical picture may change rapidly from mania to a sustained depressive disorder. In either case, suicidal ideas may appear. A sustained change to a depressive syndrome may require treatment, including the use of antidepressant drugs, which should be used cautiously to avoid precipitation of a manic relapse. Following recovery, regular follow-up is necessary to detect relapse into mania or the onset of depression. Patients should be helped to deal with or to come to terms with any precipitating causes of the episode, and with the consequences of any ill-judged actions taken during the acute illness.

Specific treatment for mania
Antipsychotic drugs

Antipsychotic drugs have an established place in the treatment of mania. The older, conventional antipsychotics are frequently used, but there is now more evidence for the effectiveness of the newer atypical antipsychotics, which are also better tolerated in the short term. An atypical antipsychotic such as olanzapine, quetiapine, or risperidone is therefore usually the first choice of treatment. Antipsychotics should generally not be used to control behaviour because the doses required for this effect are high and adverse effects are therefore more likely. A benzodiazepine such as lorazepam or diazepam should be used instead.

Lithium

Lithium is effective in mania, but less so than antipsychotic drugs, and it can be difficult to use safely in severely disturbed patients. The effect in mania may take several days to begin. Lithium is therefore used mainly in patients with milder manic episodes, especially when it is intended to continue the treatment in the long term to prevent relapse. Lithium is also used in combination with antipsychotics—caution is required when used in combination with haloperidol because extrapyramidal effects occur commonly.

Antiepileptic drugs

Valproate is effective in acute mania. It is slightly less effective than antipsychotics, but causes fewer adverse effects. Thus, it may be particularly useful in patients who are not currently taking a long-term mood stabilizer, and who have a mild manic illness without psychotic features. An advantage of valproate over lithium in the acute phase is that a high loading dose can be given, which leads to a more rapid response and shorter hospital stay. Carbamazepine is another antiepileptic drug that can be used in mania.

Electroconvulsive therapy

Although there is little evidence from randomized trials, clinical experience indicates that ECT has a powerful therapeutic effect in mania. Nevertheless, ECT is not a first-line treatment; its use is mainly in the uncommon cases when antipsychotic drugs are ineffective and the patient is so seriously disturbed that to spend time trying further medication or awaiting natural recovery is not justified.

Treatment of bipolar depression

General aspects of treatment

Depressive episodes cause more disability then manic episodes in most people with bipolar disorder. The general aspects of treatment are the same as those described above for unipolar depression, but there are important differences in both the effectiveness of treatment and the risks associated with treatment. As with the treatment of mania, the clinical status of the patient should be monitored frequently because rapid mood fluctuations are common.

Specific treatment for acute bipolar depression
Antidepressant drugs

Although there is less evidence than for unipolar depression, it appears that antidepressant drugs are reasonably effective in bipolar depression and that there are no differences in efficacy between the classes of drugs. About 5–10 per cent of patients with bipolar depression develop a manic episode following treatment with an antidepressant drug and the risk is worse with tricyclics than with SSRIs. For this reason antidepressant medication should usually be given only with the cover of an effective antimanic drug such as an antipsychotic, lithium, or valproate.

Antipsychotic drugs

There is some evidence that olanzapine, one of the atypical antipsychotic drugs, is modestly effective in bipolar depression, but is more effective when added to an SSRI.

Lithium

Lithium is less effective in depression than in mania, but it is sometimes used in less severe but recurring cases when it is used for prophylaxis after recovery from the acute episode. Also, when a depressive episode occurs in a patient who is already taking long-term lithium, one treatment option is to increase the dose of lithium.

Antiepileptic drugs

There is no good evidence that valproate or carbamazepine are effective treatments for bipolar depression. Lamotrigine, another antiepileptic, may be effective.

Electroconvulsive therapy

As in other severe or resistant depressive episodes, ECT is indicated when alternative therapies have not been effective.

Psychological treatments

Although cognitive behaviour therapy and interpersonal psychotherpy are effective in unipolar depression (see p. 111), there is very little evidence that they are effective in bipolar depression

Treatment of mixed mood episodes

Manic symptoms usually predominate over depressive symptoms in mixed states and treatment of mixed states is therefore usually the treatment of a manic episode, with antipsychotics alone or in combination with a mood stabilizer. Mood stabilizers may also be used alone. Antidepressants should not be used when manic symptoms predominate, although they may be used when depressive symptoms are prominent.

Continuation therapy

This term refers to prevention of relapse in the first few weeks and months following recovery from mania or depression (i.e. return of symptoms after initial improvement during a single episode of illness). Following resolution of **mania**, the acute phase treatment is usually continued for several weeks or months and then gradually discontinued (unless relapse prevention with the same agent is being considered, see below). Following the resolution of **bipolar depressive disorder**, it is uncertain whether antidepressants should be continued because the prolonged use of antidepressants can precipitate a manic episode.

Prevention of relapse

Bipolar disorder has a strong tendency to relapse. Following the first severe episode of mania, the risk of a serious manic relapse occurring in any year is about 10–20 per cent. The risk is greater when patients have suffered multiple previous episodes—for example, after three previous episodes, the annual risk of relapse is about 20–30 per cent.

Long-term drug treatment

Long-term drug treatment can substantially reduce the risk of relapse. There are several available treatments and the choice will depend on adverse effects and previous response to treatment. At present, the comparative efficacy of the drugs is largely unknown. *Combinations of drugs* are frequently used in practice, although there is little evidence to support this.

Lithium

Lithium reduces the risk of relapse and is more effective at preventing manic than depressive episodes. The benefits outweigh the risks of adverse events for most patients who are at least at moderate risk of relapse (those with three or more previous episodes, very severe previous episodes, or a strong family history of recurrent bipolar disorder). Because lithium treatment is associated with several adverse effects, the plasma levels should be monitored regularly (see p. 251).

Antiepileptic drugs

Valproate reduces the risk of relapse, although it is uncertain how it compares with lithium. Carbamazepine may also be useful for some patients although it is probably less effective than lithium. Lamotrigine is effective at preventing depressive relapses.

Antipsychotic drugs

Long-term treatment with antipsychotic drugs is usually reserved for patients with recurrent psychotic

---

> **BOX 8.2 CHARACTERISTIC EARLY WARNING SIGNS OF MANIC RELAPSE**
> - Reduced need for sleep
> - Increased physical activity
> - Racing thoughts
> - Elated mood
> - Irritability or rage if plans and wishes are not satisfied
> - Unrealistic plans
> - Spending recklessly

---

symptoms or for when alternative treatments have not proved effective.

Education to recognize early signs of relapse

Many patients develop characteristic **prodromal** symptoms before a relapse (see Box 8.2). These patients can be helped to recognize these symptoms and can be given an agreed plan of action to use when the prodromal signs occur. This approach can help patients avoid manic episodes but it is less certain that it helps avoid depressive episodes.

Psychological treatments

Cognitive therapy and family therapy can help prevent relapse. Cognitive therapy may work through several mechanisms:

1. Better adherence to medication due to improved understanding of the personal risks caused by the illness.

2. Early detection due to improved self-monitoring of mood.

3. Improved self-regulation of behaviour and the formulation of action plans.

Further reading

Goodwin, G. M. (2003). Evidence-based guidelines for treating bipolar disorder: recommendations from the British Association for Psychopharmacology. *Journal of Psychopharmacology* **17** (2): 149–173.

National Institute for Clinical Excellence *Depression: the management of depression in primary and secondary care.* (Draft.) www.nice.org.uk/page.aspx?o=98408.

CHAPTER 9

Schizophrenia and related disorders

Chapter contents

Diagnosis and clinical features *119*

Epidemiology *125*

Aetiology *125*

Course and prognosis *127*

Assessment and management *128*

Delusional syndromes *133*

Appendix: ICD-10 criteria for schizophrenia *135*

Schizophrenia and related disorders are characterized by psychotic symptoms such as delusions and hallucinations. There is a spectrum of severity. In **schizophrenia**, the patient suffers from psychotic symptoms and functional impairment. In **delusional disorders**, the patient experiences delusions but there is no evidence of hallucinations or any of the other symptoms characteristic of schizophrenia.

Schizophrenia can be a particularly disabling illness because of its course which, although variable, is frequently chronic and relapsing. The care of patients with schizophrenia places a considerable burden on several groups, from the patient's family through to the health and social services. General practitioners may have only a few patients with chronic schizophrenia on their lists but the severity of their problems and the needs of their families will make these patients important.

This chapter aims to provide sufficient information for the reader to be able to recognize the basic symptoms of schizophrenia and related disorders and to be aware of the main approaches to treatment.

Diagnosis and clinical features

Clinical features of schizophrenia

The clinical presentation and outcome of schizophrenia vary and schizophrenia can be a confusing illness to understand. It is best to start by considering simplified descriptions of two common presentations: (i) the acute syndrome; and (ii) the chronic syndrome. It is then easier to understand the core features as well as the diversity of schizophrenia.

The acute syndrome (positive symptoms)

The main clinical features of the acute syndrome (Table 9.1) can be illustrated by a short case study of a patient, which illustrates the following common features of acute schizophrenia (Case study 9.1).

Common features include:

* hallucinations;

* persecutory ideas;

* social withdrawal;

* impaired performance at work;

* the false idea of being referred to (a delusion of reference, see p. 7).

The term **positive syndrome** is sometimes used to refer to these features. It refers to the appearance of

---

CASE STUDY 9.1 ACUTE SCHIZOPHRENIA

A previously healthy 20-year-old male student had been behaving in an increasingly odd way. At times he appeared angry and told his friends that he was being followed by the police and secret services; at other times he was seen to be laughing to himself for no apparent reason. For several months he had spent more time on his own, apparently preoccupied with his own thoughts, and his academic work had deteriorated. When seen by the family doctor he was restless and appeared frightened. He said that he had heard voices commenting on his actions and abusing him. He also said that the police had conspired with his university teachers to harm his brain with poisonous gases and take away his thoughts, and that the police had arranged for items referring to him to be inserted into television programmes.

TABLE 9.1	The acute syndrome (positive symptoms)

Appearance and behaviour

* preoccupied, withdrawn, inactive

* restless, noisy, inconsistent

Mood

* mood change

* blunting

* incongruity

Disorders of thinking

* vagueness

* formal thought disorder

* disorders of the stream of thought

Hallucinations

* auditory

* visual

* tactile, olfactory, gustatory

Delusions

* primary

* secondary (especially persecutory)

Orientation

* normal

Attention

* impaired

Memory

* normal

Insight

* impaired

---

hallucinations and delusions in contrast to the loss of function in the chronic syndrome—the negative syndrome.

Appearance and behaviour

Many patients with acute schizophrenia appear entirely normal. Some appear awkward in their social behaviour, preoccupied and withdrawn, or otherwise odd. Others smile or laugh without obvious reason, or appear perplexed by what is happening to them. Some are restless and noisy, and a few show sudden and unexpected changes in behaviour. Others retire from company, spending much time alone in their rooms, perhaps lying immobile on the bed apparently deep in thought.

Mood

Abnormalities of mood are common. There are three main kinds:

1. **Mood change** such as depression, anxiety, irritability, or euphoria. Depressive symptoms in the acute syndrome may develop in one or more of three ways:

   * as an integral part of the disorder—caused by the same processes that cause the other symptoms such as the delusions and hallucinations;

   * as a response to insight into the nature of the illness and the problems to be faced;

   * as side effects of antipsychotic medication.

2. A reduction in the normal variations of mood, called **blunting** (or flattening) of affect. A patient with this

disorder may seem indifferent to others because of unchanging mood.

3. Emotion not in keeping with the situation, a condition known as **incongruity** of affect. A patient may, for example, laugh when told about the death of his mother.

Speech and form of thought

Speech may be difficult to follow. In the early stages, a patient's talk may be vague so that it is difficult to grasp the meaning. Later there may be more definite abnormalities (**formal thought disorder**). These abnormalities are of several kinds. Some patients have difficulty in dealing with abstract ideas (a phenomenon called **concrete thinking**), while others become preoccupied with vague pseudoscientific or mystical ideas. There is a lack of connection between the ideas expressed by the patient (**loosening of associations**). The links between ideas may be illogical, or they may wander from the original theme. In its most extreme form, loosening of association leads to totally incoherent thought and speech (**word salad**).

There may be **disorders of the stream of thought**, such as pressure of thought, poverty of thought, and thought blocking (all of which are described on p. 5).

Perception

Auditory hallucinations are among the most frequent symptoms of schizophrenia. They may be experienced as simple noises or complex sounds of voices or music. Voices may utter single words, brief phrases, or whole conversations. The voices may seem to give commands to the patient. A voice may speak the patient's thoughts aloud, either as he thinks them or immediately afterwards. Sometimes, two or more voices may seem to discuss the patient in the third person. Other voices may comment on his actions. As explained later, these last three symptoms have particular diagnostic value (see p. 123).

Visual hallucinations In schizophrenia, visual hallucinations are less frequent than auditory ones, and they seldom occur without other kinds of hallucination. A few patients experience **tactile, olfactory, gustatory**, and **somatic hallucinations**, which are often interpreted in a delusional way. For example, hallucinatory sensations in the lower abdomen may be attributed to unwanted sexual interference by a persecutor.

Abnormalities of the content of thought

Delusions occur commonly in schizophrenia. **Primary delusions** (see p. 6) occur occasionally and when present are important because they seldom occur in other disorders and are therefore of value in diagnosis. Most delusions are **secondary**, that is, they arise from a previous mental change. Delusions may be preceded by so-called **delusional mood** (see p. 7), which is seldom found in conditions other than schizophrenia, or by hallucinations. Several kinds of delusion occur. **Persecutory delusions** are common, but are not specific to schizophrenia. Less common, but of greater diagnostic value, are: **delusions of reference** (false beliefs that objects, events, or people have a special personal significance, see p. 7); **delusions of control** (the feeling of being controlled by an outside agency, see p. 8); and **delusions about the possession of thought** (the idea that thoughts are being inserted into or withdrawn from the person's mind, or 'broadcast' to other people, see p. 8).

Cognitive function

Patients with schizophrenia may have evidence of premorbid cognitive impairment and there is increasing evidence that this increases following the onset of the illness. The most severely affected neuropsychological functions appear to be executive functions (which integrate subsidiary abilities such as perception and memory), although there is little evidence for deficits specific to schizophrenia (see below).

Insight

Insight is usually impaired. Most patients do not accept that their experiences result from illness, often ascribing them instead to the malevolent actions of other people. This lack of insight is often accompanied by an unwillingness to accept treatment.

The combination of disturbed behaviour, hallucinations, and delusions is often referred to as **positive symptoms**. Schizophrenic patients do not necessarily experience all these symptoms. The clinical picture is variable, as explained later in this chapter (see pp. 123–4).

The chronic syndrome (negative symptoms)

In contrast to the 'positive' symptoms of the acute syndrome, the chronic syndrome is characterized by 'negative' symptoms (Table 9.2) of:

- underactivity;
- lack of drive;
- social withdrawal;
- emotional apathy;
- thought disorder.

The syndrome can be illustrated by a brief case study of a typical patient. This description illustrates several of the features of what is sometimes called a 'schizophrenic defect state' (Case study 9.2).

TABLE 9.2 The chronic syndrome (negative symptoms)

Lack of drive and activity
Social withdrawal
Abnormalities of behaviour
Abnormalities of movement
◆ stupor and excitement
◆ abnormal movements
◆ abnormal tonus
Speech
◆ reduced in amount
◆ evidence of thought disorder
Mood disorder
◆ blunting
◆ incongruity
◆ depression
Hallucinations
◆ especially auditory
Delusions
◆ systematized
◆ encapsulated
Orientation
◆ age disorientation
Attention
◆ normal
Memory
◆ normal
Insight
◆ variable

Impairment of volition

The most striking feature is diminished volition, that is a lack of drive and initiative. Left to himself, the patient may be inactive for long periods, or may engage in aimless and repeated activity.

Impairment of daily living skills

Social behaviour often deteriorates. Patients neglect personal hygiene and their appearance. They may withdraw from social encounters. Some behave in ways that break social conventions, for example talking intimately to strangers, shouting obscenities in public, or behaving in a sexually uninhibited manner. Some patients hoard objects, so that their surroundings become cluttered and dirty.

CASE STUDY 9.2 THE CHRONIC SYNDROME

A middle-aged man lives in a group home for psychiatric patients and attends a sheltered workshop. In both places he withdraws from company. He is usually dishevelled and unshaven, and cares for himself only when encouraged to do so by others. His social behaviour is odd and awkward. His speech is slow, and its content vague and incoherent. When questioned, he says that he is the victim of persecution by extraterrestrial beings who beam rays at him. He seldom mentions these ideas spontaneously and he shows few signs of emotion about them or about any other aspects of his life. For several years this clinical picture has changed little except for brief periods of acute symptoms, which are usually related to upsets in the ordered life of the group home.

Movement disorders

A variety of disturbances of movement occur, which are often called **catatonic**. They will be described only briefly here (they are detailed in *The Shorter Oxford Textbook of Psychiatry*). **Stupor** and **excitement** are the most striking catatonic symptoms. A patient in stupor is immobile, mute, and unresponsive, although fully conscious. Stupor may change (sometimes quickly) to a state of uncontrolled motor activity and excitement.

Patients with chronic schizophrenia sometimes make repeated odd and awkward movements. Repeated movements that **do not** appear to be goal directed are called **stereotypies**; repeated movements that **do** appear to be goal directed are called **mannerisms**. Occasionally, patients have a disorder of muscle tone that can be detected by placing the patient in an awkward posture; when the sign is present, the patient maintains this posture without apparent distress for much longer than a healthy person could without severe discomfort (**waxy flexibility**). When catatonic symptoms are prominent the illness is referred to as **catatonic schizophrenia**.

Speech and form of thought

Speech is often abnormal, reflecting thought disorders of the same kinds as those found in the acute syndrome (see above).

Affect and perception

Affect is generally blunted, and when emotion is shown, it may be incongruous. **Hallucinations** are common, and any of the forms occurring in the acute syndrome may occur in the chronic syndrome.

Thought content

In chronic schizophrenia **delusions** are common and often systematized. They may be held with little emotion. For example, patients may be convinced that they are being persecuted but show neither fear nor anger. Delusions may also be 'encapsulated' from the rest of the patient's beliefs. Thus, a patient may be convinced that his private sexual fantasies and practices are widely discussed by strangers; but his remaining beliefs are not influenced by this conviction, nor is his work or social life affected.

Cognitive function

It is now recognized that people with schizophrenia frequently suffer from a variety of cognitive impairments and that these impairments are associated with important aspects of functional outcome, such as the acquisition of social skills and the chances of successful employment. Many areas of cognitive functioning appear to be affected, the best established are deficits in learning and secondary memory, attention, and executive functioning. Verbal fluency and motor functioning also appear to be affected, although to a lesser extent.

Insight

Insight is often impaired; the patient does not recognize that his symptoms are due to illness and is seldom fully convinced of the need for treatment.

Factors modifying the clinical features

In schizophrenia several factors can interact with the disease process to modify the clinical picture.

Age of onset

The symptoms of adolescents and young adults often include thought disorder, mood disturbance, and disrupted behaviour. With increasing age, paranoid symptoms are more common, and disrupted behaviour is less frequent.

Gender

The course of the illness is generally more severe in males.

Sociocultural background

Sociocultural factors may affect the content of delusions and hallucinations. For example, delusions with a religious content are more common among patients from a religious background. Recent technological innovations are often used to explain symptoms. For example, a patient may think that his auditory hallucinations are due to nanotechnology.

Social stimulation The amount of social stimulation has a considerable effect on the type of symptoms.

Understimulation increases 'negative' symptoms such as poverty of speech, social withdrawal, apathy, and lack of drive, and also catatonic symptoms. *Overstimulation* induces 'positive' symptoms such as hallucinations, delusions, and restlessness. Modern treatment is designed to avoid understimulation; as a result 'negative' features including catatonia are less frequent than in the past. This policy can, however, result in a degree of overstimulation leading to more positive symptoms.

High emotional expression by people with whom the patient is living is one form of social stimulation that increases symptoms. Overt expressions of criticism seem to be particularly important. The more time the patient spends in the company of highly critical people, the more likely he is to relapse. This is a reason why some patients are less disturbed when living in a hostel than with their family.

Diagnosis

The diagnosis of schizophrenia is based entirely on the clinical presentation (history and examination). The only diagnostic tests used are those needed to exclude other disorders when there is clinical suspicion. Because the diagnosis is based on clinical findings, it is made more reliable when *diagnostic criteria* are used to specify patterns of symptoms that must be present to make the diagnosis. The currently most widely used diagnostic criteria are those in the International Classification of Diseases, version 10 (ICD-10) (see Appendix 9.1) and the Diagnostic and Statistical Manual of the American Psychiatric Association, version IV (DSM-IV). Currrent diagnostic criteria for schizophrenia include the following:

1. Individual symptoms that have been found to be highly specific for schizophrenia and therefore have a high *positive predictive value*. These are called **Schneider's 'first rank' symptoms** after the clinician who first described them (Table 9.3, and described more fully in Chapter 1). They occur in about 70 per cent of patients who meet the full diagnostic criteria for schizophrenia.

2. Symptoms that are more frequent but less discriminating than first rank symptoms (e.g. prominent hallucinations, loosening of association, and flat or inappropriate affect).

3. Impaired social and occupational functioning.

4. A minimum duration (6 months in DSM-IV but, unfortunately, a different period—1 month—in ICD-10).

TABLE 9.3 Schneider's 'first rank' symptoms of schizophrenia*
◆ Hearing thoughts spoken aloud
◆ 'Third person' hallucinations
◆ Hallucinations in the form of a commentary
◆ Somatic hallucinations
◆ Thought withdrawal or insertion
◆ Thought broadcasting
◆ Delusional perception
◆ Feelings or actions experienced as made or influenced by external agents
*The terms used in this list are explained in Chapter 1.

5. The exclusion of: (i) organic mental disorder; (ii) major depression; (iii) mania; or (iv) the prolongation of autistic disorder (which is a mental disorder of childhood, see pp. 291–3).

Classification of psychotic disorders that do not meet the diagnostic criteria for schizophrenia

Both ICD-10 and DSM-IV provide categories for disorders that resemble schizophrenia but fail to meet the diagnostic criteria for schizophrenia in one of the following three ways:

1. *Duration too short.* Cases lasting for less than 1 month are called acute psychotic disorders in both classifications. DSM-IV has an extra category for cases lasting less than the 6 months required in this classification for the diagnosis of schizophrenia. These cases are called **schizophreniform**. (Since ICD-10 requires a duration of only 1 month, it does not require this extra category.)

2. *Prominent affective symptoms.* These cases are called **schizoaffective** in both classifications (see p. 125).

3. *Delusions without other symptoms of schizophrenia.* These are called **delusional disorders** (in ICD-10 the term is persistent delusional disorder). Delusional disorder is described later in the chapter.

Differential diagnosis

Schizophrenia needs to be distinguished from four other types of disorder: (i) organic syndromes; (ii) psychotic mood disorder; (iii) personality disorder; and (iv) schizoaffective disorder.

Organic syndromes

In *younger patients* the most relevant organic diagnoses are:

◆ **Drug-induced states**. These states can result from the use *drugs of abuse*, especially amphetamines (see p. 201), but also phencyclidine, cocaine, ecstasy, and LSD. Cannabis intoxication may cause perceptual distortions but rarely frank psychosis. Cannabis may, however, precipitate relapse in patients with established schizophrenia. Many *prescribed drugs* can rarely cause psychotic reactions, but steroids and the dopamine agonists used in the treatment of Parkinson's disease are probably the most commonly implicated drugs.

◆ **Temporal lobe epilepsy** should be considered when the condition is brief and there is evidence of clouding of consciousness. (In a few patients, chronic temporal lobe epilepsy gives rise to a persistent state resembling schizophrenia more closely.)

In *older patients*, the organic brain diseases that should be excluded include:

◆ **Delirium**. This can be mistaken for an acute episode of schizophrenia, especially when there are prominent hallucinations and delusions. The cardinal feature of this disorder is clouding of consciousness (see pp. 219–20).

◆ **Dementia** can resemble schizophrenia, particularly when there are prominent persecutory delusions. The finding of memory disorder suggests dementia.

◆ Some other **diffuse brain diseases** can present a schizophrenia-like picture without any neurological signs or gross memory impairment; for example, *general paralysis of the insane*, a form of neurosyphilis.

To exclude organic disorders, the history taking and mental state examination should focus on cognitive impairment (including disorientation and memory deficit), which tends to be more severe in organic disorder than in schizophrenia. A thorough physical examination should be done, including a neurological examination.

Psychotic mood disorder

The distinction between mood disorder and schizophrenia depends on three main factors:

1. The degree and persistence of the mood disorder.

2. The congruence of any hallucinations or delusions to the prevailing mood.

3. The nature of the symptoms in any previous episodes (if previous episodes were predominantly mood, then current mood disorder is more likely).

Sometimes, mood and schizophrenic symptoms are so equally balanced that it is not possible to decide whether the primary disorder is affective or schizophrenic. As explained above these cases are diagnosed as **schizoaffective** disorder (see below).

Personality disorders

Differential diagnosis from personality disorder may be difficult, especially when there have been insidious changes of behaviour in a young person who does not describe hallucinations or delusions. As well as interviewing relatives, it may be necessary to make prolonged observations for first rank and other features of schizophrenia before a definite diagnosis can be reached.

Schizoaffective disorder

Some patients simultaneously have definite schizophrenic symptoms and definitive affective (depressive or manic) symptoms of equal prominence. These disorders are classified separately because it is uncertain whether they are a subtype of schizophrenia or of affective disorder. Schizoaffective disorders may require both antipsychotic and antidepressant or mood stabilizing drug treatment. When patients recover, the affective and schizophrenic symptoms improve together, and most patients lose all their symptoms, although many have further episodes. Some of these subsequent episodes are schizoaffective, but others have a more typical schizophrenic or a more typical affective form.

Epidemiology

Incidence

The annual incidence of schizophrenia is between 10 and 20 per 100 000 of the population. In men, schizophrenia usually begins between the ages of 15 and 35 years. In women, the mean age of onset of the disorder is later (Fig. 9.1). Although the incidence of schizophrenia is similar worldwide, it may be higher in certain ethnic groups (e.g. Afro-Caribbean immigrants in the UK).

Prevalence

The *point prevalence* of schizophrenia is about 4 per 1000 (much higher than the incidence because the disorder is chronic). The *lifetime risk* of developing schizophrenia is about 10 per 1000. The prevalence of schizophrenia is higher in socioeconomically deprived areas: in people who are homeless, the prevalence is 100 per 1000.

The general practitioner with an average list of 2000 may expect to have about eight patients with schizophrenia. An inner city doctor, with a large homeless population, may have considerably more cases (50–100). Although the numbers are usually small, the needs of these patients for medical care are great.

Aetiology

The aetiology of schizophrenia is uncertain, although there is evidence for several risk factors (Table 9.4). There is strong evidence for genetic causes, and good reason to believe that stressful life events may provoke the disorder. Structural changes have been found in the brains of some schizophrenic patients, particularly in the temporal lobes, but it is not yet certain how they are caused. These and some other aetiological factors will be discussed briefly; a longer account can be found in *The Shorter Oxford Textbook of Psychiatry*.

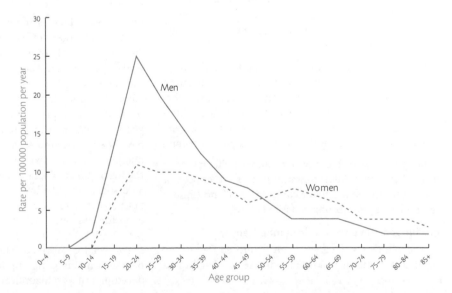

Fig. 9.1 Age- and sex-specific incidence rates for schizophrenia in men and women. (From Information and Statistics Division, NHS in Scotland, 1993.)

TABLE 9.4	Risk factors for schizophrenia	
	Risk factors	Relative risk of developing schizophrenia (%)
Predisposing		
Genetic	Monozygotic twin of a schizophrenic patient	40
	Dizygotic twin of a schizophrenic patient	15
	Child of a schizophrenic patient	10–15
	Sibling of a schizophrenic patient	10–15
Environmental	Abnormalities of pregnancy and delivery	2
	Maternal influenza (second trimester)	2
	Fetal malnutrition	2
	Winter birth	1.1
Precipitating	Chronic cannabis consumption	2

Genetic factors

There is strong evidence for the heritability of schizophrenia from three sources:

1. **Family studies** have shown that schizophrenia is more common in the relatives of schizophrenic patients than in the general population (where the lifetime risk is approximately 1 per cent). The risk is 10–15 per cent in the siblings of schizophrenics; among the children of one schizophrenic parent, 10–15 per cent; and among the children of two schizophrenic parents, about 40 per cent.

2. **Twin studies** indicate that a major part of this familial loading is likely to be due to genetic rather than to environmental factors. Among monozygotic twins, the concordance rate (the frequency of schizophrenia in the sibling of the affected twin) is consistently higher (about 40 per cent) than among dizygotic twins (about 10–15 per cent).

3. **Adoption studies** confirm the importance of genetic factors. Among children who have been separated from a schizophrenic parent at birth and brought up by non-schizophrenic adoptive parents, the likelihood of developing schizophrenia is no less than that among children brought up by their own schizophrenic parent.

Although twin studies point to genetic factors, they also indicate that environmental factors are important because, even among identical twins, half the siblings do not develop schizophrenia (see below).

Specific genes and the mode of inheritance

No specific genes have yet been identified for schizophrenia. It remains unknown whether schizophrenia is:

- monogenic (i.e. caused by a single gene);
- polygenic (i.e. caused by the cumulative effect of several genes); or
- heterogeneous (i.e. schizophrenia could be not one disorder but several, each caused by a different gene or genes).

With advances in molecular genetics, it is hoped that the gene(s) for schizophrenia will be identified in the next decade.

Environmental factors

These can predispose to the development of schizophrenia, precipitate the onset, provoke relapse after initial recovery, and maintain the disorder in persisting cases.

Predisposing factors Some factors putatively implicated in the development of schizophrenia are summarized in Table 9.4. The role of most of the environmental factors remains uncertain. Abnormalities of pregnancy (bleeding, diabetes, rhesus incompatibility, pre-eclampia), labour (uterine atony, asphyxia, emergency Caesarean section), and fetal development (low birth weight, congenital malformations, reduced head circumference) have been associated with increased risk of schizophrenia, although the size of the association is small and the mechanism of action remains obscure. There is also an association with low *social class* and this is probably both cause and effect: social deprivation increases exposure to several risk factors and it is likely that people who develop schizophrenia tend to become increasingly socially deprived. There is some evidence that heavy cannabis consumption is associated with the development of schizophrenia.

Precipitating factors of schizophrenia include stressful life events occurring shortly before the onset of the disorder.

Maintaining factors include strongly expressed feelings, especially in the form of critical comments, among family members ('high emotional expression'). High expressed emotion may lead to increased relapse rates and can be modified by family therapy.

Finally, it has been suggested that inconsistent forms of **child rearing** predispose to schizophrenia, but this is not supported by evidence. Such speculations have caused unjustified guilt in some parents.

Pathophysiology

The response of some schizophrenic symptoms to antipsychotic drugs suggests that they may have a biochemical basis. A disorder of dopaminergic function is implied by the efficacy of dopamine-blocking antipsychotic drugs, but there is little direct evidence that abnormal dopaminergic transmission is the cause of schizophrenia. Furthermore, the effect of antipsychotic drugs is not specific to schizophrenia; they reduce hallucinations and delusions in delirium, dementia, and severe depressive disorder.

Schizophrenia as a disorder of brain development

It is currently thought that schizophrenia is a **neurodevelopmental disorder** caused by one or more genes—possibly interacting with environmental factors. This idea is based on several pieces of evidence:

1. Evidence of brain abnormalities, particularly in the temporal lobes, has been consistently found in studies performing computerized tomography (CT) and magnetic resonance imaging (MRI) scans of patients with schizophrenia. These abnormalities do not appear to progress during the course of the disorder.

2. Patients with schizophrenia are more likely than controls to have dermatoglyphic abnormalities (sometimes associated with central nervous system developmental disorder) and separate 'soft' neurological signs.

3. Post-mortem studies have not found gliosis in the brains of schizophrenic patients. This means that it is likely that the brain abnormalities occurred early in life.

4. Subjects who subsequently develop schizophrenia are more likely than controls to have developmental problems during childhood.

Taken together, this evidence suggests a pathological process that takes place early in life and results in abnormal neurodevelopment, which is sometimes observable during childhood. This theory does not explain why the age of onset of schizophrenia is usually so much later or why the illness is often episodic.

Course and prognosis

The course of schizophrenia is variable:

- acute illness with complete recovery: 20 per cent;
- recurrent acute illness: 20 per cent;
- chronic illness starting acutely: 20 per cent;
- chronic illness starting insidiously: 20 per cent;
- suicide: 10–15 per cent.

In contrast to traditional views of a poor long-term prognosis in the majority of patients, it is now recognized that at least 30 per cent (and possibly as many as 50 per cent) of patients either recover completely or suffer minimal symptoms in the long term. This change to a more optimistic view of the prognosis is probably due to a combination of the increased recognition of milder illnesses and better treatment.

Patients with recurrent acute episodes often do not recover to the previous level after each relapse and so gradually deteriorate. The risk of **suicide** is high among young patients in the early stage of the disorder when insight is still present into the likely effect of the illness on the patient's hopes and plans.

TABLE 9.5 Factors predicting poor outcome in schizophrenia
Features of the illness
• Insidious onset
• Long first episode
• Previous psychiatric history
• Negative symptoms
• Younger age at onset
Features of the patient
• Male
• Single, separated, widowed, or divorced
• Poor psychosexual adjustment
• Poor employment record
• Social isolation
• Poor compliance

The best outcome is in disorders of acute onset following stress. Other predictors of outcome, some related to the illness, some to the ill person, are listed in Table 9.5. Although of some value, these predictors cannot be used to make a definite prediction for an individual patient. For this reason, advice to patients and relatives should be given cautiously, especially at the first episode of illness. The factors listed in Table 9.5 are those operating before or at the onset of schizophrenia. Factors acting after the onset are discussed next.

Life events

As noted above, stressful life events can precipitate relapses, and patients exposed to many life events generally have a less favourable course. In general, as explained above, an overstimulating environment increases positive symptoms, while an understimulating one increases negative symptoms. Prognosis depends in part on how far a balance can be achieved between these extremes.

Family life

In general, after discharge from hospital, schizophrenics returning to their families have a worse prognosis than those entering hostels. As explained above, relapse is especially likely in families where relatives make many critical comments, express hostility, and show signs of emotional overinvolvement. In such families the risk of relapse is greater if patients spend much time in contact with their close relatives (35 hours a week has been suggested as a cut-off point). Reducing this contact by arranging day care appears to improve prognosis and so may family therapy.

Cultural background

There is some evidence that the outcome of schizophrenia is better in less developed countries, where fewer demands are made on schizophrenics and there is greater family support, as part of a traditional, rural way of life.

Assessment and management

Whereas most patients with depressive disorders are treated in primary care, the majority of schizophrenic patients are treated mainly by the specialist psychiatric services. However, the first evidence of schizophrenia is usually detected by general practitioners. There is evidence that a delay in starting treatment may be associated with poorer outcome and it is important that general practitioners are familiar with the basic assessment and appreciate that referral for full assessment and management should be made as soon as possible. The importance of early intervention has recently led to the development of specific services that aim to engage the patient with services and effective interventions as quickly as possible after the onset of symptoms.

Assessment of non-urgent cases

Sometimes the patient asks for help with the symptoms of schizophrenia, but more often relatives or other people draw attention to problem behaviours that could be caused by schizophrenia. For example, a general practitioner may be asked to help a young person who is becoming increasingly withdrawn and showing odd behaviour, or an elderly woman who is reclusive and suspicious. In these situations, family doctors are in a good position to make an initial assessment because they will often know the family and the patient's background. The doctor should try to do the following:

◆ Obtain a good description of the patient's symptoms and behaviour. When possible this should be supplemented by information from an informant.

◆ Assess the patient's level of functional impairment. For example, is the patient still working? Is the patient having difficulties in his or her relationships?

◆ Make an assessment of the degree of risk the patient poses to himself and others (see pp. 172–5).

◆ Clearly inform the patient of the results of the assessment and try to persuade the patient to accept referral to the specialist mental health services.

◆ When the patient will not accept referral, the presentation should be discussed with a psychiatrist. Treatment can then sometimes be commenced, although it is advisable to maintain contact with a psychiatrist in case the situation deteriorates.

Assessment and management of acutely disturbed patients

Sometimes the family doctor's first encounter with a schizophrenic patient is during an episode of disturbed behaviour. This may occur when the patient is in the early stages of the disorder, or during a relapse of the established condition. If the patient has been or seems likely to become aggressive, special care should be taken. It is unwise to be alone with such a patient until an assessment of dangerousness has been made. On the other hand, the doctor is sometimes called to see a patient who is being restrained by several people.

An attempt should then be made to calm the patient and, if possible, remove the physical restraint while ensuring that helpers remain close at hand during the assessment.

Since not all overactive, aggressive, or otherwise disturbed behaviour is due to schizophrenia, the doctor's first task when assessing this problem is to make a provisional diagnosis. The main task is to exclude any acute organic disorder or non-psychotic disorder (such as personality disorder). At this stage the diagnosis between **schizophrenia** and **mania** may be difficult to make but the distinction does not affect the immediate management (Table 9.6).

If the cause of the behaviour disturbance appears to be a psychotic disorder, it is usually appropriate to refer for an urgent psychiatric opinion for assessment of the level of care required, including the need for hospital admission. Admission to hospital will depend on:

* the severity of the psychotic, mood, cognitive, or behavioural symptoms;

* the nature of the psychotic symptoms (e.g. command auditory hallucinations telling the patient to harm himself or others);

* the level of social support;

* the patient's insight into the illness and acceptance of need for treatment.

If the patient refuses admission to hospital when this is considered essential for his (or other people's) health or safety, compulsory powers for admission to hospital may be required (Box 9.1; see also pp. 320–1). Increasingly, alternatives to hospital admission, such as intensive community treatment, are being developed because

BOX 9.1 ETHICAL ISSUES OF COMPULSORY TREATMENT

Compulsory treatment is usually considered ethical when:

* the patient is suffering from a severe mental disorder and does not consider himself ill and/or will not consent to treatment;

* treatment is necessary for the health or safety of the patient or to protect others.

Ethical issues include:

* the nature of the psychiatric diagnosis; for example, in the USSR and China, political dissidents were considered mentally ill and compulsorily detained and treated;

* the balance between individual freedom and the protection of others;

* what is 'effective' treatment? Treatment may be defined vaguely as supportive care provided in hospital to prevent deterioration, or more specifically as a defined therapeutic intervention with known beneficial and adverse effects.

home treatment is often preferred by patients and their relatives (see Chapter 19).

Management of an acute episode of schizophrenia

If the diagnosis is uncertain, and if safe to do so, it may be desirable to withhold drug treatment for several days to allow the diagnosis to be clarified (Table 9.7).

TABLE 9.6 Assessment and management of acutely disturbed patients

Make a provisional diagnosis:
* acute organic disorder
* alcohol or drug intoxication or withdrawal
* personality disorder
* schizophrenia
* mania

Appropriate examination and blood and urine specimen (if patient permits)

Antipsychotic drug treatment if needed

Decide the need for admission to hospital (may require Mental Health Act powers)

TABLE 9.7 Hospital management of an acute episode of schizophrenia

Antipsychotic medication

Appropriate activities

Counselling for patient and family

Good response and good prognosis
* continue medication for 6 months, gradual return to work and social activities
* regular review and counselling

Incomplete response and or poor prognosis
* long-term medication (consider depot)
* counselling and support for family (reduce 'expressed emotion')
* assess needs for sheltered work or housing

When the diagnosis is sufficiently clear, antipsychotic medication is started. The antipsychotic effect may take 2–3 weeks to begin, but antipsychotics also have a calming effect, which may reduce the need for a separate sedative.

If the patient is very excited or abnormally aggressive, drug treatment may be needed for immediate behavioural control. A sedative benzodiazepine such as diazepam or lorazepam (see pp. 236–7) is usually used for behavioural control, often in combination with an antipsychotic. Escalating doses of antipsychotic drugs should not be used for behavioural control, because adverse effects may occur that discourage patients from continuing treatment in the long term.

Antipsychotic drug therapy

The most effective treatment for acute psychotic symptoms is antipsychotic drug therapy (see pp. 238–42). Most antipsychotic drugs have an immediate sedative effect, followed by an effect on psychotic symptoms (especially hallucinations and delusions), which may take up to 3 weeks to develop fully.

There are many antipsychotic drugs, which differ more in side effect profiles than in effectiveness. Equivalent doses of these drugs are shown in Table 9.8. These equivalents should only be used as a rough guide, and the manufacturer's instructions should be followed. Antipsychotic drugs should be started at a low dose and increased gradually. Second generation 'atypical' agents are often used because of the lower risk of extrapyramidal side effects. However, the decision about which drug is to be used should be tailored for the individual patient and take into account the patient's preference. For an acutely ill patient, effective treatment usually begins with olanzapine 10–20 mg or chlorpromazine 100 mg three times a day, or an equivalent dose of another drug. Depending on side effects, the dose can be increased if there is no response, but not above 900 mg of chlorpromazine a day. Prescribers should follow the manufacturer's literature or a work of reference.

TABLE 9.8 Commonly used antipsychotic drugs with the normal daily dose range

Conventional	'Atypical'
Haloperidol (2–30 mg)	Risperidone (4–16 mg)
Chlorpromazine (100–600 mg)	Olanzapine (5–20 mg)
Trifluoperazine (5–30 mg)	Sertindole (12–20 mg)
Sulpiride (400–800 mg)	Clozapine (100–900 mg)*

*Sometimes this is effective in schizophrenia resistant to conventional antipsychotics.

Choice of antipsychotic drug (see p. 242)

There are many antipsychotic drugs (Table 9.8), which are divided into two groups: the **conventional** (sometimes called first generation) and '**atypical**' (second generation) antipsychotics. The conventional antipsychotics include chlorpromazine and haloperidol. They have been available for many years and are effective but cause troublesome extrapyramidal side effects. The second group, the 'atypical' antipsychotics, cause fewer extrapyramidal side effects, but cause other adverse effects including weight gain. The atypicals include risperidone, olanzapine, and clozapine. Clozapine is currently the only drug that has been shown to be effective in illnesses that do not respond to adequate courses of conventional antipsychotics. The main problem with clozapine is that it causes agranulocytosis in < 1 per cent of cases which, rarely, may be fatal. The main side effects of antipsychotics are shown in Table 9.9.

TABLE 9.9   Side effects of antipsychotic drugs

Conventional antipsychotics

- Sedation, 70–80%
- Anticholinergic and antiadrenergic effects (including dry mouth, constipation, blurred vision, urinary retention, tachycardia), 10–50%
- Extrapyramidal side effects (parkinsonism, dystonia, akathisia, neuroleptic malignant syndrome), 60%
- Tardive dyskinesia, 4% per year of antipsychotic medication
- Endocrine effects: galactorrhoea and oligomenorrhoea
- Weight gain
- Sexual dysfunction
- Allergy

Atypical antipsychotics (e.g. risperidone, olanzapine)

- Sedation
- Weight gain
- Orthostatic hypotension
- Hyperglycaemia
- Sexual dysfunction

Clozapine

- Sedation
- Weight gain
- Hypersalivation
- Tachycardia
- Orthostatic hypotension
- Seizures, 3%
- Agranulocytosis, < 1%

The usual initial choice of drug is increasingly an atypical antipsychotic, although conventional drugs may still be used, especially when cost is an issue. Within either group, the drugs have different side effect profiles and these usually determine which drug is used. For example, chlorpromazine is suitable when sedation is desirable, and trifluoperazine is appropriate when sedation is not required. Extrapyramidal side effects occur frequently when conventional antipsychotic drugs are used and **anticholinergic medication** can be used to prevent the development of extrapyramidal symptoms including acute dystonic reactions, akathisia, or parkinsonism. However, the goal of all drug treatment should be to avoid the side effects by adjusting the dose of the chosen antipsychotic. If the patient fails to respond to at least two trials of adequate doses of the first-line antipsychotic given for an adequate duration, clozapine should be considered.

Effects of antipsychotics

Following the commencement of an antipsychotic, symptoms of excitement, irritability, and insomnia usually improve within a few days. Hallucinations and delusions may take longer to improve, often changing gradually over several weeks. If there is no improvement, a check should be made that the patient is taking the prescribed drugs. If not, the reason should be determined and an attempt made to ensure compliance. If the patient is taking the prescribed dose, this should be increased cautiously unless it is already at the top of the recommended range.

Other aspects of hospital treatment

The patient should not be left unoccupied to become absorbed in his symptoms, nor overstimulated since this prolongs the acute symptoms. Nurses and occupational therapists should work together to arrange a suitable programme of activity.

As well as drug treatment, psychological support and education about the illness and treatment are needed to help the patient accept the limitations imposed by the effects of the illness on his day-to-day life, and on his hopes for the future. With the patient's permission, similar counselling should be offered to the family.

Electroconvulsive therapy (ECT)

ECT is not used regularly in the treatment of schizophrenia but there are two important indications:

1. When there are severe depressive symptoms accompanying schizophrenia.
2. In the rare cases of catatonic stupor.

ECT is often rapidly effective in both these conditions. ECT may also be effective in acute episodes of schizophrenia, even without severe depression or stupor, but it is seldom used because drug treatment is simpler and equally beneficial. The main exception is a postpartum psychosis, when a rapid response is particularly important (see p. 115).

Drug-resistant symptoms

About 70 per cent of acute episode symptoms respond to antipsychotic drug treatment. Drug-resistant symptoms can be treated in two ways.

Alternative drug therapy Clozapine is the only agent that has clearly been shown to be effective in patients where symptoms are resistant to treatment with conventional antipsychotics (see p. 239). In practice, if a patient does not respond to two or more courses of different first-line agents, than clozapine should be considered.

Psychological treatment There is some evidence suggesting that cognitive therapy may reduce preoccupation with drug-resistant hallucinations and delusions.

Prevention of relapse

Preventing relapse in patients who recover fully from an acute episode

If the symptoms are well controlled on discharge from hospital, the dual aims of management are to continue to control symptoms with antipsychotic drugs, while making arrangements for daily living that protect the patient from too many stressors, and enable him to return as far as possible to his previous life. Even if the patient is free from symptoms, antipsychotic medication should be continued for 6 or more months, at a dose that does not produce intolerable adverse effects. For patients living with their families, family therapy aimed at reducing the number of critical comments, and improving the family's knowledge of the disorder can reduce the relapse rate.

Long-term treatment of patients who do not fully recover from an acute episode

The general aims of treatment are similar to those for patients who recover in hospital, but more attention has to be give to the social aspects of care.

The main approach to management is based on a systematic assessment of the patient's medical and social needs. Patients with schizophrenia who do not fully recover may have multiple social needs (e.g. housing and occupation), which are best met by a multidisciplinary team (see pp. 271–2). A **care plan** should be developed in which the problems are listed with the interventions proposed.

In caring for patients with chronic schizophrenia, an experienced community nurse is often one of the key professionals. The roles of the community nurse include:

♦ acting as the key worker responsible for coordinating the care plan;

♦ monitoring the patient's mental state;

♦ administering depot neuroleptic medication;

♦ monitoring compliance with medication and the presence of side effects;

♦ arranging or carrying out specific behavioural and psychological interventions;

♦ encouraging the education and support of the patient and his relatives;

♦ liaison with other care workers.

Drug therapy

Continuation therapy reduces the risk of relapse. Since adherence with medication is often poor, intramuscular depot injections are often used instead of oral medication. There are two main problems. First, 20 per cent of patients remain well without drugs and long-term conventional antipsychotic medication leads to persistent tardive dyskinesia in 15 per cent of subjects after 4 years of treatment. Therefore, if all patients receive continuation treatment, some will be exposed unnecessarily to the risk of developing side effects. Unfortunately, it is not possible to predict which patients will benefit from continuing drug treatment. The clinician and patient therefore need to work together to judge the benefit of continuation treatment by reducing the drugs cautiously when the patient has been free from symptoms for several months. Patients taking long-term continuation therapy should be assessed every 6 months for signs of tardive dyskinesia, weight gain, and hyperglycaemia (see pp. 239–41).

Second, although anticholinergic drugs reduce parkinsonian side effects, they may increase the likelihood of dyskinesia. They should not be prescribed routinely but only if there are extrapyramidal side effects that cannot be avoided by adjusting the dose of the antipsychotic drug.

Family therapy

Family psychoeducation aimed to reduce emotional involvement and criticism has been shown to reduce the rate of relapse in schizophrenic patients living with their families.

Treatment of associated depressive symptoms

Depressive symptoms in schizophrenia are common and may need specific treatment.

Antidepressants When depressive symptoms are severe, antidepressant medication can be given, although it is probably less effective in this situation than in depressive disorder. Antidepressants are also indicated in schizoaffective disorder.

Lithium may be beneficial for schizoaffective disorders, especially when there is a mixture of schizophrenic and manic symptoms (see pp. 248–9).

Psychosocial care and rehabilitation

The main aim of psychosocial care and rehabilitation is to reduce the long-term disability experienced by many patients with schizophrenia. In practice, psychosocial care is usually tailored to the individual patient's needs. Skill is required to arrange a care plan that is optimally stimulating but not too stressful. The approach is a general one including supportive care from community nurses and others. There is only limited evidence for the effectiveness of specific methods that include the following.

Social skills training uses a behavioural approach to help patients to improve interpersonal, self-care, and coping skills needed in normal life.

Employment training This includes a range of activities from help in developing the skills necessary to obtain and hold down a job, to the provision of sheltered employment or other occupational activities.

Cognitive remediation therapy aims to help the neuropsychological impairments that are often associated with schizophrenia and, hence, improve psychosocial functioning

Management of schizophrenia in primary care

In general, acute psychotic episodes should be dealt with by the specialist services because successful outcome often needs multidisciplinary team work and/or admission to hospital.

After the acute episode, general practitioners provide the majority of care for up to 25 per cent of schizophrenic patients. As well as requiring care for their psychiatric disorder, schizophrenic patients often have significant physical illness. There is evidence that less notice is taken of the physical problems of schizophrenics than of other patients. Also, drug regimens initiated by psychiatrists tend to be continued without regular reviews by the general practitioner.

A number of steps are needed to improve the care of schizophrenic patients in the community:

1. Hospital catchment areas should be based on primary care practices rather than administrative boundaries.

2. Psychiatrist and general practitioners should work closely together.

3. The responsibilities of the specialist and primary care teams should be defined clearly.

4. Clear and consistent advice should be provided to patients and carers about diagnosis, treatment, and prognosis.

5. The training of general practitioners and psychiatrists in the care of these patients should be linked.

Management of aggressive behaviour in patients with schizophrenia

Overactivity and disturbances of behaviour are common in schizophrenia. Violence to others, although often feared by lay persons, is uncommon, and homicide is rare. Nevertheless, the risk of violence should be assessed in all cases—it is greater when there are delusions of control, persecutory delusions, or auditory hallucinations.

Threats of violence should be taken seriously, especially if there is a history of such behaviour in the past, whether or not the patient was ill at the time. The danger usually resolves as acute symptoms are brought under control, but a few patients pose a continuing threat and require regular close supervision.

Treatment for a potentially violent patient is the same as for any other schizophrenic patient, although a compulsory order is more likely to be needed. While medication is often needed to bring disturbed behaviour under immediate control, much can be done by providing a calm, reassuring, and consistent environment in which provocation is avoided. A hospital with a special area with an adequate number of experienced staff is usually able to rely less on the use of large doses of medication.

Delusional syndromes

Delusional disorder

Delusional disorder is a chronic and unshakeable delusional system, developing insidiously in a person in middle or late life. The delusional system is encapsulated, and other mental functions are normal. The patient can often

work and maintain a reasonable social life. Disorders conforming strictly to this definition are rare; most eventually turn out to be an early stage of schizophrenia.

Specific delusional syndromes

The remaining delusional syndromes can be divided into two groups: those with special kinds of symptoms, and those occurring in particular situations. Of the first group, only pathological jealousy is described, and of the second group, only induced psychosis is described (the other conditions are described in *The Shorter Oxford Textbook of Psychiatry*).

Pathological jealousy

In pathological (or morbid) jealousy, the essential feature is an abnormal belief that the sexual partner is unfaithful. The condition is called 'pathological' because the belief, which may be an overvalued idea or a delusion, is held on inadequate grounds and is unaffected by rational argument. Jealousy is not classified as pathological because of strong feelings of jealousy or a violent response to a lover's infidelity; the condition is classified as pathological when the jealousy is based on unsound reasoning. Various other terms have been given to the syndrome, including sexual jealousy, erotic jealousy, morbid jealousy, psychotic jealousy, and the Othello syndrome.

Clinical features

Pathological jealousy is more common in men than women. The main feature is an abnormal belief in the partner's infidelity. This belief may be accompanied by other abnormal beliefs, for example, that the partner is plotting against the patient. The mood is variable and includes misery, apprehension, irritability, and anger.

Commonly, there is intensive seeking for evidence of the partner's infidelity; for example, by searching in diaries and correspondence, and by examining bed linen and underwear for signs of sexual secretions. The patient may follow the spouse about, or engage a private detective. Typically, the jealous person cross-questions the spouse incessantly. This may lead to violent quarrelling and paroxysms of rage in the patient, and sometimes to a dangerous assault or murder. The partner may become worn out and even make a false confession in an attempt at pacification.

Aetiology

Pathological jealousy may be secondary to other psychiatric disorders, including **schizophrenia**, **depressive disorder**, **alcoholism**, and **organic disorder**. Pathological jealousy can also arise from a **personality disorder**, in which the person has a pervasive sense of his own inadequacy, and a vulnerability to anything that might increase this sense of inadequacy, such as loss of status. In the face of such threats, the person may project blame on to the partner in the form of jealous accusations.

Prognosis

The prognosis is difficult to predict but is generally poor, depending on the prognosis of any underlying psychiatric disorder and of the patient's personality.

Assessment

Because of the risk of violence, the assessment of a patient with pathological jealousy should be particularly thorough, and specialist psychiatric advice is necessary. The spouse should be seen alone to allow a much more detailed account of the patient's morbid beliefs and actions than may be elicited from the patient. In general practice, the spouse may be the first person to seek help. The doctor should try to find out tactfully:

- the strength of the jealous person's belief in the partner's infidelity;

- the amount of resentment, and whether vengeful action has been contemplated;

- provoking factors for outbursts of resentment, accusation, or cross-questioning;

- the partner's response to such outbursts from the patient—an angry response may inflame the problem;

- the patient's response to the partner's behaviour;

- whether there has been any violence and, if there has, how it was inflicted and whether there was any injury.

Further points about assessment of risk are listed on pp. 172–5.

In addition to these specific enquiries, the doctor should take a *marital and sexual history* from both partners. It is also important to seek any evidence of an underlying psychiatric disorder (see Aetiology, above) as this will have important implications for treatment.

Treatment

The treatment of pathological jealousy is usually difficult, because the jealous person is usually uncooperative. Specialist advice is usually needed. If there is a primary disorder (see above), it should be treated. If no primary disorder is identified, an antipsychotic drug, such as trifluoperazine or chlorpromazine, given in the dosage used for schizophrenia, may reduce the intensity of the jealous beliefs and the emotional disturbance.

Open discussion of the problem may help by reducing emotional tension. The partner should be encouraged to behave in ways that least provoke the patient's jealousy, and avoiding arguments and aggressive responses to the patient's questions.

If there is no response to such treatment, or if the risk of violence is high from the beginning, inpatient care may be necessary for the jealous patient. The doctor should warn the spouse if there is a risk of serious violence. If treatment fails, it may be necessary to advise temporary or lasting separation to protect the spouse.

Induced psychosis (*folie à deux*)

An induced psychosis is a paranoid delusional system that develops in a healthy person who is in a close relationship with another person, usually a relative, who has an established, similar delusional system. The delusions are nearly always persecutory.

Induced psychosis is more frequent in women than in men. Before the induced psychosis appears, the person with the fixed delusional state has usually been dominant in the relationship, while the other person (who later develops the induced psychosis) has often been dependent and suggestible. Generally, the two have lived together for a long time in close intimacy, often cut off from the outside world. Once established, the condition persists until the two people are separated, when it usually improves gradually. This occurs sometimes without treatment but more often antipsychotic medication is required.

Further reading

McIntosh, A., Lawrie, S. (2003). *Schizophrenia* in *Clinical Evidence*. BMJ Publishing Group, London, UK.

McKenna, P. J. (1997). *Schizophrenia and Related Syndromes.* Psychology Press, Hove, UK.

A readable and comprehensive account of the aetiology, diagnosis, treatment, and prognosis.

National Institute for Clinical Excellence. (2002). *Schizophrenia: core interventions in the treatment and management of schizophrenia in primary and secondary care (NICE guideline). www.nice.org.uk/page.aspx?o=42461.*

Appendix 9.1 ICD-10 criteria for schizophrenia

(a) Thought echo, thought insertion or withdrawal, and thought broadcasting.

(b) Delusions of control, influence, or passivity, clearly referred to body or limb movements or specific thoughts, actions, or sensations; delusional perception.

(c) Hallucinatory voices giving a running commentary on the patient's behaviour, or discussing the patient among themselves, or other types of hallucinatory voices coming from some part of the body.

(d) Persistent delusions of other kinds that are culturally inappropriate and completely impossible, such as religious or political identity, or superhuman powers and abilities (e.g. being able to control the weather, or being in communication with aliens from another world).

(e) Persistent hallucinations in any modality, when accompanied either by fleeting or half-formed delusions without clear affective content, or by persistent overvalued ideas, or when occurring every day for weeks or months on end.

(f) Breaks or interpolations in the train of thought, resulting in incoherence or irrelevant speech, or neologisms.

(g) catatonic behaviour, such as excitement, posturing, or waxy flexibility, negativism, mutism, and stupor.

(h) 'Negative' symptoms such as marked apathy, paucity of speech, and blunting or incongruity of emotional responses, usually resulting in social withdrawal and lowering of social performance; it must be clear that these are not due to depression or neuroleptic medication.

(i) A significant and consistent change in the overall quality of some aspects of personal behaviour, manifest as loss of interest, aimlessness, idleness, a self-absorbed attitude, and social withdrawal.

Diagnostic guidelines. The normal requirement for the diagnosis of schizophrenia is that a minimum of one very clear-cut symptom (and usually two or more if less clear-cut) belonging to any one of the two groups listed as (a)–(d) above, or symptoms from at least two of the groups referred to as (e)–(h), should have been clearly present for most of the time *during a period of 1 month or more*. Conditions meeting such symptomatic requirements but of a duration of less than 1 month (whether treated or not) should be diagnosed in the first instance as acute schizophrenia-like psychotic disorder and reclassified as schizophrenia if the symptoms persist for longer periods.

Viewed retrospectively, it may be clear that a prodromal phase in which symptoms and behaviour—such as loss of interest in work, social activities, and personal appearance and hygiene, together with generalized anxiety and mild degrees of depression and preoccupation—preceded the onset of psychotic symptoms by weeks or even months. Because of the difficulty in timing onset, the 1-month duration criterion applies only to the specific symptoms listed above and not to any prodromal non-psychotic phase.

The diagnosis of schizophrenia should not be made in the presence of extensive depressive or manic symptoms, unless it is clear that schizophrenic symptoms antedated the affective disturbance. If both schizophrenic and affective symptoms develop together and are evenly balanced, the diagnosis of schizoaffective disorder should be made, even if the schizophrenic symptoms by themselves would not have justified the diagnosis of schizophrenia. Schizophrenia should not be diagnosed in the presence of overt brain disease or during states of drug intoxication or withdrawal. Similar disorders developing in the presence of epilepsy or other brain disease should be diagnosed as organic delusional (schizophrenia-like) disorder and those induced by drugs as psychotic disorder due to psychoactive substance use.

CHAPTER 10

Delirium, dementia, and other cognitive disorders

Chapter contents

Delirium *138*

Dementia *140*

Other organic psychiatric syndromes *143*

Neurological syndromes *144*

Epilepsy *146*

This chapter deals with organic psychiatric disorders; that is, psychiatric disorders resulting from brain dysfunction caused by organic pathology inside or outside the brain. It should be read in conjunction with Chapter 11 on psychiatry and medicine and Chapter 16 on psychiatry of the elderly. The former describes the general psychological impact of major physical disorders of all types; the latter describes the commonest causes of dementia in old age and of their management. Three types of clinical problem are described in this chapter.

1. Acute generalized impairment of brain function, **delirium**, in which the most important feature is impairment of consciousness. The disturbance of brain function is generalized, and the primary cause is often outside the brain, for example, anoxia due to respiratory failure.

2. Chronic generalized impairment, **dementia**, in which the main clinical feature is generalized intellectual impairment. There are also changes in mood and behaviour. The brain dysfunction is generalized, and the primary cause is within the brain, for example, a degenerative condition such as Alzheimer's disease.

3. **Specific syndromes**, which include disorders with a predominant impairment of memory only (amnesic syndrome), of thinking, or of mood, or personality change. We also describe a number of neurological disorders that frequently result in organic psychological complications, including a review of the psychiatric features of **epilepsy**.

TABLE 10.1	Classification of organic mental states
Global syndromes	
◆ Delirium	
◆ Dementia	
Specific syndromes	
◆ Amnesic syndrome	
◆ Organic mood disorder	
◆ Organic delusional state	
◆ Organic personality disorder	

TABLE 10.2	Clinical features of delirium
Impaired consciousness	
◆ disorientation	
◆ poor concentration	
Behaviour	
◆ overactive	
◆ underactive	
Thinking	
◆ muddled (confused)	
◆ ideas of reference	
◆ delusions	
Mood	
◆ anxious, irritable	
◆ depressed	
◆ perplexed	
Perception	
◆ misinterpretations	
◆ illusions	
◆ hallucinations (mainly visual)	
Memory	
◆ impaired	
Fluctuating course, worse in the evening	

Table 10.1 lists the main categories of psychiatric disorder associated with organic brain disease. The following sections describe these syndromes and the psychiatric consequences of a number of neurological conditions.

Delirium

Clinical features

Delirium is characterized by impairment of consciousness (Table 10.2). It is a common accompaniment of physical illness, occurring in about 5–15 per cent of patients in general medical or surgical wards, and about 20–30 per cent of patients in surgical intensive care units. It is especially common in the elderly (see Chapter 16). Most patients recover quickly, and only a few need specific treatment. Terms such as **confusional state** and **acute organic syndrome** are outdated and should be avoided.

Impairment of consciousness is the most important symptom and is recognized by disorientation (uncertainty about the time, place, and identity of other people) and poor concentration. The features *fluctuate in intensity* and are often *worse in the evening*.

Behaviour may be either overactive, with noisiness and irritability, or underactive. Sleep is often disturbed.

Thinking is slow and muddled but the content is often complex. Ideas of reference and delusions are usually transient and poorly elaborated.

Mood may be anxious, perplexed, irritable, or depressed and is often labile.

Perception may be distorted with misinterpretations, illusions (mainly visual), and visual hallucinations. Tactile and auditory hallucinations occur but are less frequent.

Memory Disturbance of memory affects registration, retention, and recall, as well as new learning.

Insight is impaired.

Amnesia On recovery there is usually amnesia. The features of delirium vary between patients, in part reflecting personality. There are two main patterns of presentation: (i) the patient is restless and oversensitive to stimuli, and may have hallucinations and delusions; and (ii) the patient is inactive and lethargic.

Aetiology

There are many causes of delirium the most important of which are listed in Table 10.3. It is more frequent among children and the elderly, among people with previous brain damage of any kind, and in conditions of low sensory input (such as isolation and low levels of illumination).

Management

Treatment is directed both to identifying and dealing with the underlying physical cause and with measures to treat the patient's anxiety, distress, and behavioural problems (Fig. 10.1).

TABLE 10.3	Some causes of delirium
Drug intoxication	
Alcohol withdrawal	
Metabolic failure	
◆ cardiac	
◆ respiratory	
◆ renal	
◆ hepatic	
◆ hypoglycaemia	
Fever	
◆ systemic infection	
Neurological causes	
◆ encephalitis	
◆ space-occupying lesions	
◆ raised intracranial pressure	
◆ following an epileptic seizure	

- Patients need *reassurance and reorientation* to reduce anxiety and disorientation; these should be repeated frequently.

- *Relatives should receive a clear explanation* of the nature of the disorder to relieve their own anxiety and to help them reassure and reorientate the patient.

- There should be a *predictable, consistent routine*. In a hospital ward there are advantages in nursing the patient in a quiet side room. At night there should be enough light to enable the patient to know easily where he is but not so much that sleep is disturbed. Relatives and friends should be encouraged to stay or to visit frequently.

- It is important to *give as few drugs as possible* since these may worsen the delirium.

- Small doses of a benzodiazepine or other hypnotic are useful to *promote sleep at night*. Benzodiazepines should be avoided during daytime as their sedative effects may increase disorientation.

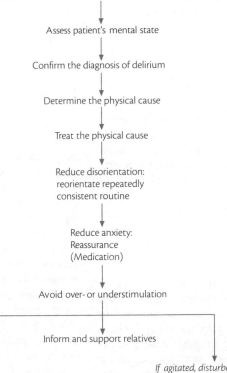

Obtain information from other informants and medical notes

↓

Assess patient's mental state

↓

Confirm the diagnosis of delirium

↓

Determine the physical cause

↓

Treat the physical cause

↓

Reduce disorientation:
reorientate repeatedly
consistent routine

↓

Reduce anxiety:
Reassurance
(Medication)

↓

Avoid over- or understimulation

↓

Inform and support relatives

If calm:
Monitor progress

If agitated, disturbed, or distressed:
Consider hypnotic at night
Consider regular medication
Monitor progress, review medication

Fig. 10.1 Treatment of delirium.

CASE STUDY 10.1 DELIRIUM

As a general hospital duty doctor you are called in the middle of the night to see a 69-year-old man who has become disturbed and distressed 3 days after major abdominal surgery. The nursing staff, who have not known the patient before, say the patient has been attempting to pull out his drip, has been shouting incoherently, and seems frightened. He has accused them of being gaolers in a prison. You look at the case notes, which contain routine medical information, but find that in the nursing notes the patient has been intermittently rather drowsy and that during the day his relatives reported that he seemed confused.
[Seek information from others and case notes]

You find it difficult to interview the patient who seems unable to concentrate on your questions and makes disconnected comments about being in prison and having been attacked by people who want to kill him. He is unable to say where he is or to tell you the date. He is bewildered and fearful. You diagnose delirium. You notice that he has pyrexia and the nurses tell you that he appears to be developing a wound infection. Consider physical treatment.
[Assess diagnosis and immediate treatment needs]

You arrange for the patient be moved to a quiet, well-lit side room. You explain to the patient that he is safe in hospital and that you will be able to help him feel better. One of the nurses takes responsibility for looking after the patient and for repeatedly reassuring him that all is well. Despite reassurance, the patient remains very agitated. Your prescribe 3 mg of haloperidol, which the patient is willing to take as syrup. You also prescribe 3 mg of haloperidol to be taken three times a day as a regular regime.
[Emphasize environmental measures; cautious use of medication for disturbed behaviour]

In the morning you review the patient who is calmer. You discuss a consistent, reassuring regime with the day nursing staff, explain to the relatives what has happened, and encourage them to spend time with the patient explaining and reassuring him about what is going on.
[Repeated explanation, involvement of relatives]

You also discuss the response of the patient and your treatment with the responsible medical team so that they are able to continue with a consistent long-term plan.
[Involve medical team in plan]

During the next few days the medical team review the patient's mental state. There is marked improvement in orientation, mood, and behaviour thus enabling a step-by-step reduction over a period of 3 days and then stopping of the regular medication.
[Review medication]

♦ When patients are particularly distressed and behaviourally disturbed, carefully monitored *antipsychotic medication* can be valuable. Following an initial dose sufficient to treat the acute situation, a regular oral dose may be given, adequate to calm the patient without causing excessive drowsiness. Haloperidol is suitable; the effective daily dose usually varies between 3 and 15 mg. If necessary, the first dose of 2–5 mg can be given intramuscularly. (See Case study 10.1.)

Dementia

Dementia is a generalized impairment of intellect, memory, and personality, without impairment of consciousness. It is an acquired disorder, as distinct from learning disability in which impairments are present from birth (see Chapter 21). Although most cases of dementia are irreversible, a small but important group are remediable. Dementia before the age of 65 is said to be presenile. Dementias of the elderly are described more fully in Chapter 16.

Clinical features

Dementia usually presents with impairment of memory. Other features include changes in behaviour, mood disorder, delusions, and hallucinations (Table 10.4). Although dementia generally develops gradually, it may come to notice after an acute deterioration caused by either a change in social circumstances or an intercurrent illness. There may also be uncharacteristic aggressive behaviour or sexual disinhibition. In a middle-aged or elderly person any social lapse that is out of character should always suggest dementia. The clinical picture depends in part on the patient's premorbid **personality**; for example, neurotic and paranoid traits may become exaggerated. People who are socially isolated or deaf are less able to compensate for failing intellectual abilities. On the other hand, a person with good social skills may maintain a social facade despite severe intellectual deterioration.

Cognitive function Disorders of cognitive function are central. *Forgetfulness* usually appears early and is promi-

TABLE 10.4	Clinical features of dementia
Cognition	
◆ poor memory	
◆ impaired attention	
◆ aphasia, agnosia, apraxia	
◆ disorientated	
Behaviour	
◆ odd and disorganized	
◆ restless, wandering	
◆ self-neglect	
◆ disinhibition	
Mood	
◆ anxiety	
◆ depression	
Thinking	
◆ slow, impoverished	
◆ delusions	
Perception	
◆ illusions	
◆ hallucinations	
Insight	
◆ impaired	

nent; difficulty in new learning is generally a conspicuous sign. *Memory loss* is more obvious for recent than for remote events. Patients often make excuses to hide these memory defects, and some confabulate. In some cases there are specific deficits of aphasia, agnosia, or apraxia. *Attention* and *concentration* are also impaired. *Disorientation* for time, and at a later stage for place and person, are almost invariable once dementia is well established (but in contrast to delirium are not usually prominent in the early stage).

Behaviour may be disorganized, restless, or inappropriate. Typically there is loss of initiative and reduction of interests. Some patients become restless and wander about by day and sometimes at night. When patients are taxed beyond their restricted abilities, there may be a sudden change to tears or anger (a '*catastrophic reaction*'). As dementia worsens patients care for themselves less well and may become disinhibited, neglecting social conventions. Behaviour becomes aimless. Eventually, the patient may become incontinent of urine and faeces.

Changes of mood In the early stages, changes of mood include anxiety, irritability, and depression. As dementia progresses emotions and responses to events become generally blunted, though there may be sudden changes of mood without apparent cause or the catastrophic reactions noted above.

Thinking slows and becomes impoverished in content. There may be difficulty in abstract thinking, reduced flexibility, and perseveration. Judgement is impaired. False ideas, often of a persecutory kind, gain ground easily and may progress to *delusions*. In the later stages, thinking becomes grossly fragmented and incoherent. Disturbed thinking is reflected in the patient's *speech*, in which syntactical errors and nominal dysphasia are common. Eventually, the patient may utter only meaningless noises or even become mute.

Perceptual disturbances (illusions and hallucinations) may develop as the condition progresses. Hallucinations are often visual.

Insight is usually lacking into the degree and nature of the disorder.

Aetiology

Dementia has many causes, of which the most important are listed in Table 10.5. Among elderly patients, degenerative disorders (notably Alzheimer's disease) and vascular causes predominate. Although these and many other causes are irreversible, when assessing a patient the clinician needs to keep in mind the whole range of causes, so as not to miss any that might be partly or wholly treatable, such as an operable cerebral neoplasm, chronic subdural haematoma, or normal pressure hydrocephalus. Table 10.6 summarizes the 'primary dementias' (i.e. diffuse diseases of the brain that can cause dementia). The first three are described in Chapter 16.

Management

Any suspicion of dementia should lead to detailed questioning about intellectual function and neurological symptoms. It is important to interview other informants, since patients are often unaware of the extent of the change in themselves. Also, details of the mode of onset and progression of symptoms may be provided more accurately by an informant. In doubtful cases, standardized procedures for assessing cognitive state may be of value, but in interpreting the results it is essential to take account of previous education and achievement. The Mini Mental State Examination (see p. 37) is used widely in assessment; it combines standard questions with tests

TABLE 10.5	Some causes of dementia

Degenerative

♦ degenerative neurological disorders causing dementia (see Table 10.6) (e.g. multiple sclerosis)

Normal pressure hydrocephalus

Intracranial tumour

Other space-occupying lesions

♦ chronic subdural haematoma

Traumatic

♦ severe head injury

Infections

♦ postencephalitis, HIV

Vascular

♦ multi-infarct dementia

Toxic

♦ alcohol

Anoxia

♦ cardiac arrest

♦ carbon monoxide poisoning

Vitamin lack

♦ vitamin B_{12}

♦ folic acid

♦ thiamine

Metabolic

♦ diabetes

Endocrine

♦ hypothyroidism

of spatial ability. The aim should be to perform the minimum of investigations to reveal the cause of the disorder, whether acute or chronic.

Computerized tomography is valuable in the diagnosis of both focal and diffuse cerebral pathology. It should be requested if there is any suspicion of organic brain disease in patients up to late middle age, or if there is any suggestion of a focal brain lesion in the elderly.

Psychological testing Specific tests of memory, learning, and other aspects of cognitive function are sometimes used by specialists to identify and quantify patients with localized brain lesions. A commonly used basic test is the *Wechsler Adult Intelligence Scale* (WAIS), which is a well-standardized test providing a profile of verbal and non-verbal abilities. It should be given by a trained tester. Organic impairment is suggested by a discrepancy between performance IQ (as an estimate of current capacity) and verbal IQ (as an estimate of previous capacity).

Aspects of differential diagnosis

Organic or functional?

It is sometimes difficult to distinguish between functional and organic psychiatric disorder, especially when an organic disorder presents with disturbances of behaviour and thinking in the absence of obvious neurological symptoms or signs. In **affective disorder** and **schizophrenia** there may be an impression of impairment of cognitive functions.

Pseudodementia

A common diagnostic problem is presented by so-called depressive pseudodementia. In this syndrome, a de-

TABLE 10.6	Degenerative neurological diseases causing dementia
Alzheimer's disease	See Chapter 16
Vascular dementia	See Chapter 16
Lewy body dementia	See Chapter 16
Frontotemporal dementias	A group of dementias (including Pick's disease) that are the second most common cause of primay dementia before old age; behavioural changes are often early
Huntington's chorea	A rare degenerative disorder, which is autosomal dominant. The pathological changes affect mainly the frontal lobes and caudate nucleus. There are choreiform movements of the face, hands, and shoulders, dysarthria, and abnormal gait. Dementia usually follows these neurological signs but may precede them. Occasionally there are persecutory delusions. A predictive test using a polymorphic DNA marker is available for members of affected families
Prion disease	A group of disorders (including Creutzfeld–Jacob disease) that cause dementia and a variety of neurological signs
Parkinson's disease	Cognitive impairment occurs in a minority of cases. It is related to the severity and duration of the disease

pressed patient complains of poor memory and appears intellectually impaired because poor concentration leads to inadequate registration and depressive mood leads to slowness and self-neglect. Characteristic features are:

◆ a history from another informant that the depressed mood preceded the memory problems;

◆ memory testing shows that the poor performance improves when interest is aroused;

◆ the patient is retarded and unwilling to cooperate in the interview; by contrast, patients with dementia are usually willing to reply to questions but make mistakes.

Conversely, *an organic disorder can present with mood disorder or behaviour change* that suggests a functional disorder. The points in favour of an organic cause are:

◆ the cognitive disorder preceded the mood or other disorder;

◆ cognitive defects occur in specific areas of intellectual function;

◆ neurological signs;

◆ the presence of symptoms seldom found in non-organic disorder, such as visual hallucinations.

It is important to consider a possible organic cause in every case of acute psychological or behavioural disturbance, especially when there are atypical features. The diagnosis of functional disorder is partly by exclusion of organic causes but also by the finding of positive evidence of psychological aetiology since organic causes may be undetectable in the early stages of disease.

Delirium or dementia?

Delirium is an acute reversible condition; dementia is a chronic disorder. As shown in Table 10.7, delirium is cha-

TABLE 10.7 Features of delirium versus dementia

Delirium	Dementia
Acute onset	Insidious onset
Fluctuating course	Stable or progressive*
Impaired consciousness	Normal consciousness
Thinking disorganized	Thinking impoverished
Perceptual disturbance common	Perceptual disturbance uncommon
Alertness usually impaired	Normally alert

*Except multi-infarct dementia.

racterized by an acute onset, fluctuating course, impaired consciousness, and disorganized thinking. Also, perceptual disturbance is more frequent and alertness more often impaired in delirium. Especially in the elderly, the two syndromes may occur together; when this happens the underlying dementia may be overlooked or the delirium may not be detected or treated. Sometimes a longstanding dementia becomes apparent only after successful treatment of a more recent delirium.

Stupor

Stupor is a rare condition in which the patient is immobile and unresponsive but has a normal level of consciousness. Stupor can occur in severe affective disorders (see p. 101) and schizophrenia (see p. 122). Lesions of the brainstem or mesencephalon can cause a similar clinical picture, although in these cases there may be some impairment of consciousness.

Management

The management of dementia is described more fully in Chapter 16 on the elderly. A minority of patients have a treatable cause. For the remainder, treatment aims to reduce disability and provide support. Whenever possible, care is outside the hospital, either with relatives or in residential accommodation. The aims of treatment are to:

◆ maintain any remaining ability as far as possible;

◆ relieve distressing symptoms;

◆ arrange for the practical requirements of the patient;

◆ support the family.

Other organic psychiatric syndromes

Brain pathology may give rise to several specific psychiatric syndromes as well as the generalized disorders described above. Sometimes these syndromes are associated with focal neurological signs, but the psychiatric syndrome may be the only abnormality (for example frontal and temporal syndromes).

Amnesic syndrome

The amnesic syndrome (otherwise known as the amnestic syndrome) is characterized by a prominent disorder of recent memory, in the absence of the generalized intellectual impairment observed in dementia or the impaired consciousness seen in delirium. The condition usually results from lesions in the posterior hypothalamus and nearby midline structures, but occasionally results from bilateral hippocampal lesions. It is

TABLE 10.8	Clinical features of amnesic syndrome

- Recent memory severely impaired
- Remote memory spared
- Disorientation in time
- Confabulation
- Other cognitive functions preserved

often described as **Korsakov's syndrome** after the Russian neurologist who first described the clinical features, or as the **Wernicke–Korsakov syndrome** because the amnesic syndrome may accompany an acute neurological syndrome described by Wernicke (**Wernicke's encephalopathy**) characterized by impairment of consciousness, memory defect, disorientation, ataxia, and opthalmoplegia.

Alcohol abuse is the most frequent cause, and seems to act by causing a deficiency of thiamine. Other causes include carbon monoxide poisoning, vascular lesions, encephalitis, and tumours of the third ventricle.

Clinical features

The central feature of the amnesic syndrome is a profound *impairment of recent memory* (Table 10.8). The patient can recall events immediately after they have occurred, but cannot do so even a few minutes afterwards. Thus, on the standard clinical test of remembering an address, immediate recall is good but grossly impaired ten minutes later. One consequence of the profound disorder of memory is an associated *disorientation in time*. Gaps in memory are often filled by *confabulation*. The patient may give a vivid and detailed account of recent activities that, on checking, turn out to be inaccurate. It is as though he cannot distinguish between true memories and the products of his imagination or recollection of events from times other than those he is trying to recall. Such a patient is often suggestible; in response to a few cues from the interviewer, he may give an elaborate account of taking part in events that never happened.

Other cognitive functions, including remote memory, are relatively well preserved. Unlike the patient with dementia, the patient with an amnesic syndrome seems alert and able to reason or hold an ordinary conversation, so that the interviewer may at first be unaware of the extent of the memory disorder.

Treatment

For cases that may be due to **thiamine deficiency**, this vitamin should be prescribed in the hope of limiting

further damage. Otherwise, there is no specific treatment and the general measures are those described above for dementia.

Course and prognosis

The course is chronic. Prognosis is better when the condition is due to thiamine deficiency, provided that thiamine treatment was started promptly. If the cause continues to act (e.g. excessive drinking that persists), the amnesia may worsen.

Organic personality disorder

Brain damage may result in **personality change** and this may be severe enough to be classified as **personality disorder**. An example is the distinctive syndrome associated with **frontal lobe damage** in which behaviour is disinhibited, overfamiliar, and tactless. Patients may be overtalkative, make inappropriate jokes, and engage in pranks. They may make errors of judgement and commit sexual indiscretions, and disregard the feelings of others. The *mood* is generally fatuous euphoria. *Concentration* and *attention* may be reduced. Measures of formal intelligence are generally unimpaired, but special testing may show deficits in abstract reasoning. *Insight* is impaired.

Organic mood disorders

Some neurological diseases (e.g. multiple sclerosis) are direct causes of mood disturbance, which may include depression, mania, or anxiety. Some endocrine disorders, for example Cushing's disease, can have the same effect. It is difficult to distinguish such disorders from emotional disorders that are a normal psychological response to physical illness, or from chance associations between mood disorder and physical disease.

Organic delusional disorder

Occasionally, brain pathology, particularly that associated with temporal lobe epilepsy, causes a delusional disorder resembling schizophrenia.

Neurological syndromes

Normal pressure hydrocephalus

In this variety of hydrocephalus there is no block within the ventricular system. Instead, there is an obstruction in the subarachnoid space.

The characteristic features are progressive memory impairment, slowness, marked unsteadiness of gait, and in the later stages, urinary incontinence. Treatment is a shunt operation to improve the circulation of cerebrospinal fluid. This procedure arrests the condition and sometimes the dementia improves. It is important to differentiate this treatable condition from the primary dementias, as well as from depressive disorder with mental slowness.

Head injury

Major head injury has both immediate effects and longer term neuropsychiatric consequences such as dementia or personality change. Some more minor head injuries cause less obvious cognitive impairments that may significantly impair functioning and behaviour for many months after the injury. Patients returning to demanding occupations or activities or who complain of difficulties following head injury require full neurological review.

Repeated minor blows to the head, such as occur in *boxing*, can lead to progressive deterioration in intellectual function. Since the clinical changes are insidious, it is important to obtain information from other informants about how current intellectual function compares with previous function and achievements. Specialist psychological assessment can be helpful.

The acute psychological effects of head injury include:

◆ *impairment of consciousness*: this occurs after all but the mildest closed head injuries;

◆ *delirium* often lasting for days or weeks after severe head injury;

◆ *post-traumatic amnesia of more than 24 hours*: this is likely to be followed by persisting cognitive impairment. Improvement usually takes place slowly over months or even years. The impairment is usually global but, after a localized injury, there may be only focal cognitive deficits affecting specific aspects of intellectual function.

Personality change is often the most serious long-term complication after severe head injury, particularly after damage to the frontal lobe. There may be irritability, loss of spontaneity and drive, some coarsening of behaviour, and occasionally reduced control of aggressive impulses. These changes often cause serious difficulties for the patient and his family.

Emotional symptoms may follow any kind of injury. Depression is frequent in those with severe physical disability following the accident. Whatever the severity of the injury, there may also be a combination of anxiety, depression, and irritability, with headache, dizziness, fatigue, poor concentration, and insomnia. This *post-*

concussional syndrome is probably due to an interaction of minor brain damage with anxiety and depression.

Assessment and management

A plan for long-term treatment should be made as early as possible after head injury. Three aspects of the problem should be assessed:

1. Neurological signs and the degree of physical disability.

2. Any neuropsychiatric problems and their likely future course.

3. Social circumstances, social support, the possibility of return to work, and the effect of the injury on the patient's responsibilities in the family.

Specialist rehabilitation should include not only physiotherapy and graded increase in physical activity, but work with the patient and family to try and minimize disabilities in everyday life and to find ways of dealing with specific cognitive deficits such as impaired memory.

Cerebrovascular disease

Among people who survive a cerebrovascular accident, about half return to a fully independent life. The rest may have psychological as well as physical problems. The psychological changes are often the more significant, preventing a return to a normal life when the physical disability has ceased to be a serious obstacle.

Cognitive defects Stroke can cause dementia as well as specific deficits of higher cortical function, such as dysphasia and dyspraxia, which may handicap the patient to a degree that is underestimated by doctors. If the stroke is repeated the dementia may progress. (The separate condition of *vascular dementia* is described on p. 222.)

Personality change Irritability, apathy, or lability of mood may occur after a cerebrovascular accident. Difficulties in coping with everyday problems is common and failure may result in a 'catastrophic reaction'. Such changes are probably due more to associated widespread arteriosclerotic vascular disease than to a single stroke, and they may continue to worsen even though the focal signs of the stroke are improving.

Depressed mood is common after a stroke. It is partly a psychological reaction to the handicap caused by the stroke but may, in part, be a direct consequence of any localized brain damage. It may contribute to the apparent intellectual impairment and is often an important obstacle to rehabilitation.

Lability of mood is frequent and may be a significant clinical problem.

Even though biological factors may contribute to aetiology, depressed mood should be treated with anti-depressant medication. Lability of mood is also frequently helped by antidepressant treatment. Practical help is frequently required by both the patient and carers.

Cerebral tumours

Many cerebral tumours cause psychological symptoms at some stage, and in a significant minority these symptoms are the first to appear. Fast growing tumours are more likely to cause a delirium, especially if there is raised intracranial pressure; slow growing tumours are more likely to present with dementia or, occasionally, depressive symptoms.

Transient global amnesia

This syndrome is an occasional but important cause of episodes of unusual behaviour, which may present as emergencies to general practitioners and casualty officers. Doctors who are not familiar with the syndrome may misdiagnose it as a dissociative disorder (see p. 94).

The condition occurs in middle or late life. There are abrupt episodes, lasting several hours, of global loss of recent memory. The patient apparently remains alert and responsive but usually appears bewildered by his inability to understand his experience. There is complete recovery, except for amnesia for the episode. The cause is unknown and there is no specific treatment.

Multiple sclerosis

Psychological symptoms occur early in the disorder, and may rarely be the presenting feature. In the established disease, *depression* and *elation* may occur, and these are sometimes severe enough to require psychiatric treatment.

Occasionally, a *rapidly progressive dementia* occurs early in the disease. In most cases, however, intellectual deterioration occurs later, is less severe, and progresses slowly. In the late stages of the disease *dementia* is common.

Epilepsy

People with epilepsy suffer from the misconceptions and prejudices of other people about epilepsy as well as from the condition itself. Such problems arise in school and, later, at work and also within the family. In caring for people with epilepsy the general practitioner should try to reduce these misunderstandings, and to

TABLE 10.9 Associations between epilepsy and psychological problems of epileptic individuals
Effects of stigma and social restrictions
Psychiatric disorder due to the cause of epilepsy
Behavioural disturbance associated with the seizure
◆ Before: tension, irritability, depression
◆ During: complex partial seizures
◆ After: automatism (rarely)
Disorders between seizures
◆ Cognitive impairment
◆ Personality disorder
◆ Paranoid disorder
◆ Sexual dysfunction
◆ Increased self-harm and suicide

support the patient and the family. Restriction of the driving of motor vehicles by epileptic individuals further limits their activities.

There are several ways in which epilepsy predisposes to psychiatric disturbance (Table 10.9).

Psychiatric disorder associated with the cause of epilepsy

When epilepsy is a consequence of brain damage, this damage may also cause intellectual impairment or personality problems.

Behavioural disturbance associated with the seizure

Before a seizure there may be a period of increasing tension, irritability, and depression lasting for hours or sometimes a few days.

During seizures of the complex partial type there may be automatic behaviour of a complicated kind. Occasionally, such seizures are prolonged for days as 'complex partial status', in which there may be an abnormal mental state, abnormal behaviour, or social withdrawal.

After the seizure there may occasionally be a prolonged period of abnormal behaviour and impaired awareness—'automatism'.

Psychiatric disorder occurring between seizures

Cognitive dysfunction The drugs used to treat epilepsy may cause impaired attention. In some patients, there is persistent abnormal electrical activity in the brain between seizures, and this activity can be associated with poor attention and memory. (For both reasons, learning problems are more common in children with epilepsy than in non-epileptic children.)

Personality Most people with epilepsy are of normal personality. When personality disorder does occur, it is not of any single kind. The causes are multiple: social limitations imposed on the epileptic person during childhood and adolescence, self-consciousness, and the reactions of other people. In cases where brain damage has caused the epilepsy, the former may contribute to the personality disorder.

Psychosis Affective disorder may be more common in people with epilepsy than in the general population.

Sexual dysfunction This problem is more common in epileptics than in non-epileptics. The causes include difficult relationships and the effects of antiepileptic medication. There may also be neurophysiological causes in some cases since sexual problems are more common with temporal lobe epilepsy than with other kinds.

Suicide and deliberate self-harm Among people with epilepsy suicide is four times more frequent, and deliberate self-harm is six times more frequent, than in the general population.

Further reading

Lishman, W. A. (1998). *Organic Psychiatry*. Blackwells, Oxford.
Although some detail is outdated, it remains the standard reference work.

CHAPTER 11

Psychiatry and medicine

Chapter contents

Epidemiology *149*

Psychological factors as causes of physical disorders *151*

Psychological complications of physical disorders *151*

Some practical problems *154*

Psychiatric services for a general hospital *155*

Some examples of psychiatric aspects of physical disorders *156*

Psychiatric aspects of obstetrics and gynaecology *156*

Physical and psychological symptoms commonly occur together and interact. Also, many psychiatric disorders cause physical symptoms, while physical symptoms and disease have psychological consequences, which include psychiatric disorder. An understanding of the psychological aspects of general medical care is important for these reasons and because:

◆ psychological factors may increase disability associated with physical illness;

◆ a psychiatric disorder may respond to treatment;

◆ untreated psychological problems may lead to the inappropriate use of medical resources and to poor compliance with medical advice.

Epidemiology

In the *general population* psychiatric disorder is two to three times more likely when physical ill health is present (Fig. 11.1). Also, disabling functional symptoms (see Chapter 7) are frequent.

In *primary care*, psychological issues are important in the management of many patients with serious acute or chronic physical illness. Functional physical symptoms are among the commonest reasons for seeking treatment and are often due to psychiatric disorder.

In *hospital practice*, psychological problems are especially frequent in accident and emergency departments, gynaecological and medical outpatient clinics, wards for the elderly, and a number of specialist units.

About a quarter of patients in medical wards (Fig. 11.2) have a psychiatric disorder of some kind.

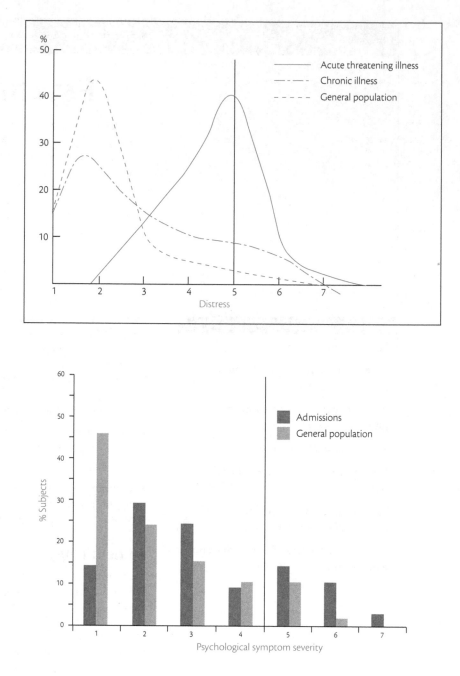

Fig. 11.1 The distribution of emotional distress in the general population and in those with physical illness. Level 5 and over indicates a diagnostic psychiatric disorder

Fig. 11.2 Frequency of psychological symptoms in consecutive women admissions to a general hospital as compared with a general population. Scores of 5 and above to the right of the vertical line indicate psychiatric disorder. (Oxford date courtesy of R. A. Mayou.)

Mood disorders are common in younger women, **organic mental disorders** in the elderly, and **drinking problems** in younger men. In outpatient clinics about 15 per cent of patients with a definite medical diagnosis have an associated psychiatric disorder, and about 40 per cent of those with no medical diagnosis have a psychiatric disorder.

Nature of the association

Psychiatric and physical disorders are both common and often occur together by chance. When they do so, they often then interact. For example, a depressive disorder provoked by business failure might make a patient less able to manage longstanding diabetes. Conversely, physical illness may exacerbate unrelated psychiatric symp-

TABLE 11.1 Associations between physical and psychiatric disorders
Psychiatric and physical disorders occurring together by chance
Psychological factors as causes of physical illness
Psychiatric consequences of physical illness:
◆ organic disorders (see Chapter 10)
◆ other disorders, especially depression and anxiety (see Chapters 8 and 6)
Psychological causes of physical symptoms (see Chapter 7)
Psychiatric disorders with physical complications:
◆ deliberate self-harm (see Chapter 13)
◆ alcohol and other substance abuse (see Chapter 14)
◆ eating disorders (see Chapter 12)

toms; for example, a virus infection could delay recovery from a depressive disorder. There are several other types of association between physical and psychological factors (Table 11.1). This chapter focuses mainly on the psychological and psychiatric consequences of physical disease, but should be read in conjunction with the other chapters referenced in Table 11.1.

Psychological factors as causes of physical disorders

It used to be thought that certain diseases—called **psychosomatic**—were caused mainly by psychological factors; asthma and ulcerative colitis are two examples. Research has not supported this idea, but there are four other ways in which psychological factors may contribute to the aetiology, presentation, and outcome of physical illness.

1. They may lead to *unhealthy habits* such as overeating, smoking, and excessive use of alcohol, which are risk factors for disease.

2. They may result in *hormonal, immunological,* or *neurophysiological changes*, which contribute to the onset or affect the course of the pathological process. It has been suggested, for example, that increased mortality among patients depressed after myocardial infarction is caused in this way.

3. They may affect the *perception* of the severity of symptoms, for example people experience pain as more severe when they are depressed.

4. Psychological factors can determine *whether a person seeks help* from a doctor about an illness; for example, a person who would not seek help for backache when in a normal mood may do so when depressed. They may

also *affect collaboration* with treatment and in this way influence outcome; for example, a depressed patient may neglect his part in the treatment of diabetes.

Psychological complications of physical disorders

Most people are remarkably resilient when ill and are able to carry on without undue distress. Even so, all physical illness has some psychological impact. In about a quarter of cases these satisfy criteria for psychiatric disorder and have a substantial effect on all aspects of outcome (Table 11.2).

Delirium is frequent in those who are severely ill (see Chapter 10). Most anxiety and depression associated physical illness is part of a psychological reaction. However, several medical disorders also cause anxiety and depressive symptoms directly, presumably through physiological mechanisms (Table 11.3). Some drugs have psychiatric side effects (Table 11.4).

Psychological reactions to illness

The usual reaction to **acute illness** is anxiety, which may be followed by depression. In up to a quarter of patients these reactions reach the diagnostic threshold

TABLE 11.2 Psychologically determined consequences of physical disorders
◆ Disturbances of mental state, some severe enough to be classified as a psychiatric disorder
◆ Heightened perception of physical symptoms and disability
◆ Impaired quality of everyday life
◆ Unnecessarily poor physical outcome
◆ Adverse effects on family and others
◆ Inappropriate or excessive consultation
◆ Poor collaboration with treatment

TABLE 11.3 Some physical disorders that cause psychiatric symptoms
Depression
Carcinoma, infections, neurological disorder, endocrine disorder
Anxiety
Hyperthyroidism, hyperventilation, hypoglycaemia, drug withdrawal
Fatigue
Anaemia, sleep disorder, chronic infection, hypothyroidism, diabetes, carcinoma, radiotherapy

TABLE 11.4 Some medications reported to cause psychiatric symptoms

- Central nervous system depressants
- Cimetidine
- Anticholinergic drugs
- Appetite suppressants
- Corticosteroids
- Corticosteroids
- Beta-blockers
- Hypotensives

for an anxiety or depressive disorder or for adjustment disorder. These responses are similar to those to other types of stress (see Chapter 5). Other reactions are also common, for example anger and the complete or partial denial of a life-threatening diagnosis. Both these responses can lead to poor collaboration with treatment.

In disabling **chronic illness**, anxiety and depressive disorders are up to twice as common as in the general population and psychological and social variables are strong determinants of other aspects of outcome (Table 11.2). The special problems of **terminal illness** are discussed in Chapter 5.

Psychiatric disorder

Although adjustment disorder, anxiety, and depression are the commonest psychiatric complications of physical illness, other psychiatric disorders may also be precipitated by physical illness (Table 11.5).

TABLE 11.5 Common psychiatric disorders in the physically ill

More common

- Adjustment disorder
- Depressive disorder
- Anxiety disorders
- Delirium

Less common

- Somatoform disorders
- Dementia
- Panic
- Phobic disorder
- Anxiety disorder
- Post-traumatic stress disorder
- Mania
- Schizophrenia and delusional disorder

Determinants of the psychological consequences of physical illness

Some illnesses and treatments are particularly threatening (Table 11.6). However, the psychological reactions depend more upon a patient's perception of the illness than to its objective nature (Table 11.7). If patients see their illness as particularly unpleasant or

TABLE 11.6 Factors associated with a particularly high risk of psychiatric problems

Severe illness

- Unpleasant, threatening, relapsing, progressive or terminal illness

Unpleasant treatment

- Some drug treatments
- Major surgery
- Chemotherapy
- Radiotherapy
- Very demanding self-care

Vulnerable patients

- Previous psychiatric problems
- Adverse social circumstances

TABLE 11.7 Determinants of the psychological impact of physical illness

Illness factors

- Pain
- Threat to life
- Duration
- Disability
- Conspicuousness to others

Treatment factors

- Side effects of medication
- Uncertainty of outcome
- Self-care demands

Patient factors

- Psychological vulnerability
- Social circumstances
- Beliefs about illness and treatment

Reactions of others

- Family
- Employers
- Doctors and others involved in care

if their ability to cope with stress is poor, then severe distress is more likely. The reactions of others may also affect patients' perceptions and their ability to cope.

Patients at high risk are especially likely to be encountered in hospital emergency departments and in a number of specialized units, such as those responsible for terminal care, cancer, severe neurological problems, and pain clinics.

Psychiatric assessment of a physically ill patient

Among severely ill patients distress is often seen as understandable and inevitable and no help is offered. This is incorrect. Most people cope remarkably well with even the most severe medical problems, *marked distress is abnormal and requires assessment and treatment*.

The psychiatric assessment of a physically ill patient is similar to that of a patient presenting solely with psychiatric symptoms (see Chapter 2), except that it requires knowledge of the nature and prognosis of the physical illness. Box 11.1 lists some screening questions.

BOX 11.1 RECOGNITION OF EMOTIONAL DISORDER IN THE PHYSICALLY ILL

Psychiatric symptoms

- How have you been feeling in yourself?
- Have you been very worried about your health?
- How have you been sleeping?
  Psychiatric history
- Are you taking any sleeping tablets or tablets for your nerves?
- Have you ever suffered from tension or nerves?
- Have you ever consulted a doctor about your nerves?

Social factors

- Any problems recently that have upset you?
- Any problems at home or at work?

Beliefs and concerns

- What do you feel is the cause of your symptoms?
- What effects do you think they will have on your life?

It is important to:

- speak to relatives who can provide extra information and also because families frequently require help themselves;
- review medical notes and referral letters as they often contain useful medical history and other information;
- be aware that some symptoms, such as tiredness and malaise, may occur in both physical and psychiatric disorder.

Management

Treatment of *acute reactions* to illness is discussed in Chapter 5. Some emotional distress is an almost inevitable accompaniment of the stress of physical illness and its treatment, although it can often be reduced by appropriate treatment. An explanation of the nature of the illness and of the proposed treatment, advice about the ways the patient can help himself, and discussion of anxieties are always useful.

As well as systematic assessment and alertness to verbal and non-verbal cues of distress, good care depends on the ability to provide and discuss information and advice with patients and their relatives. Basic psychological skills are important, including:

- knowledge of the recognition and treatment of depression;
- simple basic anxiety management skills (see p. 258);
- knowledge of the basic cognitive behavioural principles (see p. 258);
- an ability to encourage self-care.

Management of the problems of *chronic illness* is best organized as a process of 'stepped' physical, psychological, and social care, i.e. good routine care for everyone, including information and encouragement of self-care, systematic monitoring of progress, and the identification of those needing extra 'steps' of more intensive help from the medical team or psychological or psychiatric services (Table 11.8).

Psychiatric disorder

The treatment of any specific psychiatric disorder among the physically ill is similar to that of the same condition in a physically healthy person, although particular attention should be paid to adverse consequences of the side effects of antidepressant and other drugs, and to drug interactions.

TABLE 11.8 Planning the care of chronic illness

- Assessment of patient and family understanding of illness and help available
- Information about symptomatic relief and other treatment
- Explanation about who will be providing treatment, and routine and emergency contact arrangements
- Discussion of how the patient and family will be involved in care
- Practical help in everyday activities and support at home

Adjustment disorder Patients need opportunities for discussion, explanation, and problem solving.

Anxiety disorder Psychological treatment (see Chapter 18) may be required for anxiety disorders, especially if they are persistent. In the short term, brief treatment with a benzodiazepine as an anxiolytic can be helpful.

Depressive disorder Less serious depression can often be helped by support or problem-solving counselling, but more severe disorders require antidepressant medication (see Chapter 17). The choice of antidepressant may be affected by side effects and by medical contraindications; for example, tricyclic antidepressants are generally contraindicated for those with cardiac disorders, glaucoma, and prostate disorders.

Effects on families

Close relatives may suffer as much, or even more, distress than patients. It is important to include relatives in discussions about the patient's treatment, involvement in the programme of self-care, and to consider ways of helping with their own distress and any practical problems caused by the patient's illness.

Some practical problems

Acutely distressed patients

Distress, anxiety, or anger often reflects patients' uncertainties and fears about what is happening to them. It is important to try to understand the causes of the distress, to show sympathy, and to correct misunderstandings. It is always important to appear calm and to take time to understand the patient's concerns and to avoid unintentional exacerbation of problems. It is important not to show irritation and impatience. When anxiety remains severe small amounts of anxiolytic medication may be helpful.

Patients who refuse consent to medical treatment

Occasionally, patients are unwilling to accept their doctor's advice about treatment that is essential for a serious medical condition. There are many reasons for such refusal. Commonly, it is because the patient is frightened or angry, or does not understand fully what is happening. Frequently, explanation and discussion will result in informed consent (Box 11.2). Occasionally, the cause of refusal is a mental illness that interferes with the patient's ability to make an informed decision and this should be treated.

It has to be accepted that some mentally healthy patients will continue to refuse treatment even after a full and rational discussion of the reasons for carrying it out; it is the right of a conscious, mentally competent adult to do so (see Chapter 22).

Psychiatric emergencies in general hospital practice

However urgent the problem, the successful management of a psychiatric emergency, like any other medical emergency, depends greatly on a thorough clinical assessment. The aims are to:

> **BOX 11.2 MEDICOLEGAL AND ETHICAL ISSUES OF PATIENTS WHO REFUSE TO ACCEPT ADVICE ABOUT EMERGENCY TREATMENT**
>
> - *In life threatening emergencies* where it is not possible to obtain the patient's consent (impaired consciousness, evidence of psychiatric disorder which cannot be immediately assessed), opinions should be obtained from medical and nursing colleagues, and, if possible, from the patient's relatives. Detailed records should be kept of the reasons for the decision. It is essential for all doctors to know the law about these matters in the country in which they are practising.
> - If a patient has a *mental disorder that impairs the ability to give informed consent*, it may be appropriate to use legal powers of compulsory assessment and treatment of the mental disorder. The powers for compulsory treatment of a mental disorder do not give the doctor a right to treat concurrent physical illness againts the patient's wishes. Successful compulsory treatment of the psychiatric disorder may result in the patient giving informed consent for the treatment of the physical illness.

- establish a good relationship with the patient;
- to take a brief history;
- observe behaviour;
- assess the mental state.

When the patient's behaviour is very disturbed, the history may have to be obtained from other people, such as relatives or nurses. Although in managing emergencies there may not be the time or opportunity to follow the usual systematic scheme of history taking and examination, mistakes will be avoided and time saved if the assessment is as complete as the circumstances permit. Several common problems are discussed elsewhere in this book:

- deliberate self-harm (see Chapter 12);
- substance intoxication (see Chapter 14);
- acute stress reactions to trauma (see Chapter 5);
- delirium (see Chapter 10).

Acute disturbed behaviour and violence

The conditions most often leading to disturbed behaviour requiring immediate action in a general hospital or in primary care are delirium, schizophrenia, mania, agitated depression, and alcohol- and drug-related problems. Among inpatients, delirium is the most common. If the patient's behaviour is very disturbed and his manner is threatening, the first task is to assess the risk of violence (see p. 31).

When a patient is potentially or actually violent, it is essential to arrange for adequate but unobtrusive help to be available. When approaching the patient the doctor should appear calm and helpful, avoid confrontation, and try to persuade the patient to talk about the reasons for his anger.

If the patient responds so aggressively that restraint cannot be avoided, it should be accomplished quickly by an adequate number of people using the minimum of force. Single-handed attempts at restraint should be avoided. Apart from these rare circumstances, physical contact (including physical examination) should not be attempted unless the purpose has been clearly understood by, and agreed with, the patient. Extreme caution is, of course, required with a patient thought to possess any kind of offensive weapon. At such times the help of the police may be required.

Drug treatment of disturbed or violent patients

If a patient is very frightened, and simple reassurance fails, oral or parenteral diazepam (5–10 mg) is useful. If the patient is more disturbed, rapid calming can usually be achieved with 2–10 mg of haloperidol injected intramuscularly. Chlorpromazine (75–150 mg intramuscularly) is a more sedating alternative to haloperidol, but more likely to cause hypotension. When the patient is calm, haloperidol may be continued in smaller doses, usually three to four times a day, preferably by mouth, using a syrup if the patient will not swallow tablets. The dosage depends on the patient's weight and on the initial response to the drug. Careful observation by nurses of the physical state and behaviour are necessary during this treatment. Extrapyramidal side effects may require treatment with an antiparkinsonian drug.

Psychiatric services for a general hospital

General practitioners are responsible for all aspects of their patients' care: physical, psychological, and social. Similarly, in a general hospital, psychological aspects of illness are part of the consultant team's responsibilities. Sometimes, psychiatric advice is needed. In larger hospitals this advice may be from a special **liaison** (also known as **consultation liaison**) **service**. This service is staffed by psychiatrists, nurses, and psychologists, usually with a social worker. The consultation liaison service may provide:

- an emergency service for patients admitted after deliberate self-harm;
- emergency consultation for other accident and emergency department attenders;
- a consultation service for inpatients;
- outpatient care for patients referred with psychiatric complications of physical illness or functional somatic symptoms;
- regular liaison visits to selected medical and surgical units in which psychiatric problems are especially common (e.g. neurology, renal dialysis, terminal care).

In many hospitals the management of deliberate self-harm takes up most of the time of the liaision team, but in better staffed units some or all of the other functions are carried out.

Making a referral

Referral to a psychiatrist should provide basic information about:

- the medical problem;
- the reasons for the referral;
- the nature of the help required.

It is preferable, especially where problems are severe or complex, for the referring doctor to speak directly to the psychiatrist and to ask the psychiatrist to discuss later the conclusions of the assessment. Some referrals can be dealt with by discussion without the patient being seen, in other cases a single visit is enough, but sometimes continuing collaborative management will be required.

Some examples of psychiatric aspects of physical disorders

Cancer

As the most frightening of diseases, cancer causes considerable distress to patients and their families or carers. Psychologically and socially determined problems include family worries, practical difficulties, finances and work, and worries about appearance. Patients may be angry and may suffer sexual difficulties. Only a minority develop a psychiatric disorder (Table 11.9). Distress is particularly likely to occur at particular points during the patient's experience of cancer:

- at diagnosis;
- during treatment (surgery, radiotherapy, or chemotherapy);
- if terminal disease recurs.

Care should be planned to involve patients and families to prevent or minimize psychological and social problems. Most of the psychological care is provided in primary care. It is important that this includes discussion of information, which is best given in a staged manner as patients and families require it. It needs to be accompanied by practical and social support and willingness to encourage patients to talk about their worries. Specific psychological and psychiatric treatments are effective for anxiety and depression and in helping patients to cope with physical symptoms.

Surgical treatment

Most patients are anxious before major surgery; those who are most anxious before surgery are also most dis-

TABLE 11.9 Psychiatric consequences of cancer

- Emotional reaction on diagnosis or recurrence
- Anxiety
- Depression
- Anticipatory nausea with chemotherapy
- Neuropsychiatric syndromes (due to metastases, paraneoplastic syndromes)

tressed afterwards. Anxiety can be reduced by a clear explanation of the operation, its likely consequences, and the plan for postoperative care, including the effective treatment of pain. In addition, a written handout is helpful since anxious people do not remember all that they have been told. Delirium is common after major surgery, especially in the elderly.

When surgery leads to changes to the body's appearance (e.g. mastectomy) or function (e.g. colostomy) there may be additional psychological problems. These patients benefit from psychological support, which may be given by a specially trained nurse.

Screening for physical disorder or risk

Screening procedures for physical disorders, such as hypertension or early cancer, or for major risk factors, such as high blood lipid levels, are used increasingly. Screening usually causes little distress if it is explained clearly. However, a few subjects are made anxious by the screening, whether the result is positive or negative. For these people extra help is needed. Screening procedures should be designed to incorporate time to provide information, the opportunity for the discussion of anxieties, and a recognition of the small proportion of people who become anxious.

Genetic counselling

Counselling about the risk of hereditary disease is mainly given to couples contemplating marriage or planning or expecting a child. It includes providing information about risks, help with worry about increased risk, help in taking well-informed decisions about family planning (including sterilization), and treatment. Genetic counselling is usually provided in obstetric and genetic clinics, but there is also a need for advice by family doctors (Box 11.3). Ethical issues are listed in Box 11.4.

Information about increased risk is particularly distressing for parents who have experienced a previous abnormal pregnancy. Unfortunately, counselling is more effective in imparting knowledge than in changing behaviour and many couples ignore warnings that future children will be at high risk.

Psychiatric aspects of obstetrics and gynaecology

Pregnancy

Psychiatric disorder is more common in the first and third trimesters of pregnancy than in the second

BOX 11.3 BEST PRACTICE IN GENETIC COUNSELLING

In the light of current evidence, best practice for the conduct of genetic testing (presymptomatic, predispositional, and prenatal) includes the following points:

- The written protocol for the conduct of the testing programme should include how the laboratory tests are to be conducted and how communications with patients is to be managed.

- Before they decide whether to undergo a test, clear and simple information should be presented to those eligible for testing. Such information should include the advantages and disadvantages of testing, as well as the meaning of any possible test result.

- The initial offer of a test should be separated in time (a day or more) from a biological sample being taken.

- Test results should be explained and support offered to all those tested and their relatives.

- The effectiveness of a testing programme in achieving good understanding as well as facilitating behaviours that reduce risk, without high levels of emotional distress or false reassurance, needs to be assessed, not assumed.

BOX 11.4 MEDICAL AND ETHICAL ISSUES OF GENERIC COUNSELLING

- Confidentiality.
- Consent.
- Storage and use of generic information.
- Testing children: it is generally believed that it is wise to delay testing until an age which individuals can make their own decisions.
- Implications for life insurance.

BOX 11.5 SOME PSYCHOLOGICAL PROBLEMS OF PREGNANCY

Unwanted pregnancy

Most medical decisions about termination are now made by the family doctor and gynaecologist without involving a psychiatrist. In a small proportion of patients with psychiatric disorder, a specialist opinion should be obtained.

Hyperemesis gravidarum

This syndrome of severe and repeated vomiting is rare. It appears to have primary physiological causes but the psychological reaction may exacerbate the severity and duration of the symptoms and result in greater difficulty in management.

Pseudocyesis

A rare condition in which a woman believes she is pregnant when she is not and develops amenorrhoea, abdominal distension, and other changes resembling early pregnancy. It usually resolves quickly following diagnosis. It may be recurrent.

Couvade syndrome

A rare condition in which the husband of a pregnant woman experiences symptoms of pregnancy.

(Box 11.5). In the first trimester, unwanted pregnancies are associated with anxiety and depression. In the third trimester, there may be fears about the impending delivery, or doubts about the normality of the fetus. Psychiatric symptoms in pregnancy are more common in women with a history of previous psychiatric disorder, although some women with chronic psychiatric disorders may improve during pregnancy. Women with chronic psychiatric problems often attend irregularly for antenatal care and consequently have more than the average number of obstetric problems.

Treatment of psychiatric disorder during pregnancy

During pregnancy great care must be taken in the use of psychotropic drugs because of the possible risk of fetal malformations, impaired growth, and perinatal problems (Box 11.6). Abuse of *alcohol*, *opiates*, and *street drugs* may affect the fetus and should be strongly discouraged, especially in the first trimester when the risk to the fetus is greatest.

Loss of a fetus and stillbirth

Loss of a fetus during pregnancy or stillbirth has substantial and immediate psychological impact for a mother and also for the father. The loss leads to significant depression, which may continue for a several weeks. **Stillbirth** is associated with even greater distress than loss of the pregnancy at an earlier stage. The

BOX 11.6 USE OF PSYCHOTROPIC MEDICINE IN PREGNANCY AND DURING BREAST-FEEDING

Pregnancy

Avoid all medication if possible. Use only if the expected benefit to the mother is greater than the possibility of risk to the fetus.

Antidepressants There is no evidence that tricyclics or SSRIs cause fetal abnormality, but use only where there are very clear indications and in minimal dosage.

Lithium There is a risk of teratogenicity and of toxic effects on the fetus in late pregnancy. Risks are reduced by careful monitoring of levels. Ideally lithium should be avoided in the period of conception and early pregnancy, but careful represcription is possible in the final trimester. In an unplanned pregnancy during long-term therapy: discuss with parents, consider termination, careful screening for malformations. Omit perinatally.

Antipsychotics Continue in minimal dose if there are major clinical indications.

Breast-feeding

Take care with all medications.

Antidepressants Evidence is not clear but there are no definite contraindications. Avoid if possible. It is important to carefully consider the risks and benefits with the parents.

Lithium The evidence is uncertain. Breast-feeding cannot be recommended with confidence.

Antipsychotic drugs The risk is probably small, but avoid if possible.

---

distress is likely to be greatest when the pregnancy was particularly wanted, for example when there have been previous miscarriages or stillbirths.

Spontaneous abortion at any stage of pregnancy causes distress and depression is frequent.

Termination of pregnancy for medical reasons is especially likely to cause distress, depression, and feelings of guilt, which usually improve over a period of 2–3 months.

After abortion, termination, or stillbirth, mothers and fathers should be encouraged to grieve the loss as they would the death of an infant.

Postpartum mental disorders

There are three kinds of postpartum psychiatric disorder:

- maternity 'blues';
- puerperal psychosis;
- other depressive disorders of moderate severity.

The management of depressive disorder is more fully described in Chapter 8. Abuse and neglect, which also occasionally occur in infancy, are discussed in Chapter 20.

Maternity 'blues'

Between one-half and two-thirds of women delivered of a normal child experience a brief episode of irritability, muddled thinking, tearfulness, and lability of mood, which is particularly characteristic. All these symptoms reach their peak on the third or fourth postpartum day. The patient and her partner should be reassured that the condition is common and short lived. No other treatment is needed.

Puerperal psychosis

Puerperal psychosis begins, typically, 2–3 days after delivery and nearly always in the first 1–2 postpartum weeks. There are three types of psychosis:

- delirium;
- mood disorder;
- schizophrenic.

The clinical features of each of these syndromes are similar to those of the corresponding syndromes occurring outside the puerperium. Delirium used to be common before antibiotics were introduced to treat puerperal sepsis. Now it is rare in developed countries. Affective syndromes are more common than schizophrenic ones.

Puerperal psychosis occurs in about 1 in 500 births. It is more frequent among primiparous women, those who have suffered previous serious psychiatric disorder, and those with a family history of psychiatric disorder. Puerperal psychosis is not more common after complicated deliveries.

Assessment As well as taking a *history* and examining the *mental state* in the usual way, *it is essential to ascertain the mother's ideas concerning the baby*. Severely depressed patients may have delusional ideas that the child is malformed or otherwise imperfect and some patients may attempt to kill the child to spare it from future suffering. Assessment of *suicidal intent* is also important.

Treatment is as described for affective disorder and schizophrenia occurring outside pregnancy. For depressive disorders of marked or moderate severity, *ECT* is often the best treatment because its rapid effect enables the mother to resume the care of her baby quickly. When the disorder is not severe and the mother has no ideas of harming herself or the baby, treatment can be at home with appropriate help to ensure the safe care of the baby. When the disorder is more severe, or there are ideas of harm to self or baby, the mother should usually be admitted to hospital, if possible to a special mother and baby unit. If antidepressant or antipsychotic drugs or lithium have to be prescribed, then breast-feeding will have to be stopped.

Prognosis Most patients recover fully from a puerperal psychosis but a few (mostly those with a schizophrenic psychosis) remain chronically ill. At a subsequent birth, the recurrence rate for puerperal depressive disorder is between 1 in 2 and 1 in 3 (compared with 1 in 500 for those without a previous puerperal psychosis). At least half the women with a puerperal depressive disorder go on to develop a depressive disorder unrelated to childbirth.

Treatment during subsequent pregnancies Women who have had a puerperal psychosis should be referred to a psychiatrist and monitored closely during subsequent deliveries. Patients who have a history of bipolar disorder may require lithium prophylaxis, avoiding the first trimester and stopping soon after delivery.

Other puerperal depressive disorders

Postnatal depression of mild or moderate severity is much more common than puerperal psychoses, occurring in 10–15 per cent of recently delivered women. This prevalence is little different to that in the general population of young women. Tiredness, irritability, and anxiety are often more prominent than depressive mood and there may be prominent phobic symptoms.

Clinical observation suggests these disorders are caused mainly by the psychological adjustments required after childbirth, by loss of sleep, and by the hard work involved in the care of the baby. Some of these women have a history of psychiatric illness and some have experienced stressful events near the time of onset of the disorder.

There is evidence that postnatal depression adversely affects the mother/infant relationship and the cognitive and emotional development of the infant. It is not clear whether these adverse effects persist into early and later childhood.

Early detection is important and those providing care to the mother and baby need to be alert to the possibility of depression. Additional help with child care may be needed, together with counselling about any marital problems in looking after the infant. Antidepressant drugs are prescribed if there are biological symptoms of depression.

Menstrual disorders

Premenstrual syndrome

This term denotes psychological and physical symptoms starting a few days before, and ending shortly after, the onset of a menstrual period. The psychological symptoms include anxiety, irritability, and depression; the physical symptoms include breast tenderness, abdominal discomfort, and a feeling of distension. Estimates of the frequency of the premenstrual syndrome in the general population vary widely from 30 to 80 per cent of women of reproductive age, depending on the diagnostic criteria used. The cause is uncertain. Psychological factors may exacerbate distress and disability originating from physiological changes around menstruation.

Many treatments have been tried, including progesterone, oral contraceptives, bromocriptine, diuretics, and psychotropic drugs. There is no convincing evidence that any of these treatments are generally effective, and randomized trials indicate a high placebo response. Psychological support and cognitive behaviour treatment can be helpful in enabling women to cope with symptoms and the consequences in a positive way that enables them to feel more in control of their everyday life.

Menopause

Some menopausal women complain of physical symptoms of flushing, sweating, and vaginal dryness, and of headache, dizziness, and depression. Although there is a widespread belief that emotional problems are an inevitable part of the menopause, it is not certain whether psychological symptoms are more common in menopausal women than in other women of similar age. Depressive and anxiety-related symptoms around the time of the menopause could be related to hormonal changes but this has not been proved. Alternatively, or additionally, the symptoms could result from changes in the woman's role as her children leave home, her relationship with her husband alters, and her own parents become ill or die.

Oestrogens have been used but the results have been disappointing. Hormone replacement therapy (HRT) should not be seen as a treatment of depressive illness in those of menopausal age. Psychiatric disorders around the menopause should be treated as at other times of life.

Further reading

Levenson, J. L. 2004. *The American Psychiatric Publishing Textbook of Psychosomatic Medicine*. American Psychiatric Publishing Inc. Washington DC.

CHAPTER 12

Eating and sleep disorders

Chapter contents

Disorders of eating 161

　Anorexia 162
　Bulimia nervosa 165
　Obesity 166

Sleep disorders 167

Disorders of eating

Eating disorders have been increasingly conspicuous in the last 30 years. It is uncertain whether the changes in presentation reflect a true increase. Many are still clinically unrecognized and it is estimated that general practitioners recognize only 12 per cent of cases of bulimia nervosa and 45 per cent of cases of anorexia nervosa.

Anorexia nervosa and bulimia nervosa, which we describe in this chapter, are the most clearly defined subgroups of a wider range of eating disorders. Many patients present with subthreshold expressions of the two main diagnoses; others with different patterns of symptoms. These atypical disorders are classified in DSM-IV as 'eating disorder not otherwise specified' (EDNOS). Figure 12.1 shows the relationship between these disorders.

General assessment

The assessment of eating disorders requires special attention to the patterns of eating and beliefs about food. More than one interview may be needed to obtain this information and to gain the patient's confidence.

1. A thorough *history* should be taken of the development of the disorder, the present pattern of eating and weight control, and the patient's ideas about body weight.

2. In the *mental state examination*, particular attention should be given to depressive symptoms.

3. Whenever possible, the parents or other informants should be interviewed.

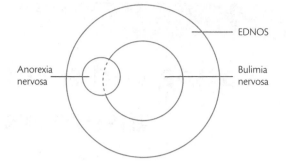

Fig. 12.1 Venn diagram illustrating the relationship between the diagnoses of anorexia nervosa, bulimia nervosa, and eating order not otherwise specified (EDNOS). (Reproduced with permission from Fairburn & Wilson (1993) *Binge eating: nature assessment and treatment.* Guilford Press, New York.)

4. Family interactions should be assessed together with their attitudes and behaviour in relation to food and meals.

Anorexia nervosa

The main clinical features of anorexia nervosa are reflected in the DSM-IV criteria:

- refusal to maintain body weight at or above 85 per cent of expected weight;

- intense fear of gaining weight or becoming fat;

- disturbance in the way body weight and shape are experienced;

- amenorrhoea in postmenarchal women.

Most patients are young women who have a distorted image of the body, believing themselves to be fat even when severely underweight. The condition generally begins with ordinary efforts at dieting by a person who was somewhat overweight at the time, and progresses to a relentless attempt to achieve an abnormally low body weight.

Epidemiology

Anorexia nervosa occurs largely among school-age girls, where the prevalence is between 0.1 and 0.5 per cent. Nearly all (95 per cent) patients are female and the condition is more common in the upper social classes and is reported to be rare in less developed countries. Many more young women have amenorrhoea and a weight loss that is less than that required to satisfy diagnostic criteria.

Clinical features

The most striking features are excessive concern with shape and weight together with a relentless pursuit of thinness, which may take several forms (Table 12.1).

TABLE 12.1	Clinical features of anorexia nervosa
Excessive concern with shape and weight	
Distorted body image	
Pursuit of thinness with consequent low body weight	
◆ dieting	
◆ avoidance of carbohydrates	
◆ self-induced vomiting	
◆ excessive exercise	
◆ purging	
Preoccupation with food (binge eating in some patients)	
Amenorrhoea	
Low mood	
Lack of sexual interest	
Consequences of starvation	
◆ emaciation	
◆ constipation	
◆ low blood pressure	
◆ bradycardia	
◆ sensitivity to cold	
◆ hypothermia	
Consequences of vomiting and laxative abuse	
◆ alkalosis	
◆ hypokalaemia	

Patients eat little and show a particular avoidance of carbohydrates. Some set daily calorie limits (often between 600 and 1000 calories). Some try to increase weight loss by self-induced vomiting (often by putting fingers in the throat), excessive exercise, or purging. Patients are often preoccupied with thoughts of food: some enjoy cooking elaborate meals for other people, and a few steal food.

Up to half of patients describe episodes of uncontrollable overeating (known as **binge eating** or **bulimia**). During binges, the patients may eat very large amounts of the foods they usually avoid, for example, a whole loaf of bread with copious jam and butter. After overeating the patient feels bloated and may induce vomiting. Binges are also followed by remorse and intensified efforts to lose weight.

Amenorrhoea is an important feature. It occurs early in the development of the condition and in about one-fifth of cases it precedes obvious weight loss. Some patients ask for help for amenorrhoea rather than for the eating disorder.

Other symptoms, especially depression, lability of mood, and social withdrawal, are all common. Lack of sexual interest is usual.

Physical consequences include emaciation and cold, blue extremities. Some patients have signs that are secondary to the low food intake, namely constipation, low blood pressure, bradycardia, sensitivity to cold, and hypothermia. Vomiting and abuse of laxatives may lead to alkalosis and hypokalaemia and these abnormalities may cause epilepsy or, rarely, death from cardiac arrhythmia.

Aetiology

Anorexia nervosa appears to result from a combination of individual genetic predisposition and social factors that encourage dieting. Many schoolchildren and female college students diet at one time or another but most stop without difficulty. Those progressing to anorexia are more likely to have low self-esteem and a preoccupation with their appearance. The prevalence of anorexia nervosa is increased in ballet students and others strongly concerned with weight and appearance. When the disorder has started, concern and overprotection by the family and arguments about food and meals may help to perpetuate it.

Course and prognosis

In its early stages, anorexia nervosa often runs a fluctuating course with periods of partial remission. The most useful *predictor of poor outcome* is a long history at the time the patient is first seen by a doctor. The long-term prognosis is variable:

- one-fifth of patients make a full recovery;
- one-fifth remain severely ill;
- three-fifths have a chronic, fluctuating course; among those with improved weight and menstrual function, some continue to have abnormal eating habits, some become overweight, and some others develop bulimia nervosa (see p. 165);
- there is a small *increased mortality* amongst severe cases, both from the effects of starvation and from suicide.

Management

There is a lack of good evidence about treatment and management, reflecting the variable severity of the disorder and also the difficulties in evaluating complex interventions in an uncommon condition. This means that current views about treatment are based mainly on clinical experience.

Family doctors play an important part in early treatment. Most patients with anorexia nervosa are very reluctant to see a psychiatrist and much depends on

---

BOX 12.1 ASSESSMENT OF EATING ISSUES: SOME TOPICS TO BE INCLUDED

- What is a typical day's eating? To what degree is the patient attempting restraint?
- Is there a pattern? Does it vary? Is eating ritualized?
- Does she avoid particular foods? And if so why?
- Does she restrict fluids?
- What is the patient's experience of hunger or of any urge to eat?
- Does she binge? Are these objectively large binges? Does she feel out of control?
- Are the binges planned? How do they begin? How do they end? How often?
- Does she make herself vomit? If so how? Does she vomit blood? Does she wash out with copious fluids afterwards?
- Does she take laxatives, diuretics, emetics, appetite suppressants? With what effects?
- Does she chew and spit? Does she fast for a day to more?
- Can she eat in front of others?
- Does she exercise? Is this to 'burn off calories'?

(Reproduced with permission from Palmer, B. (2000). *Helping People with Eating Disorders. A Clinical Guide to Assessment and Treatment*. John Wiley, Chicester.)

---

trying to establish a good relationship with the patient and the family in primary care. A thorough history should be taken, including the points in Boxes 12.1 and 12.2; particular attention should be given to depressive symptoms.

In the *physical examination* particular attention should be paid to the distribution of body hair (normal in anorexia nervosa, abnormal in pituitary failure—see below), the degree of emaciation, signs of vitamin deficiency, and the state of the peripheral circulation. A search should also be made for evidence of any other wasting disease, such as malabsorption, endocrine disorder, or cancer. Electrolytes should be measured if there is any possibility that the patient has been inducing vomiting or abusing purgatives, because of the risk of potassium depletion.

Starting treatment

If weight loss is severe, or weight is decreasing rapidly, specialist help should be obtained urgently, otherwise

BOX 12.2 ASSESSMENT OF PSYCHOLOGICAL ISSUES: SOME TOPICS TO BE INCLUDED

- What does the patient feel about her body and her weight?
- If she is restraining her eating, what is her motivation?
- Does she feel fat? Does she dislike her body? If so, in what way?
- Does she have a distorted body image? If so, in what way?
- What does she feel would happen if she did not control her weight or eating?
- Does she fear loss of control? Is she able to say what she means by this?
- Does she feel guilt or self-disgust? If so, what leads her to feel this?
- Does anything about her disorder lead her to feel good?
- If she binges, what are her feelings before, during, and after bingeing?
- What has she told others about her eating disorder—if anything?
- How does she think about her disorder? What does she make of it?

(Reproduced with permission from Palmer, B. (2000). *Helping People with Eating Disorders. A Clinical Guide to Assessment and Treatment.* John Wiley, Chicester.)

TABLE 12.2 Starting the treatment of anorexia nervosa

Assess:

- The severity of the condition (see text)
- The presence of depressive disorder
- Family problems

If there is evidence of severe weight loss or severe emotional problems, refer to a psychiatrist, otherwise proceed to:

- Take time to establish working relationships with the patient and family
- Give advice about healthy eating, and the hazards of extreme dieting
- Agree an acceptable and realistic target for weight gain, and a plan for achieving this
- Treat depressive disorder if present
- Help with personal and family problems
- Arrange regular follow-up, including monitoring of eating

treatment can be initiated by the primary care physician (Table 12.2). Success largely depends on making a good relationship with the patient, and gaining her collaboration. The patient and family should be told the nature of the disorder, the hazards of extreme dieting, and the nature and purpose of the proposed treatment. It should be made clear that the maintenance of adequate weight is an essential first priority. It is important to negotiate a reasonable dietary plan with the patient and to set this out clearly, together with a medically acceptable, but not overambitious, target weight. At the same time, help should be offered with any psychological problems. Simple supportive measures are usually enough to increase the patient's sense of personal effectiveness. When there are serious family problems that seem to be maintaining the disorder, family interviews may be helpful.

Specialist treatment

Most patients referred to a specialist will be treated as outpatients in a similar way. Rarely, the patient's weight loss is so severe as to pose an immediate threat to life. If such a patient cannot be persuaded to enter hospital (or remain there), compulsory powers have to be used. Admission to hospital may be needed if:

- the patient's weight is dangerously low (less than 65 per cent of standard weight);
- weight loss is rapid;
- there is severe depression;
- outpatient care has failed.

In hospital there should be an understanding that the patient will stay until an agreed target weight has been reached. Usually, this target has to be a compromise between the ideal weight (from height and weight tables) and the patient's idea of what her weight should be. The plan should be understood clearly by all those treating the patient. A balanced daily diet of at least 3000 calories is provided as three to four meals a day. Eating is supervised by a nurse, who has three important roles:

1. To reassure the patient that she can eat without the risk of losing control over her weight.
2. To be firm about the agreed targets.
3. to ensure that the patient does not induce vomiting or take purgatives.

It is reasonable to aim for a weight gain of between 0.5 and 1 kg each week. There is a satisfactory weight gain in hospital in about four patients out of five; the treatment of the others is very difficult and requires further long-term efforts to establish a relationship with the patient that will help her to begin to eat more and also be a basis for trying to solve other personal and social difficulties.

Treatment in hospital usually lasts between 2 and 3 months. Patients often demand to leave hospital before their treatment is finished, but with patience the staff can usually persuade them to stay. If they do leave, contact should be continued as an outpatient or in primary care. Compulsory treatment should only be considered if there is life-threatening weight loss.

Bulimia nervosa

The term bulimia refers to episodes of uncontrolled excessive eating, sometimes called binges. The clinical features are summarized in Table 12.3. As mentioned above, the symptom of bulimia occurs in some cases of anorexia nervosa, but it also occurs without preceding anorexia nervosa in a syndrome known as bulimia nervosa. DSM-IV criteria require three features:

1. Recurrent episodes of binge eating, characterized by eating a large amount of food and by a sense of lack of control over eating.

2. Recurrent inappropriate behaviour to prevent weight gain, such as self-induced vomiting, misuse of laxatives, enema, or medication, fasting, or excessive exercise.

3. Symptoms do not occur exclusively during episodes of anorexia nervosa.

TABLE 12.3 Clinical features of bulimia nervosa

Excessive concern with shape and weight
Binge eating
Behaviours to prevent weight gain
◆ dietary restraint
◆ self-induced vomiting
◆ excessive exercise
◆ purging
Normal body weight
Consequences of potassium depletion
◆ weakness
◆ cardiac arrythmia
◆ renal impairment
Other consequences of repeated vomiting
◆ swollen parotid glands
◆ pitted teeth

The balance between binge eating and behaviours to prevent weight gain is such that patients are usually of normal weight. Most patients are female and they have normal menses. Like patients with anorexia nervosa, patients with bulimia nervosa are excessively concerned with their shape and weight. Unlike patients with anorexia nervosa most bulimic patients accept the need for treatment.

It is this extreme lack of control over eating that distinguishes bulimia nervosa from anorexia nervosa. The episodes of bulimia may be precipitated by stressful events or by the breaking of self-imposed dietary rules, or they may be planned. During the episodes, enormous amounts of food are consumed: for example, a loaf of bread, a whole pot of jam, a cake, and biscuits. This voracious eating takes place alone. At first it brings a pleasurable relief from the urge to eat and other kinds of tension, but relief is soon followed by guilt and disgust. The patient induces vomiting, at first often by putting fingers in the throat, but later by an effort of will. There may be many episodes of bulimia and vomiting each day.

Depressive symptoms are common. Usually, they are secondary to the eating disorder, but a few patients have an associated depressive disorder.

Physical consequences

Repeated vomiting leads to several complications. *Potassium depletion* is particularly serious, resulting in weakness, cardiac arrhythmia, and renal damage. Urinary infections, tetany, and epileptic fits may occur. The *teeth may be pitted* by the repeated vomiting of acid gastric contents, and the *parotid glands may become swollen*.

Epidemiology

The prevalence of bulimia nervosa is between 1 and 2 per cent in women aged 15–40 years. It is more frequent in developed countries. The rapid increase in presenting cases suggests there has been a real increase in recent years, especially in young women between the ages of 15 and 24. However, it remains uncertain whether all or most of this increase could be due to an increased awareness of the disorder.

Prognosis is uncertain since there have been no long-term studies. Many patients continue with abnormal eating habits for many years, although the severity varies.

Aetiology

Unlike anorexia nervosa, genetic factors do not seem to be important, although low self-esteem and perfectionism are predisposing factors. Two important types of risk factor are those that increase the likelihood of dieting and those for psychiatric disorder in general.

Treatment

The treatment of choice is **cognitive behaviour therapy** designed to reduce dietary restraint and increase control over eating and vomiting. This treatment results in a full and lasting recovery in between one-half and two-thirds of patients. Patients keep records of their food intake and episodes of vomiting, and attempt to identify and avoid any emotional changes that regularly provoke episodes of bulimia. There is also evidence that a form of short-term psychotherapy—**interpersonal therapy**—is equally effective although slower to act.

Since specialized treatment is demanding and not widely available, there has been increasing interest in simpler and briefer forms of treatment for use in primary care. Cognitive behaviour self-help programmes appear to be effective, especially when accompanied by support and encouragement from a non-specialist (guided self-help). These programmes include educational material that aims to correct misconceptions about eating and weight control, self-monitoring of eating habits so that patients can characterize their problems, behavioural measures to help regain control over eating, and simple cognitive procedures to improve the ability to solve problems and to reduce concerns about shape and weight. Whilst there is no doubt that psychological treatments are more effective than drug therapy, antidepressant treatment may be useful where skilled therapists are not available, as an additional therapy for depressive symptoms, and where psychological treatment has failed.

Management

The assessment of bulimia nervosa is similar to that described for anorexia nervosa, but is usually easier because the patient recognizes the need for treatment. The mental state is examined for an associated depressive disorder needing treatment with antidepressant drugs. The patient's physical state should be assessed. Less severe problems can be treated in primary care (Table 12.4).

Only those patients who fail to benefit from these interventions need to be referred for specialist psychological treatment. Options for those who fail to respond to standard treatments include adding a specific serotonin reuptake inhibitor (SSRI) or changing to a different form of psychotherapy.

Obesity

Obesity is a medical condition characterized by excess body fat. It is diagnosed when the body mass index or BMI (weight in kilograms × height in m²) exceeds 30.

TABLE 12.4 Key elements of management in primary care

- Reassure that the disorder is common and that treatment is available
- Assess mood
- Diary keeping to monitor eating patterns and bulimic behaviour
- Advice about regular small meals, together with reassurance that this will not result in weight gain
- Techniques to avoid bingeing, e.g. eating in company, reducing the amount of food kept at home, distraction
- Suggestions of self-help manuals and self-help groups

Almost 20 per cent of adults in the UK meet this criteria and the figure is rising. Obesity is associated with increased mortality and severe obesity with a much greater risk. It is a chronic, lifelong problem. Obese children and adolescents are unlikely to grow out of obesity unless treated.

Most obesity is attributable to genetic factors exacerbated by social factors that encourage overeating. Psychological causes do not seem to be of great importance in most cases. There is little evidence of differences in psychopathology as compared with non-obese people, although a minority of people have major distortions of body image.

Treatment

It is important to recognize children who are overweight and give advice to them and their families; behavioural methods are often helpful.

Most mildly obese people need nothing more than advice about diet. Others, and the moderately obese, require more help. However, as many of these obese people do not eat more than other people, and of those who do, few have obvious psychological causes, it is not surprising that the long-term results of treatment are disappointing.

Treatment should aim to achieve realistic goals rather than target weights that are unlikely to be achieved and maintained. The main approaches are:

1. Diet programmes that encourage long-term changes in eating and increased activity.

2. Weight groups, whether supervised or self-help, produce short-term benefit but usually do not improve long-term results.

3. The role of the newer appetite-suppressing drugs is still unclear although they may be of use as a part of specialist treatment.

4. Behavioural methods designed to change eating habits have short-term benefits but their long-term value in uncertain.

5. Where obesity is severe, advice should be obtained from a physician with specialist experience.

6. Surgical treatment (usually gastric restriction) is probably indicated for very severe obesity (BMI > 40).

Sleep disorders

Table 12.5 lists the main types of sleep disorder; the commonest are described in this section.

Insomnia

Insomnia is complained of by between 10 and 30 per cent of the adult population. People vary in the amount of sleep they need, and many of those who complain of insomnia may be having as much sleep as others who do not complain and as much as they require physiologically. Some take 'catnaps' in the day, often through boredom, and still expect to sleep as long at night. In some, insomnia is secondary to other disorders (Table 12.5):

* painful physical conditions;
* depressive disorder;
* anxiety disorder;
* dementia;

TABLE 12.5 Classification of sleep disorders

Insomnia
* Related to a physical condition
* Associated with a mental disorder
* Associated with caffeine or alcohol
* Primary insomnia

Hypersomnia
* Narcolepsy
* Hypersomnia related to a physical condition and medication (includes sleep apnoea, neurology)
* Primary idiopathic hypersomnia

Sleep–wake schedule disorder

Parasomnia
* Nightmares
* Night terrors
* Sleepwalking

* excessive use of **alcohol**, **caffeine**, or **tobacco** (sleep may be disturbed for several weeks after stopping heavy drinking of alcohol).

In about 15 per cent of cases of insomnia, no cause can be found (**primary insomnia**).

Assessment

The diagnosis of insomnia is usually based on the account given by the patient. Occasionally, electroencephalograph (EEG) and other physiological recordings either in a sleep laboratory or at home are helpful when there is continuing doubt about the extent and nature of the insomnia. These observations often show that, despite the patient's complaint, sleeping time is within the normal range.

Treatment

When insomnia is caused by a psychiatric or physical condition, the latter should be treated. When no such cause can be found it is useful to reassure the patient and emphasize the effectiveness of simple measures (sleep hygiene):

* encourage regular habits and exercise;
* discourage overindulgence in tobacco, caffeine, and alcohol (especially before sleep);
* ensure a comfortable bed and quiet, dark bedroom;
* encourage a regular pattern of going to bed;
* avoid daytime sleep;
* provide advice on relaxation techniques for use if the patient awakes at night.

Although a hypnotic may be prescribed for a few nights at times of acute stress, demands for prolonged medication should be resisted. The withdrawal of hypnotics can lead to insomnia as distressing as the original sleep disturbance, and continued use of hypnotics can impair performance during the day and lead to dependency.

Hypersomnias

Narcolepsy

This rare disorder usually begins between the ages of 10 and 20 years. Patients are extremely drowsy and have episodes of daytime sleep lasting about 15 minutes. Most patients have sudden temporary episodes of loss of muscle tone with paralysis (cataplexy), and a quarter experience episodes of paralysis on waking from sleep (sleep paralysis), and hypnagogic hallucinations. Some patients have secondary emotional and social difficulties, which may be increased by other people's lack of understanding. Almost all cases of people with narcolepsy have the HLA type DR2 (compared with about a quarter of the general population), but it is not known how this relates to the cause of the condition.

There is no effective treatment. Patients should be referred to a specialist and encouraged to follow a regular routine with planned short periods of sleep during the day.

Idiopathic hypersomnia

Patients complain that they are unable to wake completely until several hours after getting up. During this time they feel confused and may be disorientated. They usually report prolonged and deep night-time sleep. The cause of the condition is unknown. Many patients respond to small doses of stimulant drugs. Specialist advice should be obtained.

Sleep apnoea

In this condition, daytime drowsiness occurs in association with excessive snoring and disturbed respiration at night, usually associated with upper airways obstruction. The typical patient is a middle-aged, overweight man. Treatment consists of relieving the cause of the respiratory obstruction or the obesity. If this is not successful, continuous posi-

tive pressure ventilation using a face mask may be needed.

Sleep–wake schedule disorder

It is well known that short-lived fatigue and transient difficulty in sleeping accompany the changes in bodily rhythms that occur after travel across time zones or changes in shift work. Repeated changes from day to night work may lead to persistent poor sleep, fatigue, and impaired concentration. Management consists of encouragement of greater organization of timetables and sleeping patterns. There is a role for melatonin in selected cases.

Parasomnias

Parasomnias are disturbances of behaviour occurring during sleep. These are: nightmares, night terrors, and sleepwalking. Since all are mainly problems of childhood they are discussed in Chapter 20.

Further Reading

Palmer, B. (2000). *Helping people with eating disorders. A clinical guide to assessment and treatment.* John Wiley, Chichester.
An authoritative practical guide to management.

CHAPTER 13

Suicide and deliberate self-harm

Chapter contents

Suicide and suicidal risk *170*

Deliberate self-harm *176*

Many patients deliberately take drug overdoses or harm themselves in other ways. Some die (suicide); others survive (attempted suicide, parasuicide, or deliberate self-harm). The characteristics of those who kill themselves and those who harm themselves are rather different, although they overlap. The main clinical issues are the assessment of suicide risk and the management of deliberate self-harm.

Suicide accounts for about 1 per cent of deaths. It is rare among children and uncommon in adolescents. Rates increase with age and are higher in men than in women. There are two sets of interacting causes: social factors, especially social isolation, and medical factors, among which depressive disorder, alcoholism, and abnormal personality are particularly important. The *assessment of suicide risk* depends on evaluating:

- the presence of suicidal ideas;
- the presence of psychiatric disorder;
- factors known to be associated with increased risk of suicide.

Referral to a psychiatrist is usually appropriate when the suicidal intentions are strong, associated psychiatric illness is severe, and the person lacks social support. If the risk does not seem to require hospital admission, management depends on ensuring good support, telling the patient how to obtain help quickly if needed, and ensuring that all those who need to know are informed.

Deliberate self-harm is usually by drug overdose, but may be by self-injury, lacerations, and more dangerous methods such as jumping from a height, shooting, drowning. Deliberate self-harm is commonest among younger people but has been increasing in recent years in people of all ages. Predisposing factors include childhood difficulties, adverse social circumstances, and poor health. Precipitating factors include stressful life events, such as quarrels with spouses or others in close relationships. Only a minority have a psychiatric disorder. The motives are complex and often uncertain. Frequently there is no particular wish to die.

Up to a quarter of people who harm themselves do so again in the following year and the risk of suicide during the year is about 1–2 per cent, a hundred times the risk in the general population.

Assessment must include:

• the risk of suicide;

• the risk of further deliberate self-harm;

• current medical and social problems.

Those with severe psychiatric disorder require admission and others need continuing help from a psychiatric outpatient clinic, general practitioner, or other therapist. About a quarter require no special treatment.

Suicide and suicidal risk

Most completed suicides are planned and precautions against discovery are often taken. About one in six leaves a **suicide note**. Some notes are pleas for forgiveness. Other notes are accusing or vindictive, drawing attention to failings in relatives or friends. In most cases, some warning of intention is given to relatives or friends, or to doctors. There is a history of deliberate self-harm in between one-third and one-half of completed suicides.

It is important to understand the epidemiology and causes of suicide for several clinical reasons:

1. As a basis for assessing suicidal risk.

2. To help the relatives and others in the aftermath of suicide.

3. As a guide to suicide prevention.

Epidemiology

In the UK the suicide rate has decreased over recent years (Fig. 13.1) and is about 10 per 100 000 per year (which is in the lower range of rates reported for Western countries). Suicide accounts for about 1 per cent of all deaths. However, official suicide statistics almost certainly underestimate the numbers of actual suicides because uncertain cases are not counted.

Suicide rates are highest in older people, in men, and those who are divorced or unmarried. In most countries, **drug overdoses** (especially analgesics and antidepressants) account for about two-thirds of suicides among women and about one-third of those among men. The remaining deaths are by a variety of **physical means**: hanging, shooting, wounding; drowning, jumping from high places, and falling in front of moving vehicles or trains.

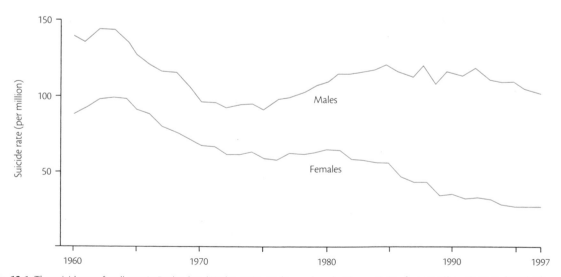

Fig. 13.1 The suicide rate for all ages in England and Wales, 1960–97. (Reproduced with permission from McClure, G. M. G. (2000). Changes in suicide in England and Wales 1960–1997. *British Journal of Psychiatry* **176**, 64–7.)

Causes of suicide

The large international, regional, and temporal variations in the prevalence of suicide reflect the importance of social causes. These causes interact with individual psychiatric and medical factors (Table 13.1). Psychiatric disorder is an important cause of suicide; in contrast it is less important in deliberate self-harm (Table 13.2).

Social causes

Social isolation Compared with the general population, people who have died by suicide are more likely to have been divorced, unemployed, or to be living alone. Social isolation is a common factor among these associations.

Stressful events Suicide is often precipitated by stressful events, including bereavement and other losses.

TABLE 13.1 Causes of suicide

Social

- Old age
- Living alone
- Lack of family and other support
- Stressful events
- Publicity about suicides

Medical

- Depressive disorder
- Alcohol abuse
- Drug abuse
- Schizophrenia
- Personality disorder
- Chronic painful physical illness and epilepsy

TABLE 13.2 Comparison of those who die by suicide and of those who harm themselves

	Suicide	Deliberate self-harm
Age	Older	Younger
Sex	More often male	More often female
Psychiatric disorder	Common, severe	Less common, less severe
Physical illness	Common	Uncommon
Planning	Careful	Impulsive
Method	Lethal	Less dangerous

Social factors influencing the method Social factors also influence the means chosen for suicide. A case that has attracted attention in a community or received wide publicity in newspapers or on television may be followed by others using the same method.

Psychiatric and medical causes

Many of the people who die from suicide have some form of psychiatric disorder at the time of death, most often a depressive illness or alcohol dependence. Some have chronic, painful physical illness.

Depressive disorder The rate of suicide is increased in patients with depressive disorder, with a lifetime risk of about 15 per cent in severe cases. Depressed patients who commit suicide differ from other depressed patients in being *older*, more often *single*, *separated*, or *widowed* and having made more *previous suicide attempts*.

Alcohol abuse also carries a high risk of suicide. The risk is particularly great among: (i) older men with a long history of drinking, a current depressive disorder, and previous deliberate self-harm; and (ii) people whose drinking has caused physical complications, marital problems, difficulties at work, or arrests for drunkenness offences.

Drug abuse also carries an increased risk of suicide.

Schizophrenia has a high risk of suicide, with a lifetime risk of about 10 per cent. The risk is particularly great in younger patients who have retained insight into the serious effect that the illness is likely to have on their lives.

Personality disorder is detected in a third to a half of people who die by suicide. Personality disorder is often associated with other factors that increase the risk of suicide, namely, abuse of alcohol or drugs and social isolation.

Chronic physical illness is associated with suicide, especially among the elderly.

Causes among special groups

Rational suicide Suicide is sometimes the rational act of a mentally healthy person. However, even if the decision appears to have been reached rationally, given more time and more information the person may have changed his intentions. For example, a person with cancer may change a decision to take his life when he learns that there is treatment to relieve pain. Doctors should try to bring about this change of mind, but some rational suicides will take place despite the best treatment.

Physician-assisted suicide has been an increasingly prominent matter of public and medical concern. It raises several important ethical and legal issues:

TABLE 13.3 Clinical issues in physician-assisted suicide

- Need to discuss medical other and opportunities to minimize pain and suffering
- Importance of understanding the patient's and family's views on death
- Importance of treating depression as a cause of the wish to die
- Need to assess the patient's competence and/or review any advance directive
- Need to provide high quality care and support to the patient and family
- Awareness of pressure on the patient from others, for instance those who may benefit financially

1. A conflict between the duty to help the patient and the duty to not do harm.

2. The competence of the patient to decide.

3. The differences between actively promoting death, withholding treatment that might prolong life, and the use of medication that as a side effect may shorten life.

Table 13.3 lists some of the clinical issues that may need to be considered, which may need to be discussed with the patient and family.

Children and young adolescents As noted above, suicide is rare among children and uncommon in adolescents, although rates in older adolescents have increased recently. In adolescence, suicide is associated with broken homes, social isolation, and depression, and also with impetuous behaviour and violence.

Doctors The suicide rate among doctors is greater than that in the general population. The reason is uncertain although several factors have been suggested, such as the ready availability of drugs, increased rates of addiction to alcohol and drugs, the extra stresses of work, reluctance to seek treatment for depressive disorders, and the selection into the medical profession of predisposed personalities.

Suicide pacts In a suicide pact, two people, usually in a close relationship in which one is dominant and the other is passive, agree that at the same time each will die by suicide. These pacts are uncommon and have to be distinguished from murder followed by suicide (occurring sometimes when the murderer has a severe depressive disorder). When one person survives, a suicide pact has to be distinguished from the aiding of suicide by a person who did not intend to die and also from an attempt to disguise murder.

Assessment of suicide risk

Every doctor will encounter at some time patients who express suicidal intentions and must be able to assess the risk of suicide (Table 13.4). This assessment requires:

- the evaluation of suicidal intentions;
- assessment of any previous act of deliberate self-harm (see p. 179);
- the detection of psychiatric disorder;
- assessment of other factors associated with an increased risk of suicide;
- assessment of factors associated with a reduced risk or suicide;
- in some cases, the assessment of associated homicidal ideas.

Evaluation of intentions Some people fear that asking about suicidal intentions will make suicide more likely. It does not, provided that the enquiries are made sympathetically. Indeed, a person who has thought of suicide will feel often better understood when the interviewer raises the issue, and this feeling may reduce the risk. The interviewer can begin by asking whether the patient has thought that life is not worth living. This question can lead to more direct ones about thoughts of suicide, specific plans, and preparatory acts such as saving tablets. Box 13.1 shows a useful standard instrument—the Beck suicide intent scale—which combines these and other informative questions.

When suicidal intentions are revealed they should be taken seriously. *There is no truth in the idea that people who talk of suicide do not enact it*; on the contrary, two-thirds of people dying by suicide have told someone of their intentions. A few people speak so repeatedly of suicide

TABLE 13.4 Risk factors for suicide

Intention	Evidence of intent to die
Psychiatric	Depression
	Schizophrenia
	Personality disorder
	Alcohol and drug dependence
Social and demographic	Older age
	Severe social and interpersonal stressors
	Isolation
Medical	Chronic painful illness and epilepsy

BOX 13.1 BECK SUICIDE INTENT SCALE

Circumstances related to suicidal attempt

1. Isolation

   0 Somebody present

   1 Somebody nearby or in contact (as by phone)

   2 No one nearby or in contact

2. Timing

   0 Timed so that intervention is probable

   1 Timed so that intervention is not likely

   2 Timed so that intervention is highly unlikely

3. Percautions against discovery and/or intervention

   0 No precautions

   1 Passive precautions such as avoiding others but doing nothing to prevent their intervention (alone in a room with unlocked door)

   2 Active precautions such as locked door

4. Acting to gain help during/after attempt

   0 Notified potential helper regarding the attempt

   1 Contacted but did not specifically notify helper regarding the attempt

   2 Did not contact or notify potential helper

5. Final acts in anticipation of death

   0 None

   1 Partial preparation or ideation

   2 Definite plans made (changes in will, giving of gifts, taking out insurance)

6. Degree of planning for suicide attempt

   0 No preparation

   1 Minimal preparation

   2 Extensive preparation

7. Suicide note

   0 Absence of note

   1 Note written but torn up

   2 Presence of note

8. Overt communication of intent before act

   0 None

   1 Equivocal communication

   2 Unequivocal communication

9. Purpose of attempt

   0 Mainly to change environment

   1 Components of '0' and '2'

   2 Mainly to remove self from environment

BOX 13.1 BECK SUICIDE INTENT SCALE (continued)

Self-report

10. Expectations regarding fatality of act

    0 Patient thought that death was unlikely

    1 Patient thought that death was possible but not probable

    2 Patient thought that death was probable or certain

11. Conception of method's lethality

    0 Patient did less to himself than he thought would be lethal

    1 Patient was not sure, or did what he thought might be lethal

    2 Act equalled or exceeded patient's concept of its medical lethality

12. 'Seriousness' of attempt

    0 Patient did not consider act to be a serious attempt to end his life

    1 Patient was uncertain whether act was a serious attempt to end his life

    2 Patient considered act to be a serious attempt to end his life

13. Ambivalence towards living

    0 Patient did not want to die

    1 Patient did not care whether he lived or died

    2 Patient wanted to die

14. Conception of reversibility

    0 Patient thought that death would be unlikely if he received medical attention

    1 Patient was uncertain whether death could be averted by medical attention

    2 Patient was certain of death even if he received medical attention

15. Degree of premeditation

    0 None; impulsive

    1 Suicide contemplated for 3 hours or less prior to attempt

    2 Suicide contemplated for more than 3 hours prior to attempt

(Reprinted with permission from Beck, A. T. *et al.* (1974). *The Prediction of Suicide.* Charles Press, Maryland.)

that they are no longer taken seriously, but some of these people do eventually kill themselves. Therefore their intentions should be evaluated carefully on every occasion.

Previous deliberate self-harm of any kind is an indicator of a substantially increased risk of suicide. Certain features of previous self-harm are particularly important predictors of suicide; these are summarized on p. 178 and in Table 13.5.

Detection of psychiatric disorder is an important part of the assessment of suicide risk. If possible an inform-

ant should be interviewed. *Depressive disorder* is highly important especially when there is severe mood change with hopelessness, insomnia, anorexia, weight loss, or delusions. It is important to remember that suicide may occur during recovery from a depressive disorder in patients who, when more severely depressed, had thought of the act but lacked the initiative to carry it out. *Schizophrenia*, *personality disorder*, and *alcohol and drug dependence* also carry an increased risk of suicide.

Assessment of social and medical general factors associated with increased suicide risk These fac-

TABLE 13.5 Factors predicting suicide after deliberate self-harm

Evidence of intent	Evidence of serious intent (see p. 179)
	Continuing wish to die
	Previous acts of deliberate self-harm
Psychiatric disorder	Depressive disorder
	Alcoholism or drug abuse
	Antisocial personality disorder
Social and demographic	Social isolation
	Unemployment
	Older age group
	Male sex

TABLE 13.6 Risk factors usually leading to the referral, in primary care, to a psychiatrist of patients at risk of suicide

- When suicidal intentions are clearly expressed
- Any change of presentation in a patient who has repeatedly self-harmed
- When associated psychiatric illness is severe
- The person lacks social support

tors have been described above and summarized in Table 13.4 and include old age, loneliness, severe and intractable current life problems, and chronic painful illness or epilepsy.

Factors that may reduce suicide risk These include the availability of good support from the family and others to assist with social, practical, and emotional difficulties.

Homicidal ideas in suicidal patients A few severely depressed suicidal patients have homicidal ideas; for example, the idea that it would be an act of mercy to kill the spouse or a child, in order to spare that person intolerable suffering. If present, such ideas should be taken extremely seriously since they may be carried into practice. It is especially important to be aware of these dangers when assessing a mother of small children.

Management of a patient at risk of suicide

The risk of suicide should be considered in any patient who is depressed or whose behaviour or talk gives any suggestion of the possibility of self-harm. In hospital, inpatient, or emergency departments, evidence of suicidal intent should normally lead to obtaining advice from a specialist. However, other medical staff need to be aware of the general principles of assessment, especially with patients who are reluctant to stay and who are medically fit. Table 13.6 summarizes the reasons for referral.

An exception to the general principle of admission when risk is judged to be high may be made when the patient lives with reliable relatives, who wish to care for the patient, understand their responsibilities, and

are able to fulfil them. In these circumstances, a psychiatric opinion is very often useful. If hospital treatment is essential but the patient refuses it, compulsory admission will be necessary.

A number of patients remain at *long-term suicidal risk* despite specialist assessment that there are no indications that hospital treatment would be of benefit. An example would be a patient with longstanding problems who has had intensive psychiatric and social help without benefit, and for whom it is evident that further hospital admission would do nothing to help with the long-term problems in everyday life. Such a decision requires a particularly thorough knowledge of the patient and his problems and should generally be made by a psychiatrist in conjunction with the general practitioner.

The four main principles of treatment are as follow.

1. **Prevention of harm**. The obvious first requirement is to prevent the patient from self-harm by preventing access to methods of harm and appropriately close observation. Most patients at serious suicidal risk require *admission to hospital*. The first requirement is the safety of the patient. To achieve this requires an adequate number of vigilant nursing staff, an agreed assessment of the level of risk, and good communication between staff. If the risk is very great, nursing may need to be continuous so that the patient is never alone. If *outpatient treatment* is chosen the patient and relatives should be told how to obtain help quickly if the strength of suicidal ideas increases, for example an emergency telephone number. Frustrated attempts to find help can make suicide more likely.

2. **Treatment of any associated mental illness** should be initiated without delay.

3. **Reviving hope**. However determined the patient is to die, there is usually some remaining wish to live. These positive feelings can be encouraged and the patient helped towards a more positive view of the

future. One way to begin this process is to show concern for the problems.

4. **Problem solving**. Initially overwhelming problems can usually be improved if they are dealt with one by one.

Help after a suicide

When a person has died by suicide, help is required by the surviving relatives and friends who may need to deal with feelings of loss, guilt, or anger. They should have a full explanation of the nature and reasons for medical and other actions to assess the suicidal risk, to treat the causes, and prevent harm. They should also have an opportunity to discuss their own feelings, including guilt that if they had behaved differently the suicide could have been prevented. Those most directly involved in the previous care of the dead person should offer to meet the relatives as soon after the suicide as possible and to meet again at a later stage if the family and friends believe it would be helpful. The relatives' distress may be considerable and may be expressed indirectly in complaints about medical care. Some relatives suffer from longstanding psychiatric or other problems that deserve treatment in their own right.

The doctor should also support other professional staff who had been closely involved with the patient. After suicide, the case should be reviewed carefully to determine whether useful lessons can be learnt about future clinical practice. This review should not be conducted as a search for a person at fault; some patients die by suicide however carefully the correct procedures have been followed.

Suicide prevention

There are three main approaches to prevention: early recognition and help for those at risk and the modification of predisposing social factors.

1. **Identifying high-risk patients**. Many people who commit suicide have contacted their doctors shortly beforehand, and many of these have a psychiatric disorder or alcohol dependence. Doctors can identify at least some of these patients as being at high risk, and offer help.

2. **Supporting those at risk**. This is mainly the responsibility of pteh rimary care and social agencies. Organizations such as the Samaritans give emergency 24-hour support to people who feel lonely and hopeless and express suicidal ideas, but it has not been shown convincingly that this support reduces suicide.

3. In addition it is possible that there are opportunities for the **modification of predisposing social factors**:

   ♦ *Reducing the means of suicide* may help reduce suicide (e.g. providing safety rails at high places, prescribing cautiously). However, people determined on suicide can find other means, such as overdoses of non-prescribed drugs.

   ♦ *Education* might be provided for teenagers about the dangers of drug overdosage and about ways of coping with emotional problems. However, there is little evidence that such education is effective.

   ♦ *Public health or social and economic policy.* Isolation and other social factors that increase the risk of suicide cannot be modified by the medical profession, they require public policy decisions.

Deliberate self-harm

Deliberate self-harm is not usually failed suicide. Only about a quarter of those who have deliberately harmed themselves say they wished to die; most say the act was impulsive rather than premeditated (Fig. 13.2). The rest find it difficult to explain the reasons or say that:

♦ they were *seeking unconsciousness* as a temporary escape or relief from their problems;

♦ they were trying to *influence another person* to change their behaviour (e.g. to make a partner feel guilty for threatening to end the relationship);

♦ that they are *uncertain* whether or not they intended to die—they were 'leaving it to fate';

♦ they were trying to get *help*.

Epidemiology

Deliberate self-harm is common and rates have risen progressively over the last 30 years. It now accounts for about 10 per cent of acute medical admissions in the UK. A further smaller number are seen by general practitioners but are not sent to hospital because the medical risks are low, or they attend emergency departments but are not admitted.

Epidemiological studies have identified the kind of people who are more likely to harm themselves and the methods that are commonly used. Deliberate self-harm is more common among four main groups:

1. *Younger adults* (Fig. 13.3): the rates decline sharply during adult life. (They are also very low in children under the age of 12 years.)

2. *Young women*, particularly those aged 15–20 years.

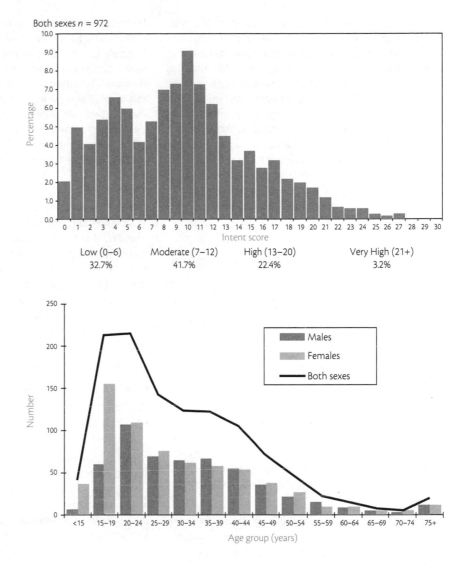

Fig. 13.2 Beck scores in deliberate self-harm attenders in 2001. (Reproduced with permission of Professor K. E. Hawton, Oxford University.)

Fig. 13.3 The age groups of deliberate self-harm patients by sex in 2001. (Reproduced with permission of Professor K. E. Hawton, Oxford University.)

3. People of *low socioeconomic status.*

4. *Divorced individuals, teenage wives,* and *younger single adults.*

Methods of deliberate self-harm

Drug overdosage In the UK, about 90 per cent of the cases of deliberate self-harm treated by general hospitals are by a drug overdose. The drugs taken most commonly in overdose are *anxiolytics, non-opiate analgesics,* such as salicylates and paracetamol, and *antidepressants.* Paracetamol is particularly dangerous because it damages the liver and may lead to delayed death, sometimes in patients who had not taken the drugs with the intention of dying. Antidepressants are taken in about

a fifth of cases: of these drugs, tricyclics are particularly hazardous in overdosage since they may cause cardiac arrhythmias or convulsions. Despite these and other dangers, most deliberate drug overdoses do not present a serious threat to life.

Use of alcohol About half the men and a quarter of the women who harm themselves have taken alcohol in the 6 hours before the act. This often precipitates the act by reducing self-restraint. Its effects interact with those of the drugs.

Self-injury In the UK, between 5 and 15 per cent of all cases of deliberate self-harm treated in general hospitals are self-inflicted injuries. Most of these injuries are *lacerations,* usually of the forearm or wrists. Most patients who cut themselves are young, have low self-esteem, impulsive or aggressive behaviour, unstable moods, difficulties in interpersonal relationships, and often problems of alcohol or drug abuse. Usually, the self-laceration follows a period of increasing tension and irritability, which is relieved by the self-injury. The cuts are usually multiple and superficial, often made with a razor blade or a piece of glass. Less frequent and medically more serious forms of self-injury include more serious lacerations, jumping from heights or in front of a moving train or motor vehicle, shooting, or drowning. These highly dangerous acts occur mainly among people who intended to die but have survived.

Causes

Deliberate self-harm is usually the result of multiple social and personal factors (Table 13.7), including national and local attitudes. Overall, rates appear to be affected by awareness of the occurrence and methods of self-harm in a population; for example, television and press reports and local knowledge of suicide and attempted suicide in the neighbourhood. Psychiatric disorder is less important than in suicide.

Social and family factors

Predisposing factors Evidence of childhood emotional deprivation is common. Many patients who harm themselves have long-term marital problems, extra-marital relationships, or other relationship problems, and may have financial and other social difficulties. Rates of unemployment are greater than in the general population.

Precipitating factors Stressful life events are frequent before the act of self-harm, especially quarrels with or threats of rejection by spouses or sexual partners.

Association with psychiatric disorder Although many patients who harm themselves are anxious or depressed, relatively few have a psychiatric disorder other than an acute stress reaction, adjustment disorder, or personality disorder. The latter is found in about one-third to one-half of self-harm patients, and dependence on alcohol is also frequent. (In contrast, psychiatric disorder is common among patients who die by suicide, see p. 171.)

The difference between factors associated with suicide and deliberate self-harm are summarized in Table 13.2.

Outcome

Since deliberate self-harm results from long-term adverse social factors and is associated with personality disorder, it is not surprising that a significant proportion of subjects have a poor overall outcome in terms of personal and social adjustment. More specifically, outcome is assessed in terms of the repetition of self-harm and suicide. Between 15 and 25 per cent of people who harm themselves do so again in the following year and 1–2 per cent commit suicide. Of those who harm themselves again:

* some repeat the act only once;

* some repeat the act several times within a period in which there are continuing severe stressful events;

* a few repeat the act many times over a long period as a habitual response to minor stressors.

The factors associated with the repetition of deliberate self-harm are shown in Table 13.8.

People who have deliberately harmed themselves have a much increased risk of later suicide (Fig. 13.4). In the year after the self-harm, the risk of suicide is about 1–2 per cent, that is about a hundred times the risk in

---

TABLE 13.7 Causes of deliberate self-harm

* Psychiatric disorder
* Personality disorder
* Alcohol dependence
* Predisposing social factors
* Early parental loss
* Parental neglect or abuse
* Long-term social problems: family, employment, financial
* Poor physical health
* Precipitating social factors
* Stressful life problems

TABLE 13.8 Factors predicting the repetition of deliberate self-harm

* Previous deliberate self-harm before the current episode
* Previous psychiatric treatment
* Alcohol or drug abuse
* Personality disorder
* Criminal record
* History of violence
* Low social class
* Unemployment
* Age 25–54 years
* Single, divorced, or separated

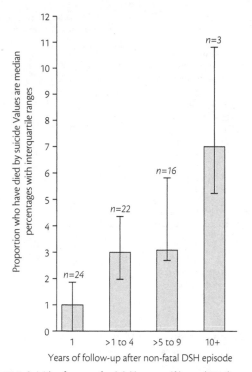

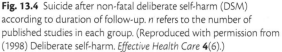

Fig. 13.4 Suicide after non-fatal deliberate self-harm (DSM) according to duration of follow-up. *n* refers to the number of published studies in each group. (Reproduced with permission from (1998) Deliberate self-harm. *Effective Health Care* **4**(6).)

the general population. The risk factors for suicide after deliberate self harm are shown in Table 13.5.

It is important to note that a *non-dangerous method of self-harm does not necessarily indicate a low risk of subsequent suicide* (although the risk is higher when a violent or dangerous method has been used).

Assessment

Every act of deliberate self-harm should be assessed thoroughly. For many patients seen in primary care, the physical consequences of the act and concern about the risk of repetition will lead to hospital referral. In other cases, referral may not be necessary; for instance, when the act was not reported until some time later, when the results are clearly not medically serious, where suicidal intent was low, and where the patient and family are known to the doctor.

All deliberate self-harm patients seen in hospital emergency departments should have a psychiatric and social assessment (Fig. 13.5). This assessment can be carried out by a psychiatrist, by general medical staff, or by psychiatric nurses or social workers with appropriate special training. All patients found on this assess-

ment to be suffering from psychiatric disorder or with a high risk of further self-harm should be seen by a psychiatrist. Since many patients who are medically fit do not wish to stay for specialist assessment, it is essential that all emergency department medical staff are competent to assess risk.

The assessment should be carried out in a way that encourages patients to undertake a constructive review of their problems and of the ways they can deal with them. If patients can then resolve their problems in this way, they may be able to do so again in the future instead of resorting to self-harm.

When to assess

When patients have recovered sufficiently from the physical effects of the self-harm they should be interviewed, if possible, where the discussion will not be overheard or interrupted. After a drug overdose, the first step is to determine whether consciousness is impaired; if it is, the interview should be delayed until the patient has recovered further and can concentrate on the questions.

Sources of information

Information should also be obtained from relatives or friends, the general practitioner, and any other person (such as a social worker) already involved in the patient's care. Such information frequently adds significantly to the account given by the patient.

Information required

What were the patient's intentions before and at the time of the attempt? Patients whose behaviour suggests that they intended to die as a result of the act of self-harm are at greater risk of a subsequent fatal act of self-harm. Intent is assessed by considering:

◆ was the act *planned* or carried out on impulse?

◆ were *precautions* taken against being found?

◆ did the patient seek *help after the act*?

◆ was the *method dangerous*? Not only should the objective risk be assessed, but also the risk anticipated by the patient, which may be different (e.g. if he believed that he had taken a lethal dose of a drug even though he had not);

◆ was there a *'final act'* such as writing a suicide note or making a will?

Does the patient now wish to die? The interviewer should ask directly whether the patient is pleased to have recovered or wishes to die. If the act suggested serious suicidal intent, but the patient denies such

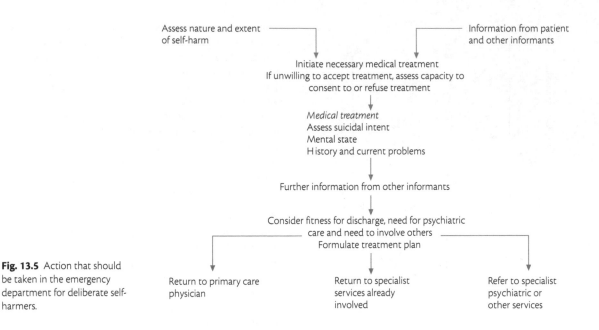

Fig. 13.5 Action that should be taken in the emergency department for deliberate self-harmers.

intent, the interviewer should try to find out by tactful but thorough questioning whether there has been a genuine change of resolve.

What are the current problems? Many patients will have experienced a mounting series of difficulties in the weeks or months leading up to the act of self-harm. Some of these difficulties may have been resolved by the time the patient is interviewed, but if serious problems remain, the risk of a fatal repetition is greater. This risk is particularly great if the problems are of loneliness or ill health. Possible problems should be reviewed systematically covering: *intimate relationships* with the spouse or another person; *relations with children and other relatives*; *employment, finance,* and *housing*; *legal problems*; *social isolation*; *bereavement*, and *other losses.*

Is there psychiatric disorder? This question is answered with information obtained from the history, from a brief but systematic examination of the mental state, and also from other informants and from medical notes.

What are the patient's resources? These include the capacity to solve problems, material resources, and the help that others can provide. The best guide to future ability to solve problems is the past record of dealing with difficulties such as the loss of a job, or a broken relationship. The availability of help should be assessed by asking about the patient's friends and relatives, and about support available from medical services, social workers, or voluntary agencies.

Is treatment required and will the patient agree to it? Of the patients referred to hospital for treatment of deliberate self-harm:

- about 1 in 10 need immediate inpatient psychiatric treatment, usually for a depressive disorder or alcohol dependency; or for a period of respite from overwhelming stressors;

- about two-thirds need care from a psychiatric outpatient team or from the primary practitioner (but many do not accept this help);

- about one-quarter require no special treatment because their self-harm was a response to temporary difficulties and carried little risk of repetition.

Management

Management (see Fig. 13.5) aims to:

- treat any psychiatric disorder;

- manage high suicide risk;

- enable the patient to resolve the difficulties that led to the act of self-harm;

- enable the patient to deal with future crises without resorting to self-harm.

The mainstay of treatment is *problem solving* (see p. 257) based on the list of problems compiled during the assessment. The patient is encouraged to consider what steps he could take to resolve each of these problems, and to formulate a practical plan for tackling them one at a time. Throughout this discussion, the therapist helps the patient to do as much as possible to help himself. When there are interpersonal problems, it is often helpful to have a joint or family discussion.

Results of treatment

Successful treatment of a depressive or other psychiatric disorder reduces the risk of subsequent self-harm. There is less strong evidence that problem solving and other psychological methods reduce repetition, although they do reduce personal and social problems. This lack of strong evidence may be due, in part, to the methodological difficulties of randomized trials in this heterogeneous population. Particular types of psychological or social problem have been shown to benefit from specific treatments, such as couple therapy for problems between couples, problem solving for practical and everyday difficulties, and cognitive behaviour treatment for longstanding personal difficulties.

Management of special groups

There are certain subgroups of patients who pose special management problems. In most cases, specialist advice should be obtained.

Mothers of young children Because there is an association between deliberate self-harm and child abuse, it is important to ask any mother with young children about her feelings towards the children; and to enquire from other informants, as well as the patient, about their welfare. If there is a possibility of child abuse or neglect, appropriate assessment action should be carried out (see p. 297). There is also an association between depression and infanticide.

Children and adolescents Deliberate self-harm is uncommon among young children, but becomes increasingly frequent after the age of 12, especially among girls. The most common method is drug overdosage; in only a few cases is there a threat to life. Self-injury also occurs, more often among boys than girls.

The motivation of self-harm in young children is difficult to determine, but it is more often to communicate distress or escape from stress than to die. Deliberate self-harm in children and adolescents is associated with broken homes, family psychiatric disorder, and child abuse. It is often precipitated by difficulties with parents, boyfriends or girlfriends, or school work.

Most children and adolescents do not repeat an act of deliberate self-harm, but an important minority do, usually in association with severe psychosocial problems. These repeated acts of deliberate self-harm carry a significant risk of suicide. Children or adolescents who harm themselves should be assessed by a child psychiatrist. Treatment is not only of the young person but also of the family.

Patients who refuse assessment and treatment Some patients try to leave hospital before emergency gastric lavage and other treatment. Others seek to do so before psychological assessment can be completed. In most countries, there is a legal power to detain those who require potentially life-saving treatment and whose competence or capacity to take an informed decision about discharge is likely to be impaired by their mental state. The doctor should obtain as much information about the mental state and suicidal risk as time allows. The patient should only be allowed to leave hospital when serious suicidal risk has been excluded.

In taking decisions about emergency treatment, the doctor is likely to be helped by relatives, inpatient medical notes, by telephoning the primary care doctor, and

---

BOX 13.2 PATIENTS WHO HARM THEMSELVES AND REFUSE TREATMENT

- There are wide differences in national procedures, practice, and legislation.

- The patient who has harmed himself and is alert and conscious should be presumed to be competent to refuse medical advice and treatment unless there is evidence to the contrary.

- The most senior experienced doctor available should be prepared to discuss the need for treatment, the alternatives, and the patient's anxieties. It is often appropriate to involve relatives. Calm, sympathetic discussion is often effective in enabling the patient to decide to consent to treatment.

- Capacity should be assessed (see p. 320), preferably by a psychiatrist.

- If the patient is competent and continues to refuse consent, the consequences should be clearly outlined to the patient and the discussion fully recorded. The patient should be allowed to go, but encouraged to return. Where possible, an alternative plan should be agreed with the patient and, if possible, relatives or friends. If the patient is assessed as being incompetent, then the reasons should be recorded fully. Emergency treatment should proceed and a compulsory order under mental health legislation sought.

any other doctor, social worker, or person who has been involved with the patient in the past. It is essential to write detailed notes and to be aware of the legal requirements about both emergency treatment and confidentiality (Box 13.2).

Frequent repeaters Some people take overdoses repeatedly, often at times of stress in circumstances that suggest that the behaviour is to reduce tension or gain attention. These people usually have a personality disorder and many insoluble social problems. Although sometimes directed towards gaining attention, repeated self-harm may cause relatives to become unsympathetic or hostile, and these feelings may be shared by professional staff as their repeated efforts at help are seen to fail. Usually, little can be done to change the pattern of behaviour. Neither counselling nor intensive psychotherapy is effective, and management is limited to providing support. Sometimes a change in life circumstances is followed by improvement, but unless this happens the risk of death by suicide is high.

Deliberate self-laceration It is difficult to help people who lacerate themselves repeatedly. They often have low self-esteem and experience extreme tension. They also often have difficulty in recognizing feelings and expressing them in words. Efforts should be made to increase self-esteem and to find an alternative, simple way of relieving tension, for example by taking exercise. Anxiolytic drugs are seldom helpful and may produce disinhibition. If drug treatment is needed to reduce tension, a phenothiazine is more likely to be effective.

Further reading

Hawton, K. E. and van Heemingen, K. (eds.). (2000). *The international handbook of suicide and attempted suicide.* John Wiley, Chischester.
Substantial and authoritative reference work with chapters by leading experts.

CHAPTER 14

Problems due to use of alcohol and other psychoactive substances

Chapter contents

Problems due to the use of alcohol *184*

Treatment of people with alcohol problems *192*

Problems due to the use of psychoactive substances *195*

This chapter is about the medical conditions caused by the use of alcohol, psychoactive drugs, and certain other chemical substances. Health problems may arise following substance use due to intoxication, withdrawal, tolerance, and dependence.

Intoxication The psychological and physical effects of the substance that disappear when the substance is eliminated.

Withdrawal Symptoms and signs occurring when the substance is reduced or stopped. The nature, time to onset, and course of the symptoms vary for different substances.

Tolerance The state in which repeated administration leads to decreasing effect.

Dependence A syndrome that includes withdrawal states, sometimes tolerance, and other features such as persistent use despite harmful effects. Dependence may be both *physical* (when physiological tolerance occurs) and *psychological*. A person is said to have a **dependence syndrome** if they have experienced three of the following six characteristics in the past 12 months:

1. A *strong desire* or sense of compulsion to take the substance.

2. *Difficulties in refraining* from using the substance, *stopping* using it, or *limiting* the amount taken.

3. A physiological *withdrawal* state when substance use has stopped or been reduced. Withdrawal symptoms may be avoided by further use of the substance.

4. Evidence of *tolerance*, a state in which increasing doses of the substance are required to produce the effect originally produced by lower doses.

5. Progressive *neglect of alternative pleasures or interests* due to the use of the psychoactive substance and in the time needed to obtain supplies, or to recover from its effects.

6. *Persistent use* of the substance *despite* clear evidence of *harm*.

Problems due to substance use are very common. Doctors in all branches of medicine need to know how to recognize and manage the various manifestations.

Problems due to the use of alcohol

Terminology

Although the term **alcoholism** is widely used in every-day speech, it has too broad a meaning to be clinically useful. It can refer to excessive consumption of alcohol, to dependence on alcohol, or to the damage caused by excessive use. The following terms define more useful categories:

- **Harmful use of alcohol** refers to a pattern of use that has caused actual mental or physical damage to the user.

- **Dangerous use** refers to a level of consumption that increases the risk of future harm (see below).

- **Problem drinking** is drinking that has caused mental, physical, or social harm but not necessarily dependence.

Central to these categories is the concept of **alcohol-related disability**, which refers to any mental, physical, or social harm resulting from excessive alcohol consumption. Both *harmful* and *dangerous use* may exist together; for example, a drinker who has already damaged his health may continue to drink heavily in a way that will cause more damage in the future. We will refer collectively to dangerous use, harmful use, and alcohol dependence as **alcohol problems**.

What is a safe level of alcohol consumption?

The relation between alcohol consumption and harm is not straightforward. Low levels of alcohol consumption may protect older people against coronary heart disease. Very high levels clearly do harm but where is the dividing line between safe and unsafe consumption? To answer this question we need a way of quantifying consumption. A widely accepted measure is in terms of

units of alcohol; one unit is 8 g of ethanol, and corresponds to the following measures in which alcohol is usually consumed:

- half a pint of beer;

- a wine glass of wine;

- a sherry glass of sherry or other fortified wine;

- a standard measure of spirits.

These measures are clinically useful but should not be regarded as precise because the strengths of different beers and wines vary.

Although it is difficult to assess the exact relationship between intake and harm, it is generally agreed that the 'safe level' of alcohol consumption is:

- men: up to **21 units** per week;

- women: up to **14 units** per week (lower because of the lower average body weight of females);

provided that the whole amount is not taken on one occasion and that there are occasional drink-free days. This level is equivalent, for example, to an average of three half pints of beer a day for a man. These limits should be modified in some patients, for example pregnant women should be advised to abstain from alcohol.

Dangerous levels of drinking (i.e. levels of consumption at which harm is likely) are:

- men: over **50 units** per week;

- women: over **35 units** per week.

Strictly speaking, levels of drinking between the safe and dangerous amounts should be called **hazardous**. In this chapter, for simplicity, we refer to all consumption greater than the safe level as *dangerous use*.

Alcohol consumption in the population

Reliable epidemiological data are difficult to obtain because people tend to underestimate both the amount they drink and the consequences of their drinking. In the General Household Survey in the UK (Fig. 14.1), the majority of the population reported safe levels of consumption with only a minority drinking more heavily. Records of the national consumption of alcohol reveal marked international variations in alcohol consumption per capita. European countries such as France and Italy have higher levels of consumption than countries such as the USA and UK—although the differences are decreasing with time. Countries with higher alcohol consumption have higher death rates from cirrhosis of the liver. Dangerous use of alcohol has increased among young women as their social roles have changed.

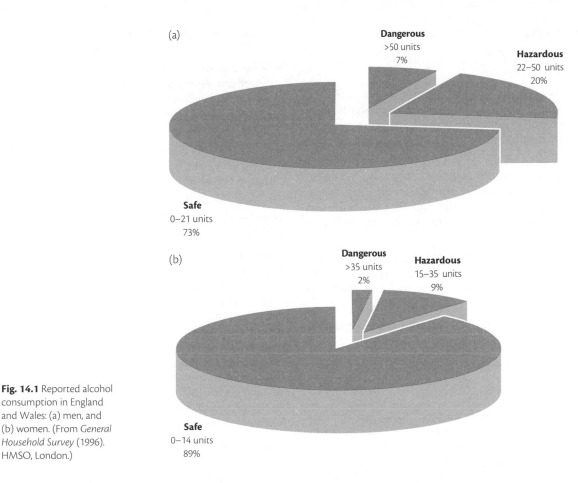

(a)

Dangerous
>50 units
7%

Hazardous
22–50 units
20%

Safe
0–21 units
73%

(b)

Dangerous
>35 units
2%

Hazardous
15–35 units
9%

Safe
0–14 units
89%

Fig. 14.1 Reported alcohol consumption in England and Wales: (a) men, and (b) women. (From *General Household Survey* (1996). HMSO, London.)

Factors associated with high alcohol consumption

Several factors are associated with the consumption of greater amounts of alcohol by individuals.

Population levels of consumption The higher the average consumption in a community, the greater the number of people who drink dangerous amounts of alcohol. This is because the consumption of alcohol in the general population is normally distributed—thus the higher average is not due to an outlying group of very heavy drinkers. This has an important practical implication. It means that population-based methods aimed at reducing everyone's level of alcohol consumption will reduce the number of people who drink dangerous amounts of alcohol (see below).

Age and sex The heaviest drinkers are among young men in their late teens and early twenties. In recent years, increased consumption of alcohol has been identified among 15–16-year-olds. Fewer women than men drink dangerous amounts of alcohol, but the rates in women are rising more quickly than in men. Women

in professional and managerial employment are most likely to drink dangerous amounts of alcohol.

Occupation The rates of dangerous consumption of alcohol are much increased among people working in occupations that provide easy access to alcohol, for example barmen, brewery workers, and kitchen porters. They are also higher among executives, salesmen, journalists, and actors, and others whose work is associated with social drinking. Doctors also have high rates of dangerous consumption.

Genetic factors Harmful drinking runs in families but this could be because of social factors. The evidence from twin studies is conflicting.

Personality factors such as anxiety and impulsiveness are suggested by clinical experience, but there is little good evidence for such an association.

Alcohol-related harm

Consumption of alcohol can lead to three types of harm (each of which is described later):

◆ physical;

◆ neuropsychiatric;

◆ social.

This harm can occur whether or not the person has become dependent on alcohol, although very high levels of consumption are likely to cause dependency. There are three main mechanisms of alcohol-related harm.

1. **Intoxication**. This includes a *direct toxic effect* on certain tissues, notably the brain and liver, and an increased *risk of accidents* (particularly road traffic accidents and accidents in the home) and *public order offences*.

2. **Chronic consumption**. This may lead to poor diet and a *deficiency of protein* and *B vitamins*, and *general neglect* that can lead to increased susceptibility to infection.

3. **Dependence**. When present, this may lead to serious withdrawal syndromes (see below).

Physical effects of alcohol abuse

The main physical consequences of dangerous use of alcohol (Table 14.1) are:

◆ **Gastrointestinal disorders**. These are common, notably gastritis and peptic ulcer; damage to the liver; oesophageal varices and carcinoma; and acute or chronic pancreatitis. Damage to the liver includes fatty infiltration, hepatitis, cirrhosis, and hepatoma.

TABLE 14.1 Physical effects of the excessive use of alcohol

Alimentary	Gastritis and peptic ulcer
	Oesophageal varices
	Oesophageal carcinoma
	Acute and chronic pancreatitis
	Hepatitis and cirrhosis
Neurological	Peripheral neuropathy
	Dementia
	Cerebellar degeneration
	Epilepsy
Other	Anaemia
	Episodic hypoglycaemia
	Haemochromatosis
	Cardiomyopathy
	Myopathy
	Obesity

A person dependent on alcohol has a ten-fold greater risk than average of dying of cirrhosis of the liver.

◆ **Disorders of the nervous system**. These include peripheral neuropathy, dementia, cerebellar degeneration, and epilepsy; as well as several less common effects on the optic nerve, pons, and corpus callosum. Neuropsychiatric disorders are described below.

◆ **Other physical disorders** include anaemia, episodic hypoglycaemia, haemochromatosis, cardiomyopathy, and myopathy.

From these and other causes, the overall **mortality rate** of subjects consuming dangerous levels of alcohol is estimated to be about twice the expected level.

Effects on the fetus

Very heavy drinking during pregnancy may cause a syndrome of facial abnormality, low weight, low intelligence, and overactivity (**fetal alcohol syndrome**). It is uncertain whether such effects are seen only after very heavy drinking by the mother, or whether lesser degrees of damage are seen after less heavy drinking. Nevertheless, it is prudent to advise pregnant women to abstain from alcohol throughout pregnancy. If they will not accept this advice, they should be counselled strongly to avoid drinking in the first trimester, and to avoid heavy drinking.

Neuropsychiatric disorders due to alcohol abuse

Alcohol-related psychiatric disabilities fall into four groups: (i) abnormal forms of intoxication; (ii) withdrawal phenomena; (iii) chronic or nutritional disorders; and (iv) associated psychiatric disorders (Table 14.2).

Abnormal forms of intoxication

As well as the familiar picture of drunkenness, people who consume dangerous amounts of alcohol persistently may develop two syndromes.

◆ **Memory blackouts** are losses of memory for events that occurred during a period of intoxication. Such episodes can occur after a single episode of heavy drinking in people who do not habitually abuse alcohol. When they occur regularly they indicate frequent heavy drinking; when they are prolonged, affecting the greater part of a day or whole days, they indicate sustained excessive drinking.

◆ **Idiosyncratic intoxication** (or pathological drunkenness) is a marked change of behaviour occurring within minutes of taking alcohol in amounts that would not induce drunkenness in most people. Often, the behaviour is aggressive. The condition is rare although apparent cases may occur after a small

TABLE 14.2 Neuropsychiatric effects of the excessive use of alcohol

Intoxication states	Memory blackouts
	Idiosyncratic intoxication
Withdrawal states	Delirium tremens
Toxic and nutritional states	Korsakov's syndrome
	Wernicke's encephalopathy
	Alcoholic dementia
Associated states	Depressive disorder
	Anxiety symptoms
	Suicide and deliberate self-harm
	Personality change
	Pathological jealousy
	Sexual dysfunction
	Transient hallucinations
	Alcoholic hallucinosis

further intake of alcohol in a person who already has a raised blood alcohol from unadmitted drinking.

Withdrawal phenomena

These are described on p. 188.

Toxic and nutritional conditions

There are three neuropsychiatric disorders of this kind: (i) **Korsakov's syndrome**; (ii) **Wernicke's encephalopathy**; and (iii) **alcoholic dementia**. (The first two are described in Chapter 10, pp. 143–4, because alcohol is not their only cause.)

Alcoholic dementia can arise after a prolonged, heavy intake of alcohol. Intellectual impairment is often associated with enlarged ventricles and widened cerebral sulci, as seen on a computerized tomography (CT) scan. After prolonged abstinence, some gradual improvement occurs in these changes, suggesting that the shrinkage is not wholly due to the loss of the brain cells. The *causes* of the dementia are uncertain but probably include a direct toxic effect of alcohol on the brain, and secondary effects of liver disease.

Associated psychiatric disorders

◆ **Depressive disorder** can be induced by prolonged dangerous use of alcohol, but depressed patients sometimes drink heavily to relieve their symptoms, so care needs to be taken to find out the sequence of changes.

◆ **Anxiety symptoms** occur commonly, especially during periods of partial withdrawal. Also, some patients with an anxiety disorder due to other causes, drink to relieve anxiety. So, as with depression, care is needed to determine the sequence.

◆ **Suicidal behaviour and deliberate self-harm** are more frequent among people who use alcohol heavily than among other people of the same age. Estimates of the proportion of harmful users of alcohol who eventually kill themselves vary from 6 to 20 per cent.

◆ **Personality change** in heavy users of alcohol often includes self-centredness, lack of concern for others, and a decline in standards of conduct, particularly honesty and responsibility.

◆ **Pathological jealousy** is an infrequent but serious complication of heavy alcohol use (see pp. 133–4.) Non-delusional suspiciousness of the sexual partner is more common.

◆ **Sexual dysfunction** is common, usually as erectile dysfunction or delayed ejaculation. The causes include the direct effects of alcohol, and a generally impaired relationship with the sexual partner as a result of heavy drinking.

◆ **Transient hallucinations** of vision or hearing are reported by some heavy drinkers, generally during withdrawal, but without all the features of delirium tremens or alcoholic hallucinosis.

◆ **Alcoholic hallucinosis** is a rare condition characterized by distressing *auditory hallucinations*, usually of voices uttering threats, occurring *in clear consciousness*. Some patients argue aloud with the voices, others feel compelled to follow instructions from them. *Delusional misinterpretations* may follow, often of a persecutory kind, so that the clinical picture can resemble schizophrenia. The condition can arise while the person is still drinking heavily, or when intake has been reduced. It is of variable duration and when chronic needs to be distinguished from a primary schizophrenic disorder.

Social damage due to alcohol

Excessive drinking can cause serious social damage including:

◆ family violence;

◆ emotional and conduct problems in the patient's children;

◆ poor work performance and sickness absence;

◆ unemployment;

◆ road accidents: in the UK about a third of drivers killed on the road have blood alcohol levels above the statutory limit, and among those killed on a Saturday night the figure is estimated to be three-quarters;

◆ crime, mainly social disorder and petty offences, but also with fraud, sexual offences, and crimes of violence including murder.

Alcohol withdrawal syndrome

Withdrawal symptoms appear characteristically on waking, after the fall in blood alcohol concentration during sleep. The earliest and commonest feature is acute *tremulousness* affecting the hands, legs, and trunk ('the shakes'). The sufferer may be unable to sit still, hold a cup steady, or do up buttons. He is also *agitated* and easily startled, and often dreads facing people or crossing the road.

Nausea, *retching*, and *sweating* are frequent. If alcohol is taken, these symptoms are usually relieved quickly; it not, they may last for several days.

As withdrawal progresses, *misperceptions and hallucinations* may occur, usually only briefly. Objects appear distorted in shape, or shadows seems to move; disorganized voices, shouting, or snatches of music may be heard. Later there may be *epileptic seizures*, and finally, after about 48 hours, **delirium tremens** may develop.

Delirium tremens

This is a severe form of withdrawal syndrome that occurs when the patient is physically dependent on alcohol. The features are:

◆ *Those seen in any delirium*: clouding of consciousness, disorientation in time and place, impairment of recent memory, illusions and hallucinations (see below), fearfulness and agitation.

◆ *Special features* of gross tremor of the hands (which gives the condition its name), autonomic disturbance (sweating, tachycardia, raised blood pressure, dilation of the pupils), and marked insomnia. There may also be fever.

◆ *Hallucinations* are characteristically visual and often frightening, involving people or animals. Auditory and tactile hallucinations also occur.

◆ *Dehydration and electrolyte disturbance* are characteristic. Blood testing shows leucocytosis, a raised erythrocyte sedimentation rate (ESR), and impaired liver function.

Delirium tremens usually last 3–4 days. As in other kinds of delirium (see pp. 138–40), the symptoms are characteristically worse at night. The condition often ends in deep and prolonged sleep from which the person awakes with no symptoms and little or no memory of the period of delirium. The *treatment* of delirium tremens (p. 193) is described for withdrawal plus the general measures for treating delirium on pp. 138–40.

Alcohol dependence syndrome

Heavy drinking can lead to an alcohol dependence syndrome with the general features described above (see pp. 183–4). The specific features of alcohol dependence are that in the late stages of dependence, due to liver damage, tolerance falls and the dependent drinker becomes incapacitated after only a few drinks. Since they can stave off withdrawal symptoms only by further drinking (**relief drinking**), many dependent drinkers take a drink on waking. In most cultures, early morning drinking is diagnostic of dependency. With an increasing need to stave off withdrawal symptoms during the day, the drinker typically becomes secretive about the amount consumed, hides bottles, or carries them in a pocket or handbag. Rough cider and cheap wines may be drunk regularly to obtain the most alcohol for the least money. A person dependent on alcohol develops a **stereotyped pattern of drinking**. Whereas the ordinary drinker varies his intake from day to day, the dependent person drinks at regular intervals to relieve or avoid withdrawal symptoms.

Course and prognosis The syndrome becomes established most often in the mid forties for men, and a few years later for women. It is now occurring increasingly among teenagers, and is sometimes seen for the first time in elderly people after retirement. Once established, the syndrome usually progresses steadily and destructively, unless the patient stops drinking or manages to bring it under control. A severely dependent person who achieves abstinence but then drinks again, is likely to relapse quickly and totally, returning to his old drinking pattern within a few days (**reinstatement after abstinence**).

Preventing alcohol-related harm

Population-based approaches

As described above (see pp. 184–5), the population mean consumption predicts the number of people with alcohol problems. The aim of population-based approaches is to reduce the average level of consumption in the population and, by doing so, reduce the amount of alcohol problems (Fig. 14.2). This can potentially be achieved in several ways:

1. *Raising the price* of alcoholic drinks by taxation.

2. *Licensing laws* to limit the hours when alcohol is available.

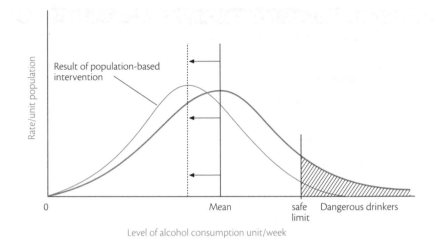

Fig. 14.2 Population-based approaches to reducing alcohol-related harm.

3. *Control of advertising and media portrayal of alcoholic drinks*. It is not certain how effective such measures would be—a ban on press and television advertising in British Columbia, Canada, made little difference.

4. *Controlling the sale* of alcohol by limiting sales in shops. It is known that the relaxation of restriction on sales can lead to increased sales, but it is not certain that increasing restriction would reduce established rates of drinking.

5. *Restrictions* on who may buy alcohol.

6. *Health education* programmes aimed especially at schoolchildren. The effectiveness of these programmes is uncertain.

Individual approaches

Individual approaches focus on identifying individuals who are consuming hazardous or dangerous amounts of alcohol and intervening with the aim of avoiding or limiting alcohol-related harm. The treatment plan for each patient should be tailored to individual needs and will depend on the amount of alcohol being consumed and whether alcohol-related harm or dependence is present.

Recognition of dangerous use

Treatment is more likely to be successful in early stages of dangerous use, and so it is important that such use of alcohol is recognized as soon as possible. General practitioners and hospital doctors are well placed to identify dangerous and harmful alcohol use: 10–30 per cent of people admitted to general hospitals have alcohol problems—the higher rates being found in accident and emergency wards. Every patient should be asked how much alcohol he drinks each week. The possibility

of dangerous levels of drinking should be considered particularly carefully in the high risk groups shown in Table 14.3.

The *medical conditions* that raise suspicion include: gastritis, peptic ulcer, liver disease, peripheral neuropathy, seizures (especially those starting in middle life), and repeated falls among the elderly. *Psychiatric conditions* with the same significance include anxiety, depression, erratic moods, poor concentration, memory impairment, and sexual dysfunction.

Questionnaires are useful methods of identifying heavy drinkers. In primary care, the **Alcohol Use Disorders Identification Test** (AUDIT) can be used

---

TABLE 14.3 Identifying alcohol problems

- Consider possible alcohol problems in the following high-risk groups:

  medical or psychiatric conditions commonly associated with excessive use of alcohol (see text)

  marital or sexual problems

  trouble with the law

  repeated absences or poor record at work

  problems with the patient's children

- Ask screening questions or use a screening questionnaire

- Ask for symptoms of alcohol dependence

- Carry out a physical examination for alcohol-related medical conditions (see Table 13.1)

- Arrange further investigations:

  alcohol diary

  laboratory tests (MCV, GGT)

GGT, gamma-glutamyltranspeptidase; MCV, mean corpuscular volume.

BOX 14.1 ALCOHOL USE DISORDERS IDENTIFICATION TEST (AUDIT)

1. How often do you have a drink containing alcohol?

   (0) Never

   (1) Monthly or less

   (2) 2–4 times a month

   (3) 2 or 3 times a week

   (4) 4 or more times a week

2. How many drinks containing alcohol do you have on a typical day when you are drinking?

   (0) 1 or 2

   (1) 3 or 4

   (2) 5 or 6

   (3) 7 to 9

   (4) 10 or more

3. How often do you have six or more drinks on one occasion?

   (0) Never

   (1) Less than monthly

   (2) Monthly

   (3) Weekly

   (4) Daily or almost daily

4. How often during the past year have you found that you were not able to stop drinking once you had started?

   (0) Never

   (1) Less than monthly

   (2) Monthly

   (3) Weekly

   (4) Daily or almost daily

5. How often during the past year have you failed to do what was normally expected of you because of drinking?

   (0) Never

   (1) Less than monthly

   (2) Monthly

   (3) Weekly

   (4) Daily or almost daily

6. How often during the past year have you needed a first drink in the morning to get yourself going after a heavy drinking session?

   (0) Never

   (1) Less than monthly

   (2) Monthly

   (3) Weekly

   (4) Daily or almost daily

BOX 14.1 ALCOHOL USE DISORDERS IDENTIFICATION TEST (AUDIT) *(continued)*

7. How often during the past year have you had a feeling of guilt or remorse after drinking?

   (0) Never

   (1)   Less than monthly

   (2) Monthly

   (3) Weekly

   (4) Daily or almost daily

8. How often during the past year have you been unable to remember what happened the night before because you had been drinking?

   (0) Never

   (1) Less than monthly

   (2) Monthly

   (3) Weekly

   (4) Daily or almost daily

9. Have you or has someone else been injured as a result of your drinking?

   (0) No

   (2) Yes, but not in the past year

   (4) Yes, during the last year

10. Has a relative or friend or a doctor or other health worker been concerned about your drinking or suggested that you cut down?

   (0) No

   (2) Yes, but not in the past year

   (4) Yes, during the last year

(From Piccinelli *et al.* (1997). *British Medical Journal* **314**, 420–4.))

(Box 14.1). In primary care, for the detection of alcohol dependence, harmful use, or dangerous intake, a cut-off score of five on this test has a sensitivity of 84 per cent, a specificity of 90 per cent, and a likelihood ratio for a positive result of 8.4. The briefer **CAGE questionnaire** is probably less sensitive but more specific—a score of three or more has a specificity of almost 100 per cent (Box 14.2).

If the screening questions raise the possibility of an alcohol problem, more detailed enquiries should be made:

- How much alcohol does the patient drink on a typical 'drinking day'? (Start by asking about the amount drunk in the second half of the day, before asking about morning drinking.)

- How does the patient feel after going without alcohol for a day or two?

- How does the patient feel on waking?

- Questions should be asked about performance at work and in family life, and about any legal problems. Relevant questions about work include extended meal breaks, lateness, absences, declining efficiency, missed promotions, and accidents.

- In appropriate cases, systematic enquiry should be made about features of the alcohol dependence syndrome and all the physical, psychological, and social disabilities described above.

There are several *laboratory tests* that may be useful in assessing the person with drinking problems:

1. **Blood alcohol** concentration estimation using a breathalyser is the most direct measure, although this does not distinguish between a single recent episode of heavy drinking and chronic abuse.

BOX 14.2 **THE CAGE QUESTIONNAIRE**

1. Have you ever felt you ought to **C**ut down your drinking?

2. Have people **A**nnoyed you by criticizing your drinking?

3. Have you ever felt **G**uilty about your drinking?

4. Have you ever had a drink first thing in the morning as an 'Eye opener'?

Two or more positive replies identifies problem drinkers; one is an indication for further enquiry about the person's drinking.

(From Mayfield *et al.* (1974). *American Journal of Psychiatry* **131**, 1121–3.)

TABLE 14.4   Treatment plan for a patient with an alcohol problem

♦ Review with the patient:
  extent of drinking
  evidence for dependence
  alcohol-related disabilities
♦ Arrange withdrawal of alcohol
♦ Treat urgent medical or psychiatric illness
♦ Set attainable goals for:
  control of drinking*
  treatment of medical disabilities
  resolution of interpersonal problems
  dealing with practical difficulties
  establishing new interests (finance, employment, the law)
♦ Try to involve partner in treatment plan
♦ Plan longer term help:
  individual or group counselling
  AA meetings
  help for the family

* Abstinence if there is evidence of harmful use.

2. **Gamma-glutamyltranspeptidase** (GGT) levels are raised in about 80 per cent of people with drinking problems

3. **Mean corpuscular volume** (MCV) is increased in about 60 per cent of people with drinking problems.

4. **Urate levels** are raised in about half of all people with drinking problems, but they are only useful as screening tests for men as they are poor discriminators in women.

If other causes of abnormality can be excluded, abnormal MCV or GGT levels strongly suggest harmful drinking. They have the advantage that values do not return to normal for some weeks after the last period of heavy drinking.

Treatment of people with alcohol problems

A thorough enquiry into drinking habits and related problems is not only a way of detecting the harmful user of alcohol; it is also a first step in treatment because it helps the patient to recognize the extent and seriousness of his problem. This recognition is needed as a means of motivating the patient to control his drinking. Without such motivation, treatment will fail. Enquiries should be persistent to uncover the extent of the problem, but not judgemental. The assessment should normally *involve the partner*, for whom it may be a first opportunity to unburden feelings and obtain help.

Treatment plan (Table 14.4)

Initial goals Treatment begins with a review of the extent of the drinking, the evidence for dependence,

the effects of the patient's heavy drinking, and the likely consequences if it continues. Any urgently needed medical or psychiatric treatment is arranged and a decision is made about withdrawal (see below). The patient should be involved in formulating the treatment plan, and if possible the partner should take part. Specific and attainable goals should be set, and the patient given responsibility for reaching them. These goals should include control of drinking, collaboration with treatment for any associated medical condition, and resolution of problems in the family, at work, and with the law. These initial goals should be short term and achievable. For example, if the amount drunk is not too great, the aim should be to reduce consumption to the safe limit in the first 2 weeks. Unrealistic goals, especially in the early stages, will lead to failure, demoralization, and a return to drinking.

Longer term goals As treatment progresses, longer term goals may be added concerned with improving marital relationships or changing the use of leisure time. Potential obstacles to progress need to be identified. For example, the patient may work in a job in which drink is readily available, or may have social relations only with people who drink heavily. The patient should be helped to overcome these problems.

Help for the family The plan will often include help for the family. The spouse or teenage children may need counselling about problems of their own that are consequent on the patient's heavy drinking. They may also need help in supporting the patient's efforts to reduce his drinking.

Abstinence versus controlled drinking

It is important to decide whether to aim for total abstinence from alcohol or for controlled drinking. Abstinence is the most appropriate goal for people with harmful use of alcohol, including dependence. However, not all such patients will accept this goal; they either refuse treatment or report abstinence while continuing to drink alcohol. For those who drink dangerous amounts of alcohol but are not dependent, an appropriate goal can be the reduction of drinking to a safe level, provided that the person:

- has not incurred serious physical consequences of drinking that require abstinence;

- is not in a job (such as heavy goods vehicle driving) that carries a risk to others;

- is not pregnant.

The target can be the usual safe limit of 21 units per week for men and 14 for women. Reduction to these limits should be in achievable stages, say 5 or 10 units a week, but the process should not be so prolonged that motivation is lost.

Treatment of special groups

Women Despite the social changes that have led women to drink more alcohol, it is still difficult for them to admit to alcohol dependency or alcohol-related problems. For this reason, treatment is often difficult. Compared with men, safe limits set in treatment should be lower (see p. 184). Drinking of alcohol by pregnant women carries risks for the fetus (see p. 186).

Doctors have higher than average rates of alcohol problems, and they too often have difficulty in admitting their problems and seeking help, especially from colleagues working in the same area. In some countries, including the UK, arrangements exist for doctors to obtain help outside their area of work, through a national scheme for sick doctors.

Withdrawal from alcohol: detoxification

When the patient is dependent on alcohol, a sudden cessation of drinking may cause severe withdrawal symptoms including delirium tremens or seizures. Since these complications may be dangerous, withdrawal (detoxification) should be carried out under medical supervision. In less severe cases, and where there is no significant physical illness or history of previous withdrawal seizures, withdrawal can be at home under the supervision of the general practitioner provided that there is someone to look after the patient. More severe cases, needing more frequent supervision and psychological support to maintain motivation, should be withdrawn in hospital or, if at home, with additional support from an appropriately trained community nurse.

Since dependent patients are unlikely to succeed in reducing alcohol gradually, it is usually best to stop the alcohol, replace it with a drug that will prevent delirium tremens or fits, and then withdraw this drug gradually. **Benzodiazepines** are the drugs of first choice. The choice of benzodiazepine should be made on the basis of speed of onset of action. For most planned withdrawals, a long-acting benzodiazepine, such as chlordiazepoxide or diazepam, is best at producing a smoother course of withdrawal and is less likely to be abused. For unplanned withdrawals, when withdrawal symptoms have already occurred, short-acting benzodiazepines may be preferable. Benzodiazepines should not be continued for longer than 14 days because the patient may become dependent on them. Chlorpromazine and other neuroleptics are *not* suitable since they may provoke seizures; *chlormethiazole is best avoided* because of cross-dependence and respiratory depression.

A suggested regimen for withdrawal is shown in Box 14.3. If withdrawal is undertaken in hospital, lower doses of benzodiazepine can be used, tailored to the emergence of withdrawal symptoms as rated by the nursing staff.

BOX 14.3 SUGGESTED WITHDRAWAL REGIMEN FOR DETOXIFICATION FROM ALCOHOL

Day 1: Chlordiazepoxide 80–100 mg in split doses

Day 2–5: Gradual and complete reduction of dose of chlordiazepoxide

- Advise on consumption of fruit juices and soft drinks

- Course of vitamins orally

- If there is a history of seizures, use phenytoin

- Monitor symptoms, blood pressure, and fluid intake

Psychological treatment

Brief interventions These consist of the following elements:

1. *Assessment* of the quantity of alcohol consumed by asking the patient to keep a diary of his consumption.

2. *Information* about the hazards of alcohol.

3. *Advice* about safe limits is effective in reducing dangerous alcohol consumption, together with problem-solving counselling (see pp. 257–8).

The patient should be encouraged to keep an on-going *diary of alcohol consumption* and of the circumstances of any relapse. Diary keeping is helpful because relapses occur in many patients and, if dealt with constructively, provide opportunities for finding out how to avoid further relapses.

Such brief interventions can be provided in primary care and general hospital settings or by a member of a specialist team.

More intensive treatment In patients who do not respond to the brief interventions described above, more intensive psychological interventions are available that are directed at: (i) sustaining motivation; (ii) avoiding relapse; and (iii) relieving psychological problems that contributed to the development of the alcohol problem in the first place. *Group therapy* is probably the most widely used treatment in specialist units because patients often accept support and advice more readily from other patients with similar problems than from doctors. Advice should be provided about *developing new activities* with the family or as hobbies or other interests. Factors that led to or maintained the alcohol problem may need specific treatment. For example, marital problems may require marriage guidance counselling; whereas difficulty in dealing with angry feelings in other relationships might require short-term psychotherapy.

Medication to maintain abstinence

Disulfiram (Antabuse: 100–200 mg/day) is used, usually in specialist practice, as a deterrent to impulsive drinking. It interferes with the metabolism of alcohol by blocking one of the enzymes involved. As a result, when alcohol is taken, acetaldehyde accumulates with consequent flushing, headache, choking sensations, rapid pulse, and anxiety. These unpleasant effects discourage the patient from drinking alcohol while taking the drug.

Treatment with disulfiram carries the occasional risks of cardiac irregularities or, rarely, cardiovascular collapse. Therefore, the drug should not be started until at least 12 hours after the last ingestion of alcohol. Disulfiram has unpleasant *side effects*, including a persistent metallic taste in the mouth, gastrointestinal symptoms, dermatitis, urinary frequency, impotence, peripheral neuropathy, and toxic confusional states. It should *not* be used in patients with recent heart disease, severe liver disease, or significant suicidal ideation.

Potential drug interactions should also be identified by consulting the manufacturer's literature or a work of reference.

Self-help groups and voluntary services

Self-help groups can be very useful in helping to maintain motivation. They also provide a valuable means of support. Patients with alcohol problems often find it easier to talk to others who have had similar problems.

Alcoholics Anonymous (AA) hold group meetings at which members obtain support from one another. If in crisis between meetings, they can obtain support from other members by telephone. Not all problem drinkers are willing to join the organization because it requires total abstinence and because the meetings involve repeated confession of each person's faults and problems. Those who remain in the organization are usually helped, and anyone with a drink problem should be encouraged to try it.

Al-Anon is a parallel organization providing support for the spouses of excessive drinkers. **Al-Ateen** does the same for their teenage children.

Councils on alcoholism are voluntary agencies that advise problem drinkers where to obtain help, provide social activities for those who have recovered, train counsellors, and coordinate services.

Hostels for homeless problem drinkers are provided in some places, often by voluntary organizations. Usually, abstinence is a condition of residence, and counselling and rehabilitation are provided.

When to obtain specialist help

Most problem drinkers can be treated in primary care using brief interventions. The general practitioner knows the patient and the family, and can carry out the treatment of the problem drinking in the context of the patient's general health, an approach that is often acceptable to the patient. The family doctor will often be able to withdraw the patient from alcohol—community alcohol teams are increasingly being developed to support general practitioners in this task.

The main reasons for referral to a specialist are:

1. Severe withdrawal symptoms, especially fits or delirium tremens, which should be treated as emergencies.

2. Planned withdrawal from alcohol when home withdrawal is inappropriate.

3. Medical or psychiatric complications requiring specialist assessment (see Tables 14.1 and 14.2).

4. Complex personal or interpersonal problems requiring more intensive psychological treatment than simple counselling.

Results of treatment

For the majority of problem drinkers, brief interventions are as effective as more intensive treatments. The results of treatment for patients with serious drinking problems are poor and the aim should therefore be on the early detection and treatment of alcohol problems. It is important to maintain a helpful and non-judgemental attitude. Relapses should be viewed constructively and further help offered. The general practitioner is in a good position to watch patiently, waiting for opportunities to help.

In the early stages of dangerous drinking, the patient is more likely to have the *characteristics related to good outcome*:

♦ good insight;

♦ strong motivation;

♦ a supportive family;

♦ a stable job;

♦ the ability to form good relationships;

♦ control of impulsivity;

♦ the ability to defer gratifications.

Problems due to the use of psychoactive substances

The term **psychoactive substance** is often used instead of the term **drug** because some people use substances that are not generally regarded as drugs, for example, organic solvents or mushrooms with psychedelic properties. We use the term psychoactive substance when the broad meaning is required, while retaining the word drug for other purposes. The substances that are used commonly fall into six groups:

1. Opioids.

2. Anxiolytics and hypnotics.

3. Stimulants.

4. Hallucinogens.

5. Cannabis.

6. Organic solvents.

In this chapter, we focus on the harmful effects of these substances to the user's health. The use of many of these substances is illegal in many countries. The use of others (e.g. nicotine) is legal despite the harmful medical consequences of smoking. It is important to distinguish between **harmful** use and **illegal** use of substances. The clinician's role should be directed at the former—to help the user overcome dependence and to avoid the adverse health consequences of psychoactive substance use.

Epidemiology of psychoactive substance use

The extent of supply and consumption of drugs is often concealed because the possession of many drugs is illegal or socially unacceptable. Therefore, there are no reliable estimates of the extent of drug consumption in the population. In the UK, indirect information has been collected about drug-related offences, hospital treatment, and cases reported to government agencies but none of these sources are reliable. Similar difficulties are encountered in different countries, so that no accurate international comparison can be made.

In the UK, at least 25 per cent of schoolchildren have used illicit substances or solvents on at least one occasion by the age of 16 years. In most developed countries, the extent of psychoactive substance use seems to be increasing.

Causes of the harmful use of psychoactive substances

Four kinds of cause are important:

1. The *pharmacological properties* of the substances themselves (see below).

2. The *availability of the substances*. The availability of most psychoactive substances is limited in one way or another. Psychoactive substances are usually obtained in one of three ways:

   ♦ prescribed by doctors (e.g. benzodiazepines);

   ♦ purchased legally (e.g. nicotine, alcohol, and, for adults, solvents);

   ♦ purchased illegally: this category includes most of the other drugs discussed in this chapter plus nicotine, alcohol, and solvents under certain age limits. Control of the availability of such drugs depends on political action and requires extensive activity by the police and other enforcement agencies to detect and control the importation and distribution of drugs.

3. *Personal factors* may determine why one person who has access to a drug uses it harmfully, while another with similar access does not. They include:

   ◆ *personal vulnerability*: a lack of personal resources needed to cope with the challenges of life. This problem is often manifest in teenage years as difficulty in accepting authority, truancy or underachievement at school, or delinquency;

   ◆ *disorganized family background*.

4. *Social pressures* are important. Some social groups disapprove of drug taking, and this shared value helps to restrain its members. In other groups, drug taking is condoned or even encouraged, and it gives a young person status among his peers.

Types of dependence

Not all people who use psychoactive substances become dependent on them. Dependence may be pharmacological or psychological.

Pharmacological dependence is caused by changes in the receptors and other cellular mechanisms affected by the substance. Substances vary in the degree to which they cause pharmacological dependence: opioids and nicotine readily cause it, cannabis and hallucinogens are less likely to do so.

Psychological dependence operates partly through conditioning. Some of the symptoms experienced as a substance is withdrawn (e.g. anxiety) become conditioned responses that reappear when withdrawal takes place again. Cognitive factors are also important—patients expect unpleasant symptoms and are distressed by the prospect. For this reason, reassurance is an important part of the treatment of patients who are withdrawing from drugs.

Harm related to the use of substances

Substance-related harm may be due to:

1. The toxic properties of the substances themselves (see below).

2. The method of administration (e.g. problems due to the intravenous use of substances, Box 14.4).

3. The social consequences of regular use of substances (Box 14.5).

BOX 14.4 THE HARMFUL EFFECTS OF INTRAVENOUS DRUG TAKING

Some drug abusers administer drugs intravenously in order to obtain an intense and rapid effect. The practice is particularly common with opioids, but barbiturates, benzodiazepines, and amphetamines are among other drugs that may be taken in this way. Intravenous drug use has important consequences—some local, some general.

Local effects include:

◆ thrombosis of veins;

◆ infection at the injection site;

◆ damage to arteries.

General effects are due to transmission of infection, especially when needles are shared. They include:

◆ bacterial endocarditis;

◆ hepatitis;

◆ HIV infection.

BOX 14.5 SOCIAL HARM DUE TO THE USE OF PSYCHOACTIVE SUBSTANCES

There are three reasons why drug abuse has undesirable social effects.

1. **Chronic intoxication** may affect behaviour adversely, leading to a poor work record, unemployment, motoring offences, failures in social relations, and family problems including the neglect of children.

2. **The need to finance the habit**. Most illicit drugs are expensive and the abuser may cheat or steal to obtain money. Women may adopt prostitution putting themselves at risk of sexually transmitted diseases and other problems

3. **The creation of a drug subculture**. Drug users often keep company with one another, and those with previously stable social behaviour may be under pressure to conform with a *group ethos* of antisocial or criminal activity.

Diagnosis of dependence on substances

It is important to diagnose dependence early, at a stage when tolerance is less established, behaviour patterns are less fixed, and the complications of intravenous use have not developed. Dependent people may come to medical attention in several ways.

1. They may declare that they are dependent on a substance.

2. They may request drugs for medical reasons. Some patients conceal their dependency, asking instead for opioids to relieve pain or for hypnotics to improve sleep. General practitioners and hospital emergency department staff should be wary of such requests from patients whom they have not met before, and if possible should obtain information about previous treatment (if necessary by telephone) before prescribing.

3. They may ask for help with the complications of substance use such as cellulitis, pneumonia, hepatitis, HIV/AIDS, or accidents; or for the treatment of a drug overdose, withdrawal symptoms, or an adverse reaction to a hallucinogenic drug.

4. Their dependence might be detected during treatment of an unrelated illness.

A doctor who is not used to treating substance-dependent people should remember that the patient may be trying to deceive him. Some patients overstate the dosage in the hope of obtaining extra supplies to use themselves, give to friends, or sell. Others take more than one substance but do not admit it. It is important to check the patient's account for internal inconsistencies and to seek external verification whenever possible (e.g. by obtaining permission to contact another doctor who has treated the same patient).

Evidence of intravenous use Clinical signs that suggest that drugs are being injected include:

♦ needle tracks and thrombosis of veins, especially in the antecubital fossa;

♦ scars of previous abscesses;

♦ concealing the forearms with long sleeves even in hot weather.

Intravenous drug use should be considered in any patient who presents with subcutaneous abscesses, hepatitis, or HIV/AIDS, whether or not the person is asking for help with substance use.

Behavioural changes may suggest problem use. These include repeated absence from school or work, occupational decline, self-neglect, loss of former friends, and joining the 'drug culture'. Petty theft and prostitution are other indicators.

Laboratory tests should be used whenever possible to confirm the diagnosis. Most substances can be detected in the urine, the notable exception being lysergic acid diethylamide (LSD). Specimens should be examined as quickly as possible, with an indication of the interval between the last admitted drug dose and the collection of the urine sample. The laboratory should be provided with as complete a list as possible of drugs likely to have been taken, including those prescribed, as well as those obtained in other ways.

Principles of prevention

There are two main strategies of prevention of harm related to the use of psychoactive substances:

1. **Reducing use**. This includes:

♦ *limiting availability*;

♦ *health education*, particularly in schools, but also centred on locations with widespread drug use, such as certain clubs;

♦ *media campaigns*;

♦ *tackling social causes* such as poor social conditions, unemployment among young people, and lack of leisure facilities.

However, there is little evidence than any of these measures are effective. Indeed, some health education and media campaigns may actually increase the extent of use.

2. **Reducing harm** associated with use of substances. The harm reduction approach became more accepted in the 1980s in response to the spread of HIV/AIDS through intravenous drug use and sexual intercourse. The main features of this approach include:

♦ the *education* of drug users about the dangers of intravenous use; such advice is often more effective when given by ex-drug users than by doctors;

♦ schemes for *providing clean syringes and needles* in exchange for used ones in the hope of reducing the sharing of contaminated ones;

♦ the prescription of *oral maintenance drugs* to avoid the use of intravenous drugs;

♦ the free supply of *condoms* to reduce sexual transmission.

These approaches are controversial since some of the measures can be seen to condone drug taking, but the danger of HIV infection is now generally considered greater than that of increasing drug abuse.

Principles of treatment and rehabilitation
(Table 14.5)

The first part of treatment consists of:

1. *Assessment* of the type, amount, and route of substance use, and the evidence for dependence.

2. Provision of *information about the dangers* of continued use.

3. *Assessment of the motivation* of the user to change his own behaviour.

4. *Clarification of the goals* of treatment. These goals include: a defined period of abstinence; breaking contact with people who use substances and attempting to establish new relationships; starting to deal with debts or personal problems; and to take up new hobbies or interests so that time previously spend on obtaining and taking drugs does not remain unfulfilled.

The next step of treatment is to *withdraw the substance*. If the person is severely dependent or if withdrawal effects could be serious (e.g. seizures during withdrawal from barbiturates) withdrawal should be in hospital.

TABLE 14.5 Treatment plan for a person using drugs harmfully
◆ Review with the patient:
the type of drug(s) and amounts taken
intravenous usage and its dangers, especially HIV
evidence of dependence
consequences of drug taking:
◆ caused by the drug
◆ related to intravenous use
◆ social and psychological
the patient's personal and social resources and problems
◆ Arrange withdrawal
◆ Treat urgent medical or psychiatric complications
◆ Set attainable short- and medium-term goals for:
abstaining from drugs
parting from the drug culture
dealing with personal and financial problems
establishing new interests
◆ Plan longer term help:
individual or group counselling
help for the family

Otherwise it can be at home under close supervision. Withdrawal is achieved by reducing the dose progressively over a period of 1–3 weeks, depending on the initial dose. With opioids and benzodiazepines it is usual to begin by replacing the substance with an equivalent dose of a longer acting compound of the same type, and then withdraw that substance. (A longer acting compound is chosen because withdrawal effects are less acute.) As noted above, psychological factors contribute to dependence, and strong and repeated reassurance is an important part of treatment.

Maintenance programmes

Maintenance refers to the continued prescribing of a substance, usually an opioid drug, for a person who is unwilling to withdraw, combined with help with social problems and a continuing effort to bring the person to accept withdrawal. Maintenance is therefore more than merely providing drugs. The rationale for this procedure is to minimize harm in the following ways:

1. To *remove the need to obtain 'street' drugs*, and thereby reduce the need to steal, engage in prostitution, or associate with other drug users.

2. To *stop intravenous use*, thus reducing the spread of HIV.

3. To *provide social and psychological help* to bring the person to the point at which he will be willing to give up drugs.

Unfortunately, the available evidence does not suggest that these aims are achieved regularly: many patients continue in their previous way of life, many continue to take street drugs as well as the prescribed methadone, and few become willing to give up drugs. Despite these drawbacks, this treatment is in use in the hope that it may have some effect in reducing intravenous usage thereby limiting the spread of HIV.

Some patients on maintenance therapy attend a succession of general practitioners in search of supplementary supplies of drugs, posing as temporary residents. The doctor should not prescribe but should help the patient to return to the clinic where he is in treatment.

Rehabilitation

People who have abused drugs for a long time may need considerable help in making social relationships and in obtaining and retaining a job. When these problems are severe, treatment in a therapeutic community can be helpful.

Effects and harmful use of specific substances

Opioids

This group of drugs includes morphine, heroin, codeine, and synthetic analgesics such as pethidine and methadone. As well as the desired effect of euphoria these drugs produce analgesia, respiratory depression, constipation, reduced appetite, and low libido. These drugs can be taken by mouth, intravenously, or by smoking. The most widely abused of these drugs is **heroin**, which has a particularly powerful euphoriant effect. Although some people take heroin intermittently without becoming dependent, with regular usage dependence develops rapidly, especially when the drug is taken intravenously.

Tolerance develops rapidly, leading to increasing dosage. When the drug is stopped, tolerance diminishes so that a dose taken after an interval of abstinence has a greater effect than it would have had before the interval. This loss of tolerance can result in dangerous—sometimes fatal—respiratory depression when a previously tolerated dose is resumed after a drug-free interval, for example, after a stay in hospital or prison.

Withdrawal The symptoms due to withdrawal from opioids are shown in Table 14.6. With heroin, these features usually begin about 6 hours after the last dose, reach a peak after 36–48 hours, and then wane. These symptoms cause great distress, which drives the person to seek further supplies but seldom threatens the life of a person in reasonable health.

Prognosis After 7 years only one-quarter to one-third of opioid-dependent people will have become abstinent, and between 10 and 20 per cent will have died from

TABLE 14.6 Symptoms of the opioid withdrawal syndrome
◆ Intense craving for the drug
◆ Restlessness and insomnia
◆ Muscle and joint pain
◆ Running nose and eyes
◆ Sweating
◆ Abdominal cramps
◆ Vomiting and diarrhoea
◆ Piloerection
◆ Dilated pupils
◆ Raised pulse rate
◆ Instability of temperature control

causes related to drug taking. Deaths are from accidental overdosage—often related to loss of tolerance after a period of enforced abstinence—and from medical complications such as infection with HIV. When abstinence is achieved, it is often related to changed circumstances of life, such as a new relationship with a caring person.

Pregnancy The babies of opioid-dependent women are more likely than other babies to be premature and of low birthweight. Also, they may show withdrawal symptoms after birth, including irritability, restlessness, tremor, and a high-pitched cry. These signs appear within a few days of birth if the mother was taking heroin, but are delayed if she was taking methadone, which has a longer half-life. Later effects have been reported, these children being more likely as toddlers to be overactive and to show poor persistence. It is uncertain whether these late effects result from the unsuitable family environment provided by these mothers, or from a lasting effect of the exposure to the drug.

Treatment of opioid dependence

Treatment of crisis Heroin-dependent people present in crisis to a general practitioner or casualty doctor in three circumstances:

1. *Seeking the prescription of drugs* either by requesting them directly or by feigning a painful disorder. Although withdrawal symptoms are very unpleasant, they are not usually dangerous to an otherwise healthy person. Therefore, it is best not to offer drugs unless this is the first step of an agreed withdrawal or maintenance programme. (In the UK, only specially licensed doctors may legally prescribe heroin or certain related drugs to a drug-dependent person as maintenance treatment.)

2. *Drug overdose* requiring medical treatment, directed particularly to any respiratory depression produced by the drug.

3. *Complication of intravenous drug usage* such as an acute local infection, necrosis at the injection site, or infection of a distant organ, usually the heart or liver.

Planned withdrawal of opioids (detoxification) The general principles of drug withdrawal have been outlined above. When heroin is withdrawn, psychological management is particularly important. Withdrawal is usually undertaken by substituting methadone (a longer acting drug) for heroin. The main steps are shown in Box 14.6.

Continued prescribing (maintenance) The principles of maintenance treatment for opiate dependence have

BOX 14.6 THE PLANNED WITHDRAWAL OF OPIOIDS (DETOXIFICATION)

- When the starting dose is very high, withdrawal should be in hospital.

- It is often difficult to judge the starting dose because patients often take adulterated preparations of heroin (and may lie about the amount taken). For this reason treatment should be discussed with and often carried out by a specialist in drug dependence.

- The starting dose of methadone is usually 10–20 mg daily, which is increased in 10–20 mg steps until there are no signs of intoxication or withdrawal. The usual daily dose is 40–60 mg.

- The initial dose is reduced by about a quarter every 2 or 3 days, but a slower rate may be needed. However, very slow withdrawal should be avoided because it may lead to continued prescribing.

- The regimen should be agreed with the patient as a contract that he will accept throughout the treatment.

- Urine tests for drugs should be carried out weekly after withdrawal until the doctor is confident that the patient is remaining drug-free.

been discussed. *Methadone* is prescribed and dispensed daily, usually in a liquid preparation formulated to discourage efforts to inject it. The equivalent dosage is difficult to determine since street drugs are adulterated to a varying degree. The treatment should be initiated by a specialist, although care can be shared with the primary care physician. There is some evidence that *drugs with a longer half-life*, such as buprenorphine and levamethadyl acetate hydrochloride (LAAM) may be at least as effective as methodone. These drugs have the advantage that they can be taken less often than every day.

Rehabilitation This follows the general lines described on p. 198.

Results of treatment Although about 90 per cent of opioid-dependent patients can withdraw successfully, about 50 per cent will recommence use by 6 months following withdrawal.

Anxiolytic and hypnotic drugs

The most frequently used drugs in this group are now benzodiazepines. The most serious health problems are presented by barbiturates, which, although seldom used therapeutically, are widely available as street drugs. Other currently used drugs of this kind include chlormethiazole and glutethimide.

Barbiturates

Barbiturates are taken by mouth and intravenously. Some elderly people are dependent on barbiturates prescribed originally many years ago as prescribed hypnotics. Younger dependent people use illegal supplies of barbiturates, and some dissolve capsules and inject intravenously—a particularly dangerous practice leading to phlebitis, ulcers, abscesses, and gangrene.

Intoxication The symptoms of barbiturate intoxication resemble those of alcohol:

- slurred speech;

- incoherence;

- drowsiness;

- depression of mood.

Younger intravenous users are often unkempt, dirty, and malnourished. *Nystagmus*, a useful diagnostic sign, is often present. Urine should be examined to investigate the possible simultaneous abuse of other drugs. Blood levels are generally useful only in acute poisoning.

Tolerance develops to barbiturates, although less quickly than to opioids. Tolerance to the psychological effects of barbiturates is greater than tolerance to their depressant effects on respiration, so increasing the risks of unintentional fatal overdosage.

Withdrawal The abrupt withdrawal of barbiturates from a dependent person can be followed by a withdrawal syndrome resembling that occurring with alcohol (see p. 188), with a *high risk of seizures*. With longer acting drugs, the withdrawal syndrome may be delayed for several days after the drug has been stopped; for this reason observation should be prolonged if dangerous consequences are to be avoided. The syndrome of barbiturate withdrawal begins with anxiety, restlessness, disturbed sleep, anorexia, and nausea. It may progress to tremulousness, disorientation, hallucinations, vomiting, hypotension, pyrexia, and to major seizures. If the withdrawal syndrome is not treated, some patients die.

When drugs are withdrawn as part of treatment, the patient should be supervised closely in hospital, unless: (i) the starting dose is small; and (ii) there is no history of epilepsy. Phenothiazines should be avoided because they may lower the seizure threshold. Unless it is certain that the dosage is small, the advice of a specialist should be obtained.

Benzodiazepines

Benzodiazepines cause symptoms of *intoxication* similar to those of barbiturates (see above). *Tolerance* and *dependence* develop when the drugs are prescribed continuously for a long period. The exact period is uncertain, but 6–8 weeks is widely accepted as the limit that is without risk.

The **benzodiazepine withdrawal syndrome** is characterized by:

◆ irritability;

◆ anxiety;

◆ disturbed sleep;

◆ nausea;

◆ increased perceptual sensitivity;

◆ tremor;

◆ sweating;

◆ palpitations;

◆ headache;

◆ muscle pain.

Seizures may occur when the dose of benzodiazepine taken has been high.

Planned withdrawal of benzodiazepines

The withdrawal symptoms are less pronounced with long-acting (e.g. diazepam) than with short-acting benzodiazepines (e.g. lorazepam), so a short-acting drug should be replaced with a long-acting drug in the equivalent dose before starting withdrawal.

When benzodiazepines are withdrawn therapeutically, the dose should be reduced very gradually: by about 10 per cent every 2 weeks. If withdrawal symptoms appear during withdrawal, the dose can be increased slightly, and then reduced again by a smaller amount than before. As the dose decreases, it may not be possible to achieve the required dose reduction with the strengths of tablets available. At this stage the drug can be taken on alternate days or a liquid preparation (e.g. diazepam elixir or nitrazepam syrup) can be used.

Anxiety management techniques (see p. 261) help to reduce the distress caused by withdrawal symptoms. They have the advantage that they should reduce the need for anxiolytic medication if anxiety recurs in the future. Self-help groups (e.g. Tranx) can also be a valuable source of support during withdrawal.

Stimulant drugs

The stimulant drugs abused most often are amphetamines, cocaine, and 'ecstasy'.

◆ **Amphetamine sulphate** is taken by mouth or by intravenous injection.

◆ **Free-base amphetamine** (made by heating amphetamine sulphate) is usually smoked and absorbed through the lungs from which is absorbed rapidly.

◆ **Cocaine hydrochloride** is taken by sniffing into the nose (where it is absorbed through the nasal mucosa) or by injecting.

◆ **Free-base cocaine** ('crack') is usually smoked to give a rapid and intense effect.

◆ **Ecstasy** (3,4-methylenedioxymethamphetamine, MDMA) is taken orally. It has been used increasingly since the 1980s, especially at dances ('raves') and clubs. It produces an intense feeling of well-being and increased energy.

These drugs produce an elevation of mood, overactivity, overtalkativeness, insomnia, anorexia, and dryness of the mouth and nose. The pupils dilate, the pulse rate and blood pressure increase, and, with large doses, there may be cardiac arrythmia and circulatory collapse. The overactivity can cause dehydration; overhydration can occur if the user drinks large amounts of water to overcome the dehydration. Occasionally, patients complain of an unusual feeling under the skin, as if insects were there ('formication').

The *prolonged use* of large quantities of these drugs may result in disturbances of perception and thinking. Particularly with amphetamines, a **paranoid psychosis** may occur, closely resembling the paranoid form of schizophrenia, with persecutory delusions, auditory and visual hallucinations, and sometimes aggressive behaviour. Usually, the condition subsides within a week or two of stopping the drug, but occasionally persists for months. In some of these prolonged cases the diagnosis proves to be schizophrenia, not drug-induced psychosis. **Depression** may also follow long-term use of stimulants. Ecstasy may be neurotoxic when taken repeatedly.

Stimulant drugs do not readily induce *tolerance*. The *withdrawal syndrome* is often troublesome and consists of low mood and reduced energy.

Treatment of overdosage requires sedation and the management of any hyperpyrexia or cardiac arrythmia. Paranoid symptoms can be controlled with an antipsychotic drug.

Hallucinogens

This group of drugs includes synthetic compounds such as **lysergic acid diethylamide (LSD)** and naturally occurring substances found in species of mushroom (e.g. *Psilocybe semilanceata*). Synthetic and naturally occurring **anticholinergic drugs** are also abused for their hallucinogenic effects.

The drugs produce distortions or intensifications of sensory perception, sometimes with 'cross-over' between sensory modalities so that, for example, sounds are experienced as visual sensations. Objects may seem to merge, or move rhythmically; time appears to pass slowly; and ordinary experiences may seem to have a profound meaning. The body image may be distorted or the person may feel as if outside his body. These experiences can be pleasurable, but at times they are profoundly distressing and lead to unpredictable and dangerous behaviour. The physical effects of hallucinogens are variable: LSD can cause a rise in heart rate and dilation of the pupils.

Frightening experiences can usually be controlled by strong reassurance; otherwise an anxiolytic such as diazepam should be given. Antipsychotic drugs are also effective, but those with anticholinergic effects (such as chlorpromazine) must *not* be given if the patient has taken phencyclidine (PCP), which has anticholinergic properties, or an anticholinergic drug such as benzhexol.

'Flashbacks' are recurrences of experiences occurring originally during intoxication with hallucinogens, the recurrence occurring weeks or months after the drug was last taken. The experience may be distressing and require reassurance and treatment with an anxiolytic drug. Although flashbacks may recur, they subside eventually.

Phencyclidine

PCP or 'angel dust' is a synthetic hallucinogen with particularly dangerous effects. Intoxication with this drug can be prolonged and hazardous, with agitation, aggressive behaviour, and hallucinations, together with nystagmus and raised blood pressure. With high doses, there may be ataxia, muscle rigidity, and convulsions; and in severe cases, an adrenergic crisis with heart failure, cerebrovascular accident, or malignant hypothermia. In treatment, chlorpromazine should be avoided since it may increase the anticholinergic effects of PCP. Instead, haloperidol or diazepam may be given.

Cannabis

Cannabis, which derives from the plant *Cannabis sativa*, is consumed in two forms. The dried vegetative parts of the plant form marijuana ('grass'); the resin secreted by the flowering tops of the female plant form cannabis resin. In many parts of the world, cannabis is consumed widely, much as alcohol is consumed in the West. In most Western societies the use of cannabis, although illegal, is widespread. Cannabis is currently being investigated as a therapeutic agent for multiple sclerosis and other chronic and painful disorders.

The effects of cannabis vary with the dose, the user's expectations, and the social setting. Like alcohol, cannabis seems to exaggerate the pre-existing mood, whether euphoria or dysphoria. It produces a feeling of enhanced enjoyment of aesthetic experiences, and distorts experiences of time and space. Cannabis intoxication can lead to dangerous driving. The physical effects of cannabis include reddening of the conjunctiva, dry mouth, and tachycardia.

Cannabis does not produce a *withdrawal syndrome*; and although *psychological dependence* can develop, physical dependence does not seem to occur.

It is not certain whether cannabis causes a **psychosis**. Some patients develop an acute psychosis while consuming large amounts of cannabis, recovering quickly when the drug is stopped. In these cases it is uncertain whether cannabis caused the psychosis, or the increased use of cannabis was a response to the early symptoms of a psychosis with a different cause. Fortunately, this uncertainty seldom causes practical problems since the clinical management is unaffected: the drug should be stopped, the progress of the symptoms observed, and chlorpromazine or another antipsychotic drug prescribed if symptoms do not subside within a week.

Organic solvents

The use of volatile solvents occurs mainly among teenagers, usually as occasional experimentation. Serious problems arise in a minority who use solvents regularly, and any user may take an accidental overdose or become asphyxiated while taking the substance.

The solvents used most often are cleaning fluids, adhesives, and aerosols. Petrol and butane and other substances may also be used. The substance is inhaled from a partially closed container in which the concentration can build up, or from an impregnated cloth, or plastic bag. The main features of solvent intoxication are shown in Table 14.7.

Psychological dependence occurs but physical dependence is unusual. Chronic heavy users may develop a transient psychosis. Some of these substances have

TABLE 14.7	Clinical features of solvent intoxication

- Slurring of speech
- Disorientation
- Uncoordination of gait
- Nausea and vomiting
- Coma
- Visual hallucinations (often frightening)

neurotoxic effects with resultant peripheral neuropathy and cerebellar dysfunction. Overdosage can be fatal, resulting from the direct effects of the drug, or from asphyxia or the inhalation of vomit.

Treatment is along the general lines of that for the harmful use of drugs described on pp. 198–9, with an emphasis on improving any personal or family problems contributing to the abuse.

Further reading

Edwards, G., Marshall, J. & Cook, C. C. H. (1997). *The Treatment of Drinking Problems; a Guide for the Helping Professions*, 3rd edn. Cambridge University Press, Cambridge.
A comprehensive account of the practical treatment of the problems due to the use of alcohol.
Gossop Drug Addiction and its Treatment.
Robson, P. (1999). *Forbidden Drugs*, 2nd edn. Oxford University Press, Oxford.
Reviews the effects of each group of illegal drugs, and considers why people take them and discusses the nature of addiction and approaches to treatment.

CHAPTER 15

Problems of sexuality and gender

Chapter contents

Sexual behaviour in the population 206

Sexual dysfunction 207

Disorders of sexual preference 211

Disorders of gender identity: transsexualism 213

Psychological problems of homosexual people 214

Problems of sexuality and gender are common. Doctors may be asked to give advice about four types of problem:

1. **Sexual dysfunction**—impaired or dissatisfying sexual enjoyment or performance.

2. **Abnormalities of sexual preference**—unusual sexual interests and activities that are preferred to heterosexual intercourse.

3. **Disorders of gender identity**—in which the patient feels as if they are of the sex opposite to their biological sex.

4. **Psychological problems encountered by homosexual people**.

Of these, the first group are the most common. In this chapter, we describe the common sexual disorders and outline their treatment. After studying the chapter, the reader should:

◆ know the clinical features of the most common sexual problems;

◆ be able to take a history of a sexual problem;

◆ understand how to formulate a sexual problem.

We assume that readers will have learnt about the physiology of the sexual response elsewhere—if not, we recommend reading the appropriate chapters of Bancroft's *Human Sexuality and its Problems* (Oxford University Press, 1988). The main stages of the physiology of the sexual response are summarized in Tables 15.1 and 15.2. Doctors should also be aware of

TABLE 15.1 Male sexual responses

	Excitement	Plateau	Orgasm	Resolution
Penis	Erection	Erection maintained	Urethra contracts repeatedly	Gradual detumescence
Scrotum	Skin thickens, testes raised	Testes raised further	No change	Return to normal
Prostate, seminal vesicles	–	–	Contract with emission of seminal fluid to urethra	Return to normal
Pulse and blood pressure	Increase	Further increase	Further increase	Return to normal
Respiration	–	Rate increases	Rate increases further	Return to normal

TABLE 15.2 Female sexual responses

	Excitement	Plateau	Orgasm	Resolution
Breasts	Nipple erection in some	Enlargement, areolar engorgement	No change	Return to normal
Labia	–	Engorgement	No change	Return to normal
Clitoris	Head swells	Head withdraws	No change	Return to normal
Vagina	Lubrication, expansion, distension of inner two-thirds	Outer third swells. Inner two-thirds distends further	Contractions of outer third	Return to normal
Uterus	Body and cervix raised	Further elevation	Contractions	Position returns to normal; os gapes open
Pulse and BP	Slight elevation	Further increase	Increase continues	Return to normal
Respiration		Rate increases	Rate increased further	Return to normal

BOX 15.1 ETHICAL PROBLEMS IN THE TREATMENT OF SEXUAL PROBLEMS

When sexual problems are the main topic of the consultation, there is a risk that the professional relationship will become sexualized. Codes of good medical practice contain an absolute prohibition of sexual relationships between doctors and their patients because of the potential for exploitation.

There is a risk that the doctor may allow their own views regarding sexual behaviour to have an unwarranted influence on their care of the patient.

the ethical problems in assessing and treating sexual problems (Box 15.1).

Sexual behaviour in the population

Some knowledge of 'normal' sexual behaviour will help a doctor assess a patient's presenting problem. The age of first intercourse is dropping over time. This is probably due to a combination of a trend to earlier sexual maturity and a relaxation of social attitudes towards sexuality. Surveys suggest that about 20 per cent of females and about 30 per cent of males experience heterosexual intercourse before the age of 16 years. More than 80 per cent of both sexes have experienced sexual intercourse by the age of 20 years. Earlier age of first intercourse is associated with lower social class, lower levels of education, and lack of religious affiliation. The earlier first intercourse occurs, the less likely it is to be accompanied by adequate contraceptive use and the more it is felt by the subject, on retrospect, to have been too early.

When surveyed, over half of adults reported having engaged in vaginal intercourse in the preceding week and more than half report having experienced oral sex in the preceding year. Ninety-six per cent of men and 97 per cent of women reported mostly or exclusively **heterosexual** (erotic thoughts and feelings directed towards a person of the opposite sex) experience and attraction. One per cent of men and 0.25 per cent of women reported mostly or exclusively **homosexual** (erotic thoughts and feelings directed towards a person of the same sex) experience and attraction. However, 6 per cent of males and 3 per cent of females reported some homosexual experience in addition to their mainly heterosexual orientation. Homophobic attitudes were widespread—a survey in 1994 suggested about two-thirds of the population believe that homosexuality is always or mostly wrong.

Sexual dysfunction

It is difficult to establish the prevalence of sexual problems in the population because of the difficulties involved in carrying out surveys of people's sexual behaviour. The commonest kinds of problems presenting to a sexual dysfunction clinic are shown in Table 15.3 and the terms are explained below.

Assessment of sexual dysfunction

Patients with sexual problems initially often complain about other symptoms because they feel too embarrassed to reveal a sexual problem directly. For example, a patient may ask for help with anxiety, depression, poor sleep, or gynaecological symptoms. It is therefore important to ask routinely a few questions about sexual functioning when assessing patients with non-specific psychological or physical symptoms.

In a full assessment, the interviewer should begin by explaining why it will be necessary to ask about intimate details of the patient's sexual life and should then ask questions in a sympathetic, matter of fact way

---

BOX 15.2 ASSESSMENT OF A SEXUAL PROBLEM

- Define the problem:
  - its nature;
  - is it recent or longstanding;
  - whether it has occured with this partner only.
- Assess the sexual drives of both partners.
- Enquire about the couple's relationship and social relationships in general.
- Discuss their sexual development including traumatic experiences.
- Previous and present psychiatric and medical illness and treatment; pregnancy, childbirth, and abortion(s); alcohol and drug use.
- Assess the mental state, especially for depressive disorder.
- Assess motivation for treatment.
- Physical examination and any relevant laboratory tests.

(Box 15.2). Whenever possible both sexual partners should be interviewed, at first separately and then together.

The assessment should cover the following issues:

- *The problem.* Has the problem been present from first intercourse, or did it start after a period of normal sexual functioning? Each partner should be asked, separately, whether the same problem has occurred with another partner, or during masturbation.

- The *strength of sexual drive* should be assessed in terms of the frequency of sexual arousal, intercourse, and masturbation.

- *Motivation* for treatment should be assessed, starting with questions about who took the initiative in seeking treatment and for what reason.

- Assess each partner's *social relationships* with the other sex, with particular reference to shyness and social inhibition.

- Enquiries should be made about the partners' *feelings for one another*: partners who lack a mutual caring relationship are unlikely to achieve a fully satisfactory sexual relationship. Many couples say that their marital problems result from their sexual problems, when the

---

TABLE 15.3 Relative frequency of sexual problems presenting to a sexual dysfunction clinic

Women	
Low sexual desire	50%
Orgasmic dysfunction	20%
Vaginismus	20%
Dyspareunia	5%
Men	
Erectile dysfunction	60%
Premature ejaculation	15%
Delayed ejaculation	5%
Low sexual desire	5%

Adapted from Hawton, K. (1985). *Sex Therapy: a Practical Guide*. Oxford Medical Publications, Oxford University Press, Oxford.

BOX 15.3 PHYSICAL EXAMINATION OF MEN WITH SEXUAL DYSFUNCTION

Is there evidence of diabetes mellitus or adrenal disorder?

+ Hair distribution; gynaecomastia.

+ Blood pressure, peripheral pulses.

+ Fundi for retinopathy.

+ Reflexes, especially the ankle relex.

+ Peripheral sensation.

Are there any abnormalities of the genitalia?

+ *Penis:* congenital abnormalities, foreskin, pulses, tenderness, plaques, infection, urethral discharge.

+ *Testicles:* size, symmetry, texture, sensation.

TABLE 15.4 Physical disorders and drugs causing low sexual desire

Physical disorders	Drugs
Hypogonadism	Hypnotics
Angina and previous myocardial infarction	Anxiolytics
Epilepsy	Antipsychotics
Renal failure and dialysis	
Hypothyroidism	
Mastectomy	
Oophorectomy	
Colostomy	
Ileostomy	

causal connection is really the reverse. Tactful questions should be asked about commitment to the partner and, when appropriate, about infidelity and fears of sexually transmitted disease, including HIV.

+ Assess *sexual development* and *sexual experience*, paying particular attention to experiences such as child abuse, incest, or sexual assault that may have caused lasting anxiety or disgust about sex. Enquiry should be made about homosexual as well as heterosexual feelings.

+ In the *medical history*, the most relevant things to look for are previous and present psychiatric and chronic physical disorders and their treatment; pregnancy, childbirth, and abortion(s); use of alcohol or drugs, such as selective serotonin reuptake inhibitors (SSRIs).

+ In the *mental state examination* look especially for evidence of depressive disorder.

+ A *physical examination* is important because physical illness often causes sexual problems (Box 15.3; Table 15.4). The physical examination of women may require specialist gynaecological help. Further investigations may be necessary depending on the findings from the history and examination (e.g. if diabetes is suspected as a cause of sexual disorder).

Specific sexual disorders

Low sexual desire

This problem may occur in both sexes, but is commoner in women. In some cases, sexual desire has always been low (**primary low sexual desire**): this may be the extreme of the range of biological variation, or it may be due to fears originating from adverse experiences in childhood, such as sexual abuse. In other cases, sexual desire has been normal in the past but has become impaired (**secondary low sexual desire**): the causes then include general problems in the relationship between the partners, physical disorders (Table 15.4), and depressive disorder (in which lack of sexual desire may continue for some weeks after other symptoms have resolved).

Treatment

Treatment is of the cause if one can be identified. The relationship between the partners may improve with couple therapy (see p. 266); a depressive disorder should be treated in the usual way (see p. 109); and fear or guilt caused by adverse experiences in early life may respond to brief dynamic psychotherapy (see p. 262). Low sexual drive cannot be increased by giving hormones.

Male erectile dysfunction

Erectile dysfunction is the inability to reach erection or sustain it long enough for satisfactory coitus. **Primary erectile dysfunction** is rare and usually has a physical basis, such as neurological damage or leakage from the penile cavernous bodies.

The common causes of **secondary erectile dysfunction** are:

+ anxiety about sexual performance;

+ alcohol abuse;

+ drug side effects (Table 15.5);

+ diabetes;

+ arteriosclerosis;

TABLE 15.5 Physical disorders and drugs causing erectile dysfunction

Physical disorders	Drugs
Diabetes mellitus	Antihypertensives
Arteriosclerosis	Beta-blockers
Hyperprolactinaemia	Diuretics
Pelvic autonomic neuropathy	Cimetidine
Rectal surgery	Tricyclic antidepressants
	MAOIs*
	Antipsychotics

MAOI, monoamine oxidase inhibitor.

- other physical illness (Table 15.5);
- age-related diminution of sexual function.

Assessment of erectile dysfunction should identify whether it is invariable (suggesting a physical or drug cause) or present only in some circumstances (suggesting a psychological cause). Questions should be asked about erections on waking from sleep and during masturbation—if they are present, a physical cause is unlikely.

Treatment

Treatment of erectile dysfunction should combine psychological approaches with physical approaches as appropriate. If the disorder is caused by a drug or other physical cause, these should be stopped or treated if possible. Psychological treatment includes the use of sexual therapy techniques (see below) and anxiety management. Physical treatments of erectile dysfunction include drug treatment with sildenafil (a potent inhibitor of phosphodiesterase type V), intracavernosal injections of smooth muscle relaxants (e.g. papaverine or prostaglandin E_1), vacuum devices, and, occasionally, surgical insertion of semirigid rods.

Conditions with discomfort or pain

Pain on intercourse occurs mainly among women, either as vaginismus or as dyspareunia.

Vaginismus

Vaginismus is a painful spasm of the vaginal muscles during intercourse. This spasm may be due to aversion to intercourse or may result from painful scarring after episiotomy or other procedures. The condition may be made worse by an inexperienced or inconsiderate partner. Generally, the spasm begins when the man attempts penetration, but in severe cases it occurs even if the woman attempts to insert her own finger into the vagina. In such severe cases no intercourse can take place.

Treatment

It should be explained to the patient that vaginismus is a form of muscle spasm that can be overcome by relaxation exercises. A graduated behavioural approach to treatment is used. At first, diagrams and mirrors are used to improve the patient's understanding of sexual anatomy and response. Once the woman is familiar and comfortable with her genitals, she is encouraged to introduce the tip of her finger into the vagina. She gradually inserts the whole of her finger and, once she can do this without discomfort, she should try inserting two fingers. In many women, this process will allow the woman to overcome the vaginismus. In situations where the woman finds it difficult to transfer from finger to penile penetration, graduated dilators can be used.

Vaginismus should be distinguished from **lack of vaginal lubrication**, which is usually due to lack of sexual arousal, but may also be due to drug side effects and physical disorders (e.g. diabetes). It is more common following the menopause. *Treatment* consists of removing the cause or using additional lubrication.

Dyspareunia

Dyspareunia is pain on intercourse (Table 15.6). When the pain arises after even partial penetration of the vagina, it may result from impaired lubrication with vaginal secretions (due to aversion to intercourse or inadequate foreplay) or from painful scarring. When pain is felt only during deep penetration, it may be due to pelvic pathology such as endometriosis, pelvic inflammatory disease, ovarian cyst, or tumour. Pain on deep penetration may also result from diminished lubrication in the later stages of prolonged intercourse.

Treatment of dyspareunia depends on the cause. When it is the result of psychological factors causing

TABLE 15.6 Physical disorders causing pain

Pain	
Dyspareunia	Episiotomy
	Endometriosis
	Pelvic inflammatory disease
	Pelvic cysts or tumours
Painful ejaculation	Urethritis
	Prostatitis

impaired sexual arousal, sexual therapy techniques can be used. Referral to a gynaecologist should be made if simple measures are ineffective.

The corresponding disorder among men involves **painful ejaculation**, an uncommon disorder usually caused by urethritis or prostatitis, but occasionally without detectable cause.

Orgasmic dysfunction

In men, orgasmic dysfunction is premature ejaculation or retarded ejaculation; in women it is inhibited orgasm.

Premature ejaculation

Premature ejaculation is habitual ejaculation before penetration or shortly afterwards, so that the woman gains no pleasure. It is common among young men during first sexual encounters, and usually improves with increasing sexual experience. The partner can assist by interrupting foreplay whenever the man feels himself becoming highly aroused (**stop–start technique**). This process prolongs the period during which the man can be highly aroused, but not ejaculate.

Retarded ejaculation

Retarded ejaculation may be part of a general psychological inhibition about relationships with women. It can also be caused by drugs, notably *antipsychotic drugs and monoamine oxidase inhibitors*. If the condition is caused by drugs, the dose should be reduced if practicable. When the causes are psychological, psychotherapy can be tried although its results are uncertain.

Inhibited female orgasm

Inhibited female orgasm during intercourse is frequent although most women can achieve it through clitoral stimulation. In one survey, a quarter of women said they had not experienced orgasm during the first year of marriage. Whether treatment is requested depends on what the couple regards as abnormal. Failure of female orgasm may be due to the man's incapacity to arouse his partner or show her affection and is a likely cause if the woman can experience orgasm by masturbation. Other causes are tiredness, depressive disorder, physical illness, and the effects of medication.

Treatment

Treatment begins by dealing with any remediable cause. If no such cause is found, the woman is helped to express her sexual needs to the partner, and he is encouraged to respond to them (using sex therapy if necessary, see below). If the relationship between the couple is poor, couple therapy may be used (see p. 266).

Sexual dysfunction among people with physical handicaps

Physically handicapped people have sexual problems arising from several sources, including: (i) direct effects of the handicap on sexual function (e.g. impairment of the autonomic nerves to the genitalia in disease of the spinal cord); (ii) general effects such as tiredness and pain; (iii) fears about the deleterious effects of intercourse on the handicapping condition; and (iv) lack of information about the sexual activities that are possible for people with the disability. It is helpful if the general practitioner can provide disabled individuals with an opportunity to raise any sexual difficulties. When necessary, treatment is provided by adapting methods already described for treating sexual dysfunction in non-handicapped people.

Psychological treatment of sexual dysfunction

Specific treatment recommendations are given above in the sections on individual disorders. Many disorders will respond to the steps outlined. However, the treatment of a broad range of sexual dysfunctions may need more structured psychological treatment. In this form of treatment the couple is seen together whenever possible. There are three stages: (i) improving communication; (ii) education; and (iii) 'graded activities'.

Improving communication has two main aims: (i) to help the couple to talk more freely about their problems; and (ii) to increase each partner's understanding of the wishes and feelings of the other. These aims may be appropriate to various kinds of problems. For example, a woman may believe that her partner should know instinctively how to please her during intercourse; she may then interpret his failure to please as lack of affection rather than as the result of her not communicating her wishes to her partner. Alternatively, the man may wish the woman to take a more active role in intercourse but be unable to say this to her. A further aim of this stage of treatment is to enable the couple to achieve a general relationship that is more affectionate and satisfying.

Education focuses on important aspects of the male and female sexual responses; examples are the longer time that is needed for a woman to reach sexual arousal, and the importance of foreplay, including clitoral stimulation, in bringing about vaginal lubrication. Suitably chosen books on sex education can reinforce the therapist's advice. Educational counselling is often the most important part of the treatment of sexual dysfunction, and it may need to be repeated when the couple have made some progress with the graded activities described next.

'**Graded activities**' begin by negotiating with the couple a mutually agreed ban on full sexual intercourse. The couple are encouraged instead to explore the pleasure that each can give the other in tender physical contact. The partners are encouraged to caress each other but not to touch the genitalia at this stage. When they can achieve caressing in a relaxed way that gives enjoyment to each partner, the next stage is genital foreplay without penetration. When genital foreplay can be enjoyed by both partners, the next stage is the resumption of full intercourse in a gradual and relaxed way, in which the partner with the greater problem sets the pace. During this stage a graduated approach starts with 'vaginal containment', in which the penis is inserted gradually into the vagina without thrusting movements. When this graded insertion is pleasurable for both partners, movement is introduced; usually by the woman at first. At each stage, each partner is encouraged to find out and provide what the other enjoys. The couple are advised to avoid checking their own state of sexual arousal. Such checking is common among people with sexual disorder, and has the effect of inhibiting the natural progression of sexual arousal to orgasm. Each partner should be encouraged to allow feelings and physical responses to develop spontaneously whilst thinking of the other person.

Hormones have no place in the treatment of sexual dysfunction *except* in cases where there is a primary hormonal disorder. The overall *results* of sex therapy are that about a third of cases have a successful outcome and another third have worthwhile improvement. Patients with low sexual drive generally have a poor outcome.

Disorders of sexual preference

Disorders of sexual preference are sometimes known as **paraphilias**. A sexual preference can be said to be abnormal by three criteria:

1. Most people in a society regard the sexual preference as abnormal.

2. The sexual preference can be harmful to other people (e.g. sadistic sexual practices).

3. The person with the preference suffers from its consequences (e.g. from a conflict between sexual preference and moral standards).

Doctors may be concerned with these conditions in three circumstances. They may be asked for help by the

TABLE 15.7	Abnormalities of sexual preference
Abnormalities of the sexual object	
◆ sexual fetishism	
◆ transvestism	
◆ paedophilia	
Abnormalities of the sexual act	
◆ exhibitionism	
◆ voyeurism	
◆ sexual sadism	
◆ sexual masochism	

person with the abnormal sexual preference; they may be approached by the sexual partner; or they may be asked for an opinion when a person has been charged with an offence against the law—for example, exhibitionism or a sexual act with a child. (These offences, and others unrelated to abnormal sexual preference, are considered in Chapter 22.)

Disorders of sexual preference are divided into: (i) abnormalities of the sexual 'object'; and (ii) disorders of the sexual act (Table 15.7). The *aetiology* of these conditions is not known, and the various theories will not be discussed. They may, however, be associated with the presence of other disorders including depression, alcohol abuse, and dementia. *Treatment* is described after the descriptions of the disorders, on p. 212.

Disorders of preference of the sexual object

Fetishism

In this condition, an inanimate object is the preferred or only means of achieving sexual excitement. Almost all fetishists are men and most are heterosexual. Among the many objects that can evoke arousal in different people, common examples are rubber garments, women's underclothes, and high-heeled shoes. The smell and texture of these objects is often as important as their appearance in evoking sexual arousal. Some fetishists buy the objects, but others steal them and so come to the notice of the police. Sometimes the behaviour is carried out with a willing partner or with a paid prostitute, but often it is a solitary accompaniment of masturbation.

Fetishistic transvestism

In this condition, the person repeatedly wears clothes of the opposite sex as the preferred or only means of sexual arousal. It can be thought of as a special kind of fetishism. Nearly all fetishistic transvestites are men. The clothing varies from a single garment to a complete set of clothing. Cross-dressing nearly always begins after puberty. At first, the clothes are worn only in private; a few people, however, go on to wear the clothes in public, usually hidden under male outer garments, but occasionally without precautions against discovery. A few transvestites wear a complete set of female garments; the condition then has to be distinguished from transsexualism (see p. 213). The essential difference is that transvestites are sexually aroused by wearing the clothing, while transsexuals are not.

Paedophilia

Paedophilia is repeated sexual activity or fantasy of such activity with prepubertal children as the preferred or only means of sexual excitement. Most paedophiles are men. Few paedophiles seek the help of doctors; those who do are mostly middle aged although the behaviour has often started earlier. From the ready sale of pornographic material depicting sex with children, it is likely that paedophilic fantasies are not rare, although paedophilia as an exclusive form of sexual behaviour is infrequent.

The child is usually above the age of 9 years but prepubertal, and may be of the same or opposite sex to the paedophile. The sexual contact may involve fondling, masturbation, or full coitus with consequent injury to the child.

Disorders of preference of the sexual act

The second group of disorders of sexual preference involves variations in the behaviour carried out to obtain sexual arousal. Generally, the acts are directed towards other adults but sometimes towards children (e.g. by some exhibitionists or sadists).

Exhibitionism

In this condition, sexual arousal is obtained by exposure of the genitalia to an unprepared stranger. Nearly all exhibitionists are men. The act of exposure is usually preceded by a period of mounting tension, which is released by the act. Usually, the exhibitionist seeks to shock or surprise a female. Most exhibitionists fall into two groups. The first consists of men with inhibited temperaments who generally expose a flaccid penis and feel much guilt after the act. The second consists of men with aggressive personality traits who expose an erect penis while masturbating, and feel little guilt afterwards. In Britain, exhibitionists who are arrested are charged with the offence of **indecent exposure** (see p. 325).

When exhibitionism begins in middle or late life, the possibility of organic brain disorder, depressive disor-

der, or alcoholism should be considered since these conditions occasionally 'release' this pattern of behaviour. In other people, the exhibitionism may start during a period of temporary stress.

Voyeurism

Voyeurism is observing others as the preferred and repeated way of obtaining sexual arousal. Most voyeurs are inhibited heterosexual men. Some voyeurs spy on couples who are having intercourse, others on women who are undressing or naked.

Sexual sadomasochism

Sadomasochism is a preference for sexual activity that involves bondage or inflicting pain on another person. If the individual prefers to receive such stimulation, the disorder is called **masochism**. If the individual prefers to administer such stimulation, the disorder is called **sadism**. Beating, whipping, and tying are common forms of such activity. Sometimes the acts are symbolic and cause little actual damage, but occasionally the acts cause serious injuries from which the partner may die.

Mild sadomasochistic behaviour is common and is considered to be part of the range of normal sexual activity. The disorder should be diagnosed only if sadomasochistic activity is the most important source of gratification or necessary for sexual stimulation.

Management of disorders of sexual preference

All cases of this kind should be referred to a specialist if possible, although the referring clinician should first assess the problem as follows.

Assessment (Table 15.8)

The first step is to identify the problem and record its course. The second step is to *exclude any mental disorder* that may have released the sexual behaviour in a person who previously experienced sexual fantasies but did not act on them. It is particularly important to seek

TABLE 15.8 Assessment of abnormalities of sexual preference

- Identify the problem and its course
- Exclude any associated mental disorder (especially depressive disorder, alcoholism, and dementia)
- Assess normal sexual functioning
- Consider the role of the abnormal sexual behaviour (see text)
- Assess motivation for treatment

these causes when the abnormal sexual behaviour appears for the first time in middle or late life.

The third requirement is to *assess normal sexual functioning* since one of the main aims of treatment is to strengthen this. Whenever possible, the patient's sexual partner should be interviewed. If normal sexual behaviour is inadequate, appropriate treatment is given (see p. 210).

Next, an assessment is made of the *role of the abnormal behaviour* in the patient's life. As well as providing sexual arousal, such behaviour may be used as a way of coping with loneliness, depression, or anxiety. If so, the patient should be helped to find adaptive ways of coping with these states.

Finally, *motivation for treatment is assessed.* Often the patient has been urged to attend by another person, usually the wife or the police. In such cases the patient may have no wish to change. Other patients seek help when they become temporarily depressed or guilty, either because the sexual behaviour has caused a problem, or for some other reason. Such people may lose their motivation quickly when their mood returns to normal.

Treatment

Sexual counselling may help with any problems in forming relationships with the opposite sex. Any sexual dysfunction should be treated, using the methods described on p. 210.

The patient should be encouraged to use distraction to control any fantasies of the abnormal sexual behaviour during masturbation, since such fantasies are likely to reinforce and maintain the sexual disorder. He should also stop the use of any pornographic materials used to stimulate these fantasies.

Counselling should be used to help with any problems consequent to giving up the deviant sexual behaviour. Often, leisure time has been spent in seeking out abnormal sexual stimuli, and new interests may need to be developed. When the sexual behaviour has been used to cope with depression or anxiety, the patient should be helped to develop more adaptive ways of coping.

Antiandrogens and oestrogen have been used to reduce sexual drive, especially in patients whose abnormal sexual behaviour is potentially dangerous to other people. The benefits of such treatment have not been clearly established.

Some people with abnormal sexual preferences appear before the courts. Sanctions such as a suspended sentence or probation order sometimes help a patient to control his behaviour, provided that he is motivated to help himself.

Disorders of gender identity: transsexualism

In this rare disorder, the person has the conviction of being of the sex opposite to that indicated by the external genitalia. The person wishes to alter the external genitalia to resemble those of the opposite sex, and to live as a member of that sex. Most transsexual people are men; most women who cross-dress and imitate men are homosexual. In male to female transsexual people, the conviction of being a woman usually dates from before puberty, but medical help is not requested until early adult life, when most have begun to dress as women. Unlike transvestites, they report no sexual arousal from cross-dressing; and unlike homosexual men who dress as women, they do not seek to attract people into a homosexual relationship.

Transsexual men may take a series of steps to become more like women. They practise female styles of speaking, gesturing, and walking; they remove body hair by electrolysis; they attempt to increase breast tissue by taking oestrogen or by obtaining a surgical implant; and they may seek an operation to remove the male external genitalia and form an artificial 'vagina'. Requests for such operations are often made in a determined and persistent way reflecting the person's great distress and may be accompanied by threats of suicide or self-mutilation if surgery is not provided. Since such threats are carried out occasionally, with serious consequences, a specialist opinion should be obtained.

It might be thought that a logical treatment of transsexualism would be a psychological procedure to alter the person's beliefs about his gender identity. No form of psychotherapy, however, has been shown to succeed in this aim. In any case, most transsexual patients reject this approach, hoping instead to alter their bodies to conform more closely with the gender they feel is theirs. In a few specialist centres operations with this purpose are carried out on selected patients (gender reassignment). Good results have been reported, but there is no high quality evidence of the long-term effectiveness of the procedure. Decisions about such treatment are therefore taken on an individual patient basis after thorough assessment, and are made jointly by an experienced psychiatrist and surgeon, in consultation with the general practitioner.

Psychological problems of homosexual people

As described earlier (see p. 206), there is no sharp dividing line between homosexual and heterosexual people. About 1 per cent of men and 0.25 per cent of women are exclusively homosexual throughout their lives, while a further proportion are overtly homosexual or bisexual for a few years but subsequently are predominantly heterosexual. This bisexual potential is greatest in adolescence, after which most people settle permanently into one or other sexual role. Homosexuality is not a psychiatric disorder, but some homosexual people experience sexual and emotional problems for which they seek medical help. These problems are the subject of this section.

Homosexual men consult doctors with four main kinds of problem:

1. A sexually inexperienced young man who has homosexual thoughts and feelings may ask for advice on whether he is homosexual. The doctor should find out whether the young man has heterosexual as well as homosexual thoughts and feelings, and whether he has decided how he would prefer to develop. If the man has heterosexual feelings and wishes to develop them, he should be advised to avoid situations that stimulate homosexual feelings, and should be helped to develop social skills with women.

2. The second kind of problem is presented by young men who have realized correctly that they are predominantly homosexual and who ask for counselling about the implications for their lives. Such young men should be helped to think out the implications themselves, and may be put in touch with a self-help group of homosexuals.

3. The third problem is presented by the established homosexual who becomes depressed or anxious because of difficulties in his sexual relationships. Again, counselling is appropriate as for problems in heterosexual relationships.

4. The fourth problem is presented by the homosexual who is concerned about HIV and AIDS. Such a patient requires appropriate medical investigation, treatment, and counselling.

Homosexual women ask for advice less often than homosexual men; when they do seek help, it is usually about problems in their relationship with the partner —often jealousy or depression. Married homosexual women may ask for advice about their relationships with the husband and family, or about dysfunction in heterosexual intercourse. Counselling is the appropriate treatment.

Further reading

Bancroft, J. H. J. (1988). *Human Sexuality and its Problems*, 2nd edn. Churchill Livingstone, Edinburgh.
A comprehensive account of normal and abnormal sexual behaviour.
Hawton, K. (1985). *Sex Therapy: a Practical Guide.* Oxford University Press, Oxford.
Although dated, this book still provides a clear and practical account of simple kinds of therapy suitable for use by the non-specialist.
Johnson, A. E., Wadsworth, J. & Field, J. (1994). *Sexual Attitudes and Lifestyles.* Blackwell, Oxford.
A large UK survey of sexual experience and attitudes in the general population.

CHAPTER 16

Psychiatry of the elderly

Chapter contents

Psychiatric disorder in the elderly 216

Specific psychiatric disorders 219

Delirium 219
Dementia 220
Depressive disorder 225
Mania 227
Paranoid syndromes 227
Anxiety, minor mood disorder, and
   personality disorder 227
Abuse of alcohol and drugs 228

Physical abuse of the elderly 228

Figure 16.1 shows how the age structure of the population is changing; the proportion of older people in less developed countries is increasing much faster than it is in developed countries. As many illnesses, such as most of the dementias, occur more frequently with increasing age, all countries will be faced with the problem of

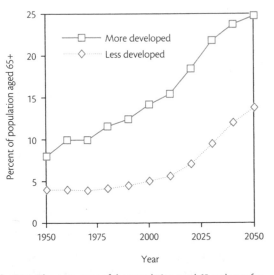

Fig. 16.1 The percentage of the population aged 65 and over for more developed and less developed countries. (Data from 1996 United Nations population estimates and projections; from Jorm, A. F. (2000).) The ageing population and epidemiology of mental disorders among the elderly. In New Oxford Textbook of Psychiatry. Eds M. Gelder, J. J. Lopez-Ibor, and N. C. Andresen. Oxford University Press, Oxford.

managing large numbers of mentally ill older people. The proportion with cognitive impairment will double in the UK in the next 50 years and will increase even more dramatically in less developed countries.

Older people with mental health problems present particular challenges, which the practice and organization of old age psychiatry services have to take into account. Elderly patients are often physically as well as mentally frail and this affects presentation and course. On the other hand, they have the advantage of a lifetime's experience of responding to fortune and adversity.

When considering psychiatric disorder in the elderly, the clinician must be able to collect and integrate information from a variety of sources, and to produce a mangement plan that takes account of psychological, physical, and social needs as well as the psychological. This plan is likely to involve the cooperation of several professionals. It is in this clinical complexity that much of the challenge and fascination of old age psychiatry lies.

Epidemiology

Psychiatric disorder, like medical illness, is especially prevalent in the elderly (Fig. 16.2). This is reflected in

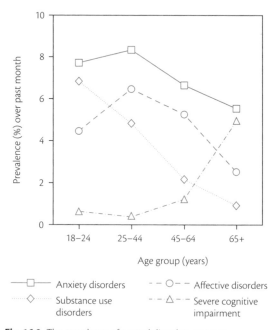

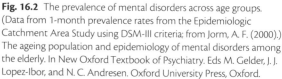

Fig. 16.2 The prevalence of mental disorders across age groups. (Data from 1-month prevalence rates from the Epidemiologic Catchment Area Study using DSM-III criteria; from Jorm, A. F. (2000).) The ageing population and epidemiology of mental disorders among the elderly. In New Oxford Textbook of Psychiatry. Eds M. Gelder, J. J. Lopez-Ibor, and N. C. Andresen. Oxford University Press, Oxford.

the large proportion of time spent on the care of the elderly in primary care and the high proportion of hospital inpatient and outpatient attenders who are aged 65 or older. Although psychiatric disorders in old age have some special features, they do not differ greatly from the psychiatric disorders of younger adults.

Normal ageing

The following changes are seen in normal ageing.

Structural changes in the brain With advancing age, the weight of the brain decreases, the quantity of nerve processes declines, and there is a minor and selective loss of cells. Senile plaques are increasingly common, and ischaemic lesions are present in the brains of about half of normal subjects aged over 65.

◆ **Psychological changes** From mid life there is a decline in intellectual functions, as measured with standard intelligence tests, together with deterioration of short-term memory and slowness. Also, there may be alterations in personality and attitudes, such as increasing cautiousness, rigidity, and 'disengagement' from the outside world.

◆ **Social difficulties** Many elderly people have lower incomes and poorer accommodation than younger people. Most live at home—about half with their spouse, and about one in ten with their children. Some of those who live alone are very isolated. These unsatisfactory social circumstances are typical of most Western countries, but in some cultures, for example the Chinese, the elderly are esteemed and most can expect to live with their children.

◆ **Use of medical services** The elderly consult their family doctors more often than younger people and they occupy one-half of all general hospital beds. These demands are particularly great in those aged over 75. Treatment is often made difficult by the presence of more than one disorder and by increased sensitivity to drug side effects.

Psychiatric disorder in the elderly

The elderly suffer from all the psychiatric disorders described in other chapters of this book, but dementia and delirium are particularly common. Since the prevalence of dementia increases with age (Fig. 16.3), there has been a disproportionate increase in the demand for psychiatric care for the elderly, and this trend is likely to continue. Although mild in this age group, depression is the most frequent problem seen in primary care; dementia is the most serious.

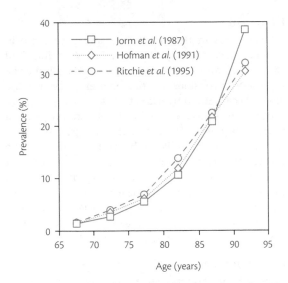

Fig. 16.3 Prevalence rates for dementia across age groups: data from 3 meta-analyses. From Jorm, A. F (2000). The ageing population and epidemiology of mental disorders among the elderly. In New Oxford Textbook of Psychiatry. Eds M. Gelder, J. J. Lopez-Ibor, and N. C. Andresen. Oxford University Press, Oxford.

Assessment

General principles

Many elderly patients can be assessed in exactly the same way as younger people. However, even more careful consideration needs to be given to medical factors

---

TABLE 16.1 Role of the primary care physician in elderly patients

Assessment

♦ Reach the correct diagnosis and detect any remediable pathology

♦ Assess the patient's functional state and encourage optimum functioning

♦ Review medication

♦ Assess the role of the primary health care team in providing services

Management

♦ Coordinate social support and make appropriate referrals to other agencies

♦ Identify the early stage of chronic disorders and help the patient and carers come to terms with the diagnosis and prognosis

♦ Anticipate and avert crises by assessing social and domestic circumstances

♦ Monitor the needs of carers and support them

---

and social circumstances (Table 16.1). After making a diagnosis there are three important practical issues that always need to be considered:

1. Can the patient's care be managed at home?

2. If so, what additional help is needed by the patient and family?

3. Can the patient manage his financial affairs?

Whenever possible the doctor should *interview any relatives or friends* who can give information about the patient and may be involved in care, especially if there is any possibility of intellectual impairment. The reasons for the request for treatment should be considered carefully, since this may reflect changes in the attitudes of the family and neighbours to the patient's longstanding problems rather than any change in the medical condition. When a specialist opinion is required it is often better to arrange this at the patient's home where patients can be observed in their usual surroundings.

History

The following specific information should be obtained during the assessment:

♦ timing of onset of symptoms and their subsequent course;

♦ a description of behaviour over a typical 24 hours;

♦ previous medical and psychiatric history;

♦ living conditions and financial position;

♦ ability for self-care and to manage finances and deal with hazards such as fire;

♦ any behaviour that may cause difficulties for carers or neighbours;

♦ the ability of family and friends to help;

♦ other services already involved in the patient's care.

Examination and investigation

Physical examination When there are medical indications, a thorough physical examination should be carried out, including an appropriately detailed neurological assessment with particular attention to vision and hearing.

Physical investigations If an organic cause of the psychiatric disorder is suspected, investigation may be required, guided by the diagnostic possibilities suggested by the history.

Psychological assessment Simple tests such as the Mini Mental State Examination (see p. 37) are valuable

BOX 16.1 ETHICAL AND LEGAL ISSUES IN THE ELDERLY

- Confidentiality in relation to information from carers.

- Confidentiality of information about financial circumstances.

- Consent to treatment:

  - capacity to consent to physical and psychological treatment;

  - advance directives;

  - decisions 'not to treat'.

- Management of financial affairs:

  - nominating another to take responsibility (Power of Attorney);

  - procedures to enable others to take responsibility.

- Entitlement to drive a car.

but must be used as part of a wider clinical examination. Regular clinical review and screening are valuable for older people. This should include a search for possible psychiatric disorder, especially for early dementia and depressive disorder.

Principles of treatment

National policies for the provision of services for the elderly differ widely. There are varying emphases on social policies to provide sheltered accommodation and care in the community. Most problems are managed in primary care but more complex problems require close links with multidisciplinary psychiatric services, with geriatric medicine, and with social and voluntary services offering help in the community.

Whatever the nature of services, the treatment of psychiatric disorders in the elderly resembles that of the same conditions in younger adults, although there are some differences in emphasis:

- it is more often necessary to treat concurrent physical disorders;

- special caution is needed in drug dosages;

- social measures and services are even more important;

- families need to be involved and supported, even more than with younger patients;

- it is essential to be aware of legal and ethical issues (Box 16.1).

Ethical issues

Ethical issues in the elderly are similar to those in younger people but problems relating to impaired capacity are much more common (Box 16.1). It may be necessary to consider practical matters as well as the ability to consent to treatment.

Advance directives ('living wills') are accepted in many countries as a means of enabling people to indicate how they would like to be treated if they lose the capacity to take decisions. They respect the principle of autonomy and are seen as helpful by many doctors. However, there can be practical problems. It must be clear that the person was competent when the directive was drawn up and interpretation needs to be flexible to take account of particular medical situations.

Place of treatment

Although it may often seem easier to treat more severe problems in hospital, *treatment at home* is usually preferable because most elderly people want to be at home and usually function better there. Plans should be responsive to changing needs, and discussed regularly with the family or other carers to ensure that home care does not place an unreasonable burden on them. *Short stays in hospital* may be needed for acute problems and to allow a holiday for the carers. *Long-term care* in a home or hospital is needed for a minority of the elderly.

Treatment of physical illness

Any physical disorder causing *organic mental disorder* should be treated if possible. The treatment of other *physical disorders* may benefit the mental state in a non-specific way. *Mobility* should be encouraged, and is often helped by physiotherapy. A good *diet* should be ensured.

Psychotropic medication

Drug-induced morbidity is common among elderly patients who may develop side effects at lower doses than do younger people. Some drugs may cause mental symptoms as side effects; most often these are drugs that are:

- used to treat cardiovascular disorders (hypotensives, diuretics, and digoxin);

- acting on the central nervous system (antidepressants, hypnotics, anxiolytics, antipsychotics, and antiparkinsonian drugs).

Many elderly people sleep poorly, and some take hypnotics regularly. Such drugs should be avoided as they may cause daytime drowsiness, confusion, falls, incontinence, and hypothermia. If a hypnotic is essential, the minimum effective dose should be used, the side effects monitored carefully, and the course of treatment made as short as possible. Dichloralphenazone, chlormethiazole, and medium- or short-acting benzodiazepines are used as hypnotics for the elderly.

Elderly patients may not take drugs as prescribed, especially when they are living alone, have poor vision, or are confused. For this reason, the drug regimen should be as simple as possible, medicine bottles should be labelled clearly and easy to open, and the patient should be provided with memory aids (e.g. by containers with separate compartments for the drugs to be taken at each time of day). If possible, drug taking should be supervised by one of the carers or by a community nurse, both of whom need to be adequately informed of the drug regimen.

It is prudent to start treatment with small doses and increase these gradually to find the minimal effective dose. Response to the medication should be reviewed regularly. Despite the need for caution in prescribing, elderly patients should not be denied effective drug treatment, especially for depressive disorders.

Psychological treatment

Discussion and problem solving are as important in the care of the elderly as in the care of younger patients, and joint interviews with partners or carers are often valuable.

Memory aids Patients with memory disorder may be helped by simple measures such as the use of notebooks and alarm clocks to aid memory. In residential accommodation the use of colour coding of doors and similar features of design can help to reduce disorientation.

Interpretative psychotherapy is seldom appropriate for the elderly.

Social measures

Many patients can be helped to remain independent by attendance at a *club or day centre* as a way of encouraging self-care, domestic skills, and social contacts. *Domiciliary occupational therapy* may help patients who cannot travel to a day centre. More severely impaired patients may benefit from *residence* in an old people's home provided that their individual needs and dignity are respected. Table 16.2 summarizes social provision.

Involving and supporting families and carers

Families should be able to discuss problems and receive advice about the patient's care (Table 16.3). For exam-

TABLE 16.2 Social measures that should be considered in the care of elderly patients
Psychosocial treatments
◆ Encourage self-care
◆ Social contacts
Legal and financial advice
◆ Financial
◆ Driving
◆ Estimating capacity
Social services
◆ Domiciliary
◆ Day care
◆ Residential and nursing care
Voluntary services

TABLE 16.3 Support for the carers of elderly patients
Good prompt care for patients
◆ Early identification of dementia
◆ Comprehensive medical and social assessment of identified cases
◆ Timely referrals between agencies, for example from general practitioner to old age psychiatrist
◆ Continuing reviews of each patient's needs and back-up for carers
◆ Active medical treatment for any intercurrent illness
Information and help for carers
◆ Provision of information, advice, and counselling for carers
◆ Regular help with household and personal care tasks
◆ Regular breaks for carers, for example by providing day care and respite care for the patient
◆ Appropriate financial support
◆ Permanent residential care if this becomes necessary

ple, if the patient is incontinent, relatives can be helped by the provision of laundry services. Day care or holiday admissions can allow carers periods of respite. With such help, many relatives can undertake the care of elderly people without undue burden.

Although most families care effectively for their elderly members, occasionally they *neglect* or even *abuse* the elderly person, or misuse their property. Elderly women are more often affected than elderly men, and those who have psychiatric disorder may be at greater risk. Although not common, vigilance is required to recognize problems.

TABLE 16.4	Clinical features of delirium

- Acute onset
- Fluctuating orientation
- Fluctuating alertness and disturbed sleep
- Impaired recent memory
- Abnormal perceptions, especially visual illusions or hallucinations
- Perplexity or suspiciousness
- Irritability and agitation

TABLE 16.5	Immediate treatment of delirium

Obtain information from informants and medical notes

Look for and treat the causes

Maintain the patient's general physical condition

Provide an appropriate environment:

- visual: adequate lighting, spectacles
- auditory: repeated, frequent explanations, hearing aids, minimal disturbance from others

Maximize familiarity with the environment:

- aid orientation by outside view, clock, etc.
- visits by relatives
- regular routine

Consistent nursing:

- minimize medical interventions
- avoid conflict
- minimum number of staff involved

Limited use of psychotropic drugs (see text)

TABLE 16.6	Causes of dementia

- Alzheimer's disease
- Vascular dementia
- Lewy body disease
- Mixed causes (e.g. Alzheimer's and vascular)
- Parkinson's disease
- Vitamin B_{12} deficiency
- Normal pressure hydrocephalus
- Hypothyroidism

Specific psychiatric disorders

Delirium

Delirium is more fully described in Chapter 10 but the *clinical features* are summarized in Table 16.4. Among elderly patients the central feature, impairment of consciousness, may not always be obvious, especially when the onset is gradual. When this happens, delirium (a reversible disorder) may be misdiagnosed as dementia (an irreversible disorder). It is not uncommon for delirium to occur in patients with established dementia, resulting in considerable deterioration in cognitive function. The commonest causes of delirium in the elderly are infections of the urinary tract, chest, skin, or ear, cardiac failure, iatrogenic side effects of drugs, and cerebrovascular ischaemia.

In the absence of an obvious medical cause for delirium, look for occult urinary or other infection, or constipation. It is important not to miss alcohol-related cases, prescribed drug side effects or withdrawal, and head injury. Although the mental state improves when the cause of delirium is removed, many of the causes of delirium threaten life, and mortality is high.

Treatment (see Chapter 10) is directed to the cause of the delirium but, until this has taken effect, drugs may be needed to control symptoms of agitation, disturbed behaviour, and psychotic behaviour (Table 16.5). The best choice is generally a small dose of an antipsychotic drug such as haloperidol that relieves symptoms without increasing confusion. If sleep is poor or disturbed, a hypnotic can be useful—chlormethiazole or dichloralphenazone are often used, rather than benzodiazepines.

Dementia

Dementia is common in the elderly. Most sufferers live at home, and in the UK about a quarter live alone. A primary care doctor with 2000 patients can expect to care for about 20 people with dementia. The main account of the syndrome of dementia is given in Chapter 10. This section is concerned with special points about dementia in the elderly. There are three common causes of dementia in this age group:

1. Alzheimer's disease.

2. Vascular dementia.

3. Lewy body disease.

Other causes are listed in Table 16.6.

Alzheimer's disease

Prevalence The prevalence in developed countries of moderate and severe Alzheimer's disease is about 5 per cent of individuals aged 65 years and over, and 20 per

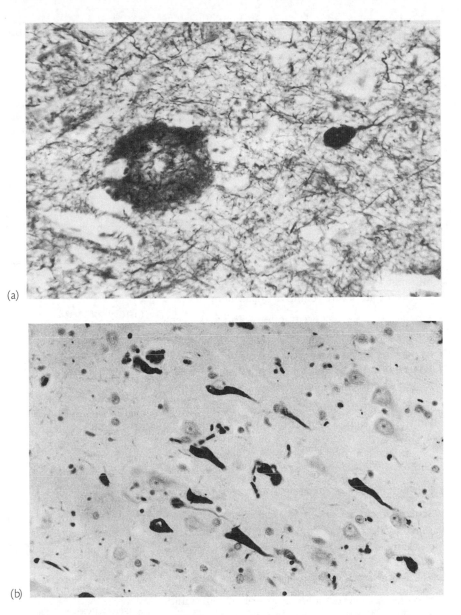

(a)

(b)

Fig. 16.4 (a) Amyloid plaque and neurofibrillary tangle from the brain of a patient who died of Alzheimer's disease. The plaque shows denser outer staining with an inner core. (b) Characteristic flame-shaped neurofibrillary tangles from the brain of a patient who died from Alzheimer's disease. The tangles are stained with an antibody to hyperphosphorylated tau protein. (Reproduced by permission of Professor Margaret Esiri.)

cent of those aged over 80 years. Therefore, as life expectancy increases in developing countries so the number of patients with Alzheimer's disease increases. About 80 per cent of these demented people live in the community rather than institutions. It is more common in women.

Pathology The brain is shrunken, with widened sulci and enlarged ventricles. There is cell loss, shrinkage of the dendritic tree, proliferation of astrocytes, and increased gliosis. Senile *plaques* and *neurofibrillary tangles* occur throughout the cortical and subcortical grey matter (Fig. 16.4).

Aetiology Genetic factors play a role, especially in those with early onset of the disease. Pedigree studies of a small number of families have suggested inheritance that is consistent with autosomal dominance. First degree relatives of those with late onset Alzheimer's disease have a risk of developing the disorder that is three times that of the general population. However, most cases appear to be clinically sporadic without a family history. Recent evidence does not support the suggestion that excessive aluminium is a cause, and other hypotheses about the role of slow viruses or abnormal immune mechanisms have not been confirmed.

Clinical features Doctors are seldom consulted in the early stages of the disorder; help is often requested after a sudden worsening associated with an intercurrent physical illness.

* The earliest feature is usually minor *forgetfulness*, which may be difficult to distinguish from the effects of normal ageing.

* *Disorientation* is usually an early sign and may be evident for the first time when the person is in unfamiliar surroundings, for example on holiday.

* The *mood* varies—it may be predominantly depressed, euphoric, flattened, or labile.

* Many patients are *restless* by day, and some *sleep poorly* at night, waking disorientated and distressed.

* *Social behaviour declines* and self-care may be neglected, although some patients maintain a good social facade despite severe cognitive impairment.

* *Personality change* may occur, often with an exaggeration of less favourable traits.

* In the later stages of the disorder, the above features progress, and signs of *parietal lobe dysfunction* (such as dysphasia or dyspraxia) may occur.

Course There is a progressive decline. Incidental physical illness may cause a superimposed delirium resulting in a sudden deterioration in cognitive function from which the patient may not recover fully. Death occurs usually within 5–8 years of the first signs of the disease.

Treatment is considered later (see p. 225).

Vascular dementia

Vascular dementia is slightly more common among men than women. It begins usually in the late sixties or seventies, often more suddenly than Alzheimer's disease, sometimes after a cerebrovascular accident.

Pathology Vascular dementia is associated with multiple infarcts of varying size caused by thromboembolism from extracranial arteries or arteriosclerosis in the main vessels. The brain is atrophic and the ventricles are dilated.

Clinical features The symptoms are characteristically fluctuating, and episodes of confusion are common, especially at night. Fits or episodes indicating cerebral ischaemia occur at some stage in many cases. There may be neurological signs. In some cases emotional and personality changes may be apparent before impairment of memory and intellect.

Diagnosis The diagnosis from Alzheimer's disease is difficult to make with certainty unless there is a clear

TABLE 16.7 Clinical features of Alzheimer's disease and vascular dementia

Alzheimer's disease	Vascular dementia
Insidious decline	Stepwise progression
Poor memory	Patchy impairment of cognitive function
Progressive disorientation	Poor memory
Mood change	Episodes of confusion
Restless activity	Mood change
Insomnia	Personality change
Decline in social behaviour	Seizures
Personality change	Neurological signs (see text)
Dysphasia, dyspraxia	

history of stroke or neurological localizing signs (Table 16.7). Suggestive features are patchy defects of cognitive function, stepwise progression of the condition, and the presence of hypertension and of arteriosclerosis in peripheral or retinal vessels.

Prognosis From the time of diagnosis the lifespan averages 4–5 years, although the variations are wide. About half the patients die from ischaemic heart disease, while others die from cerebral infarction or renal complications.

Lewy body disease

The name refers to the characteristic pathology, namely Lewy bodies in the cerebral cortex and substantia nigra. It is a progressive dementing illness that can sometimes be distinguished from Alzheimer's by its fluctuating course, the occurrence of hallucinations (especially visual), delusions, and signs of parkinsonism. There may be repeated falls and transient disturbances of consciousness.

Differential diagnosis of dementia in the elderly

General aspects of the diagnosis of dementia are discussed in Chapter 10. In the elderly, dementia must be differentiated from three other disorders:

1. **Delirium**. This is suggested by impaired and fluctuating consciousness, and by perceptual misinterpretations and visual hallucinations (Table 16.8).

2. **Mood disorders** (see Chapter 8).

3. **Paranoid states** (see p. 227).

It is important to *consider treatable causes* of dementia (Table 16.9) even though they are rare.

TABLE 16.8 Some clinical features distinguishing delirium and dementia

Feature	Delirium	Dementia
Clinical course		
◆ Mode of onset	Acute or subacute (hours or days)	Chronic (usually several years)
◆ Fluctuations	Frequent and rapid (in hours)	Slow changes (months)
Conscious level		
◆ Attention	Markedly reduced	Reduced in severe cases
◆ Arousal	Increased or decreased	Usually normal
◆ Alertness	Reduced in severer cases	Normal
Cognitive changes		
◆ Delusions	Fleeting, poorly systemized	If present, often consistent
◆ Hallucination	Common (usually visual)	Infrequent (both visual and verbal)
◆ Orientation	Usually impaired	Impaired in proportion to severity
Motor features		
◆ Abnormal movements	Tremor and myoclonus	Usually absent
◆ Psychomotor activity	Usually abnormal: increased or decreased	Usually normal
◆ Dysgraphia	Usually present	Absent in mild cases
◆ Autonomic features	Abnormalities often present	Normal (except that postural hypotension is common)

TABLE 16.9 Treatable causes of apparent dementia

- ◆ Depressive pseudodementia
- ◆ Delirium
- ◆ Slow-growing operable cerebral tumour
- ◆ Hypothyroidism
- ◆ Normal pressure hydrocephalus
- ◆ Vitamin B_{12} or folic acid deficiency
- ◆ Renal failure
- ◆ Severe anaemia

TABLE 16.10 Early assessment of dementia in primary care

- ◆ Alertness to evidence (usually from a relative) of decline in intellectual function (memory, judgement) or everyday behaviour (self-care)
- ◆ Depression, agitation, paranoid symptoms
- ◆ Clinical testing, orientation, and memory testing
- ◆ Mini Mental State Examination
- ◆ Assess functional impairment (e.g. taking medication, telephoning, managing budget, travel in cars and on public transport)

Assessment

The assessment should always include a thorough search for treatable causes of delirium superimposed upon dementia. About 10 per cent of those first thought to have dementia will have a treatable cause (Table 16.9). Table 16.10 summarizes the ways of achieving early diagnosis in primary care.

The aims of assessment are:

- ◆ to identify rare treatable conditions that may present as dementia;
- ◆ to diagnose any condition that may exacerbate dementia (e.g. a superimposed delirium);
- ◆ to diagnose of the cause of dementia;
- ◆ to obtain the information needed to plan continuing care.

Early diagnosis is important because it enables planning with the patient and with all those involved in care. Information from carers about the impairment caused by the dementia is essential (Table 16.11). Because impairments develop gradually they are often attributed at first to normal ageing. Important clues to dementia are:

- ◆ general forgetfulness;
- ◆ misplacing items;
- ◆ forgetting the names of close family members;
- ◆ increased anxiety or depression.

TABLE 16.11 Information to be sought from carers about dementia patients

- Forgetfulness
- Memory lapses
- Personality changes
- Failure to recognize people
- Failure to cope with previous routine tasks
- Lack of self-care and reduction in personal standards
- Giving up previous interests and hobbies
- Emotional changes: anxiety, depression, irritability, lack of care, and concern
- Nocturnal confusion
- Disorientation for time and place
- Difficulty in speech
- Extent to which changes have been gradual or have suddenly worsened

TABLE 16.12 Assessment of functional capacity in dementia patients

- Continence
- Dressing
- Self-care
- Cooking ability and nutrition
- Shopping/housework
- Degree of orientation in the home
- Capacity to manage financial affairs
- Formal and informal supports
- Social contacts
- Safety in the home

TABLE 16.13 Reasons for referral of dementia patients to a hospital consultant

- Early diagnosis of a possible dementia and the cause
- Detection of reversible conditions mimicking dementia
- Specialist advice about management, including advice on drug treatment
- Uncontrollable agitation
- Assessment and management of challenging behaviours
- Access to specialist services

Questions about the patient's functional capacity may reveal defects in self-care, ability to cope with familiar tasks, and emotional changes (Table 16.12). Table 16.13

BOX 16.2 ASSESSMENT OF COMMON PROBLEMS

Aggression

- Is it verbal or physical?
- To whom is it directed and when—is there a reason?
- What resources are available?
- Should drugs be used?

Incontinence

- What kind and how often?
- Are there contributing medical factors (e.g. drugs)?
- What means of coping with the problem are available (e.g. pads or laundry services)?

Wandering

- Frequency?
- What is the degree of danger?

Refusal of services

- How do the risks balance against the choices of the individual?
- What alternative sources of help are available?
- When should the situation be reassessed?

Refusal to accept admission to residential care

- What other ways could there be to limit risks of wandering and self-neglect?
- Is additional community support available?
- Are compulsory procedures appropriate?
- Can some one be appointed to take on legal powers for financial and other matters?

summarizes the common reasons for referral for a specialist opinion and Box 16.2 the points to be considered when assessing common problems found in dementia.

Examination and investigation

The mental state examination should include a systematic assessment of cognitive functions. A full physical examination and investigation is required in:

- patients with a rapid onset of fluctuating cognitive impairment and for those with unusual patterns of cognitive impairment and clear consciousness;

◆ patients with onset under the age of 75 years.

Specific investigations are usually not indicated in those with insidious onset of the typical pattern of dementia over the age of 75.

To determine the cause of dementia, biochemical or other physical investigations may be indicated. According to the diagnostic possibilities, these may include: blood count and film, erythrocyte sedimentation rate (ESR), VDRL serology, thyroid function, urea and electrolytes, liver function, vitamin B_{12}, chest X-ray, skull X-ray, electrocardiogram (ECG), and electroencephalograph (EEG). A scan is indicated when a localized lesion is suspected.

Treatment of dementia in the elderly

The first step is to *treat any treatable physical disorder* causing the dementia in the hope of arresting or possibly reversing it to some extent. If the physical disorder has caused an associated delirium, the mental state may improve considerably with treatment of the physical disorder. Even minor medical problems, such as constipation and urinary infection, may worsen the behavioural problems of a demented person (Table 16.14).

In early dementia, all those involved should consider what the patient should be told about the diagnosis. The patient may wish to know and there may be important reasons for early plans for future care, avoidance of unsuitable activities (such as driving), and planning family life and financial matters.

Psychological and social treatment For elderly demented patients psychological and social treatments are similar to those for younger patients (see Chapter 10).

Care Whenever feasible, patients should be *cared for at home*, especially when family and friends can contribute to their care. If necessary, help can be provided by a community psychiatric nurse or social worker. *Day care* may be needed to help the patient and their family.

TABLE 16.14 Management of dementia
◆ Treat any primary disorder
◆ Treat the cause of superimposed delirium
◆ Treat even minor medical problems (see text)
◆ Involve and support relatives
◆ Arrange practical help in the home
◆ Arrange help for carers (e.g. 'holiday admissions')
◆ Medication for night- and daytime restlessness
◆ If home care fails, arrange residential or hospital care

TABLE 16.15 Role of the primary care team in dementia patients
◆ Investigate treatable causes (present in about 10 per cent)
◆ Exclude coincident conditions: especially depression, delirium, paranoid disorder symptoms, and concurrent physical illnesses
◆ Minimize associated disabilities
◆ Decide whether to refer to consultant (see Table 16.13)
◆ Manage and coordinate access to other resources
◆ Help carers by providing information and advice, especially about the emotional and behavioural changes that have taken place or may do so

Inpatient care may be needed to tide over a crisis, or to enable the family to have a period of rest or a holiday. If the patient cannot be managed at home, *residential care* may be appropriate in an old people's home. The role of the primary care team is summarized in Table 16.15. In most cases, *long-term care in hospital* is required only when intensive nursing is needed

Drug treatment Medication should be used with care as the side effects may be greater than the benefits. It is occasionally appropriate to consider *sedative drug treatment*, such as the use of thioridazine or promazine, for restlessness when it is exhausting both for carers and the patient. *Antipsychotic drugs* may be required to control paranoid delusions, and *antidepressants* may be indicated when depressive symptoms are prominent.

Central cholinesterase inhibitors are of specific benefit for approximately one-half of patients with mild/moderate dementia of Alzheimer's disease, delaying deterioration and resulting in some improvement in cognitive function for up to a year. They should only be prescribed by specialists and the response should be carefully monitored. A second generation of drugs is being developed and they can be expected to be available in the next few years.

Management of behavioural disturbance Non-drug interventions are the most important. They include identifying and remedying any medical or environmental causes, providing extra support for carers, and considering environmental changes. Medication is most useful for specific psychiatric causes of disturbance such as depression, anxiety, or psychotic symptoms. Sleep disturbance is best managed by avoiding caffeine and other stimulants, trying to increase daytime activity and reducing daytime sleep. Antipsychotic drugs are widely used in the management of disturbed behaviour, but there is little convincing evidence to support their use for non-specific indications. Such therapy should be a last resort for severe problems.

Depressive disorder

Depressive disorders are common in later life with a prevalence of about 10–15 per cent for those aged 65, of which a quarter are severe. Many of these disorders are found in people who have had a depressive disorder at an earlier age; first depressive illnesses decline in incidence after the age of 60, and are rare after the age of 80. The incidence of **suicide** increases steadily with age and is usually associated with depressive disorder.

Clinical features

There are no fundamental differences between depressive disorders in the elderly and those in younger people, but some symptoms are more common in the elderly. Anxiety and hypochondriacal symptoms are frequent. Depressive delusions of poverty and physical illness are more common among severely depressed patients, as are hallucinations of an accusing or obscene kind.

A few retarded, depressed patients have conspicuous difficulty in concentrating and remembering but there is no corresponding defect in clinical tests of memory function (**pseudodementia**). The possibility of a depressive disorder should be considered whenever an elderly patient develops apparent cognitive impairment, anxiety, or hypochondriacal symptoms.

Course

Untreated depressive disorders in the elderly often have a *prolonged course*, some lasting for years. With treatment, most patients improve considerably within a few months, but about 15 per cent do not recover completely even after vigorous treatment. Long-term follow-up of recovered patients shows that relapse is frequent. Suicide is more likely than in younger people.

The factors predicting a better prognosis are:

* onset before the age of 70;
* short duration of illness;
* good previous adjustment;
* no concurrent disabling physical illness;
* good recovery from previous episodes.

Aetiology

In general, the aetiology of depressive disorders in late life resembles that of similar disorders occurring in earlier life (see Chapter 8), except that genetic factors

TABLE 16.16 Clinical features of dementia and pseudodementia

Dementia	Pseudodementia
Prolonged progressive course	Course of weeks or months
Impaired orientation	Normal orientation
Mood changes secondary	Begins with mood symptoms
Memory impaired, may confabulate	Unwillingness to answer
Progressive course	May be diurnal variation
May be past history of mood disorder	

may be less important. Neurological and other physical illnesses seem to be more frequent among depressed elderly patients than among younger ones, and may act as provoking or maintaining factors.

Differential diagnosis

Depressive disorder has to be differentiated from a number of other states:

Dementia The most difficult differential diagnosis is between depressive pseudodementia and dementia, and a specialist opinion is often required (Table 16.16). The distinction depends on a detailed history from other informants, and careful observation of the mental state and behaviour of the patient. In *depressive pseudodementia*, mood disturbance usually precedes other symptoms and the depressed patient's lack of interest and unwillingness to answer can usually be distinguished from the demented patient's true failure of memory. In depression, there may be diurnal variation and a past history of mood disorder. The diagnostic problem is made more difficult because dementia and depressive disorder sometimes coexist.

Paranoid disorder When paranoid ideas are prominent in a depressive disorder, it has to be differentiated from a paranoid disorder. In a depressive disorder, the patient usually believes that the supposed persecution is justified by his own wickedness; in a paranoid disorder he usually resents it as unjustified. Depressive symptoms usually follow the onset of paranoid disorder, but it is often difficult to be certain of the sequence.

Anxiety disorder A depressive disorder with symptoms of agitation may be mistaken at first for an anxiety disorder. It is essential to look for characteristic pessimism and other symptoms of low mood.

Management

In most respects the treatment of depressive disorders is the same for the elderly as for people of other ages (see Chapter 8). Suicide risk should be assessed (see p. 172).

Antidepressant drugs are effective in the elderly, but should be used cautiously and adjusted according to side effects and response. Some psychiatrists use tricyclic antidepressants as the first choice; others prefer specific serotonin reuptake inhibitors (SSRIs) . The latter are particularly useful for those who find the side effects of tricyclic antidepressants intolerable, for those with cardiac arrhythmias or epilepsy, and for those where the risk of delirium is high (e.g. patients with dementia). To reduce side effects, the starting dose is about half the usual dose for younger patients, and the drug may be given more than once a day. Although it is appropriate to start cautiously, it is important to achieve a full therapeutic dose. After recovery, antidepressant medication should be reduced slowly and then continued in reduced dose for at least 2 years. Patients with a history of recurrent depression require long-term continuation treatment.

Electroconvulsive therapy (ECT) is useful for the small minority of patients with severe and distressing agitation, life-threatening stupor, or failure to respond to drugs. Special care is needed with the anaesthesia. It may be necessary to space out treatments at longer intervals than in younger patients to reduce post-treatment memory impairment.

Mania

Unlike depressive disorder, mania does not increase in incidence with age. Hence, in old age mania is much less frequent than depressive disorder, accounting for 5–10 per cent of affective disorders. In the elderly, depressive symptoms are often present with the manic symptoms, and the condition is frequently recurrent. Treatment of the acute illness is similar to that for younger patients (see Chapter 8), although with special caution over the side effects of drugs. Lithium prophylaxis is valuable but blood levels should be kept at the lower end of the therapeutic range used for younger patients, and should be monitored with special care.

Paranoid syndromes

Paranoid syndromes, with persecutory beliefs, delusions, or hallucinations, may be due to:

* dementia;
* mood disorder;
* schizophrenia and delusional disorder (sometimes referred to as late paraphrenia);
* paranoid personality disorder.

The commonest syndromes are those secondary to dementia or mood disorders.

Schizophrenia and delusional disorder may begin in old age or may have begun earlier in life and continued into old age. In the elderly, the symptoms are generally less florid and the behaviour less disturbed than in young patients. The same aetiological factors have been identified as in younger adults, but evidence of previously suspicious personality, social isolation, and deafness seem to be particularly important.

Differential diagnosis

In the elderly, **schizophrenia and delusional disorders** are diagnosed by the same criteria as in younger patients. In **dementia** there is cognitive impairment, and visual hallucinations may occur. In **mood disorder**, the mood disturbance is more profound than in other paranoid states, and the persecutory delusions are usually associated with ideas of guilt. In **paranoid personality disorder** there is lifelong suspiciousness and distrust, with sensitive ideas but no delusions.

Treatment

In general, the treatment of these disorders in the elderly is similar to that for younger people (see Chapter 9). Outpatient treatment may be possible, but admission to hospital is often required for adequate assessment and treatment. Most patients require antipsychotic medication but the dosage is usually less than that needed for younger adults, for example, 2–5 mg of trifluoperazine three times a day or haloperidol 1–10 mg once daily. As with younger patients a depot preparation should be considered. Any sensory deficit, such as deafness or cataract, should be assessed and, if possible, treated. Attendance at a day hospital or day centre may be needed to avoid social isolation, ensure adequate supervision, and prevent relapse. (See Case study 16.1.)

Patients with long histories in younger life will require continuing specialist care that takes account of the changing circumstances of old age.

Anxiety, minor mood disorder, and personality disorder

Anxiety and minor mood disorder are as common in the elderly as in younger people, but occur rarely for the first time in old age. There is often a predisposing

---

CASE STUDY 16.1 PARANOID SYMPTOMS

The son of an 82-year-old widow comes to your surgery to say that he is concerned about his mother. He has noticed, over a period of months, that his mother has complained of increasingly numerous events in which neighbours and other people have apparently shouted abuse from outside her house and persecuted her. She believes that they have stolen objects and that they have moved her furniture around. She thinks that there is a complex conspiracy that involves a number of her neighbours and which is intended to drive her out of her own home. The son has realized that many of the allegations are a fantasy and unbelievable and has tried to persuade his mother to seek help. However, she has maintained that she is perfectly well and that the problem lies with her neighbours' behaviour.

[Importance of information from relative]

You have known the patient for many years and have occasionally visited her to treat minor ailments. You say that you will visit her home and say that you are making one of your regular visits to the older patients in your practice. When you arrive, the patient is initially somewhat suspicious but lets you in and tells you about her beliefs that she is being persecuted. When you express some doubt, it is clear that she will not be dissuaded from these beliefs.

[Home visit; maintaining relationship]

You feel that it is unlikely that she would agree to a visit from a psychiatrist and that you should try and establish the diagnosis. While your patient is upset about what has been happening, it is also apparent that when she discusses her own family and other issues she is cheerful and retains her usual sense of humour. You conclude she is not suffering from a depressive illness. At the same time, it is apparent that her memory of past events and of previous discussions with you is excellent and that she has a good knowledge of current events. It is clear that she is not suffering from dementia. She is not deaf. You conclude that she is almost certainly suffering from primary paranoid disorder.

[Differential diagnoses: dementia, depression, primary paranoid disorder]

You conclude that medication would be appropriate and you are eventually able to persuade your patient that she should try some new tablets to treat the very considerable distress that she reports in association with the persecutory symptoms. You prescribe Stelazine 5 mg per day and arrange to visit her again. When you return to your surgery, you consult the local psychiatrist for the elderly and agree that the present plan is appropriate and that, if necessary and the patient consents, a psychiatric consultation could be arranged at a later stage.

[Negotiating acceptable treatment]

Two weeks later you are pleased to find that the patient is no longer describing the persecutory symptoms, which she says have stopped several days previously (although she apparently still believes that they were genuine). She agrees that the medication has been helpful for her distress and is willing to continue for the time being. You suggest that you will check on the medication when you see her for her usual blood pressure review.

[Regular review of patient; link with family]

---

personality disorder. Common precipitating factors are physical illness, retirement, bereavement, and change of accommodation. Among the elderly these syndromes are usually of a non-specific kind, with anxiety, depressive, and hypochondriacal symptoms. Specific obsessional, phobic, and conversion disorders are less common. It is important to identify anxiety that is secondary to depressive disorders in early dementia.

Personality disorder may cause difficulties for elderly patients and their families. Paranoid traits may become accentuated with the social isolation of old age, sometimes to the extent of resembling a paranoid disorder. Personality disorder in the elderly often leads to isolation and occasionally to self-neglect, which can be extreme.

Treatment The treatment of emotional and personality disorders in old age is similar to that in younger adult life. It is essential to treat any physical disorder. Social measures are usually more useful than psychological treatment, but psychotherapy and behavioural treatments should not be ruled out because of age alone.

Abuse of alcohol and drugs

Although excessive drinking declines with increasing age, the problem is still significant among the elderly. Sometimes the excessive drinking began at a younger age and sometimes begins in old age, often as a response to loneliness, boredom, or unhappiness. The management of the problem in the elderly is similar to that for younger people (see Chapter 17).

The overuse of prescribed drugs, especially hypnotics, analgesics, and laxatives, is common and it may be difficult to distinguish between deliberate overuse and that consequent on poor memory for the correct dosage or for the time when the last dose was taken.

Physical abuse of the elderly

Cruelty and physical maltreatment of elderly people may occur by carers at home or in residential care. It is especially likely where there is a long history of disturbed relationships, where carers are ignorant, unsympathetic, or overwhelmed by the behavioural difficulties, and, occasionally, for financial exploitation. Clinicians need to be aware of the possibility of physical abuse and be prepared to intervene in whatever way will prevent continuing abuse and to deal with underlying problems.

Further reading

Jacoby, R. & Oppenheimer, C. (2002). *Psychiatry in the Elderly*, 3rd edn. Oxford University Press, Oxford. *A comprehensive work of reference.*

CHAPTER 17

Drugs and other physical treatments

Chapter contents

General considerations 231

Review of drugs used in psychiatry 233

Other physical treatments 252

This chapter is about the use of drugs and electroconvulsive therapy (ECT). Psychological treatment is considered separately in Chapter 18. This is a convenient way of dividing the subject matter of a book, but in practice these *physical treatments are always combined with psychological treatment*, most often supportive or problem-solving counselling, but also one of the specific methods described in Chapter 18.

The account in this chapter is concerned with practical therapeutics rather than basic pharmacology, and it will be assumed that the reader has studied the pharmacology of the principal types of drug used in psychiatric disorders. (Readers who do not have this knowledge should consult a textbook, for example, *The Oxford Textbook of Clinical Pharmacology and Drug Therapy* by D. G. Grahame-Smith and J. K. Aronson.) Nevertheless, a few important points about the actions of psychotropic drugs will be considered, before describing the specific groups of drugs.

New drugs are introduced every year. Chapter 3 contains advice about finding a review of evidence about the effectiveness of new drugs.

General considerations

Pharmacokinetics of psychotropic drugs

To be effective, psychotropic drugs must reach the brain in adequate amounts. How far they do this depends on their absorption, metabolism, excretion, and passage across the blood–brain barrier.

Absorption Most psychotropic drugs are absorbed readily from the gut, but absorption can be reduced by intestinal hurry or a malabsorption syndrome.

Metabolism Most psychotropic drugs are metabolized partially in the liver on their way from the gut via the portal system to the systemic circulation. The amount of this so-called *first pass metabolism* differs from one person to another, and is altered by certain drugs, taken at the same time, which induce liver enzymes (e.g. barbiturates) or inhibit them (e.g. monoamine oxidase inhibitors, MAOIs). Although first pass metabolism reduces the amount of the original drug reaching the brain, the metabolites of some drugs have their own therapeutic effects. Because many psychotropic drugs have active metabolites, the *measurement of plasma concentrations of the parent drug is generally a poor guide to treatment*. Such measurement is used routinely only with lithium carbonate, which has no metabolites (see pp. 248–9).

Distribution In the plasma, psychotropic drugs are bound largely to protein. Because they are lipophilic, they pass easily into the *brain*. For the same reason they enter into *fat stores* from which they are released slowly, often for many weeks after the patient has ceased to take the drug. They also pass into *breast milk*—an important point when a breast-feeding mother is treated.

Excretion Psychotropic drugs and their metabolites are excreted through the kidneys, so smaller doses should be given when renal function is impaired. Lithium is unique among the psychotropic drugs in being filtered passively in the glomerulus and then partly reabsorbed in the tubules by the mechanism that absorbs sodium. The two ions compete for reabsorption so that when sodium levels fall, lithium absorption rises and lithium concentrations increase—potentially to a toxic level.

Drug interactions

When two drugs are given together one may either interfere with the other, or enhance its therapeutic or unwanted effects. Interactions can take place during absorption, metabolism, or excretion; or at the cellular level. For psychotropic drugs, most pharmacokinetic interactions are at the stage of liver metabolism, the important exception being lithium for which interference is at the stage of renal excretion. An important pharmacodynamic interaction is the antagonism between tricyclic drugs and some antihypertensive drugs (see Box 17.3). When prescribing a psychotropic drug and another drug, the manufacturer's literature or a work of reference should be consulted to determine whether the drugs interact.

Drug withdrawal

When some drugs are given for a long period, the tissues adjust to their presence and when the drug is withdrawn there is a temporary disturbance of function until a new adjustment is reached. This disturbance appears clinically as a withdrawal syndrome. Among psychotropic drugs, anxiolytics and hypnotics are the most likely to induce this effect (see p. 237)

General advice about prescribing psychotropic drugs

Use well-tried drugs When there is a choice of equally effective drugs, it is generally good practice to use the drugs whose side effects and long-term effects are understood better. Also, well-tried drugs are generally less expensive than new ones. Clinicians should become familiar with a few drugs of each of the main types—antidepressants, antipsychotics, and so on. In this way they will become used to adjusting dosage and recognizing side effects.

Change drugs only for a good reason If there is no therapeutic response to an established drug given in adequate dosage, it is unlikely that there will be a better response to another drug from the same therapeutic group. The main reason for changing medication is that side effects have prevented adequate dosage. It is then appropriate to change to a drug with a different pattern of side effects; for example, from an antidepressant with strong anticholinergic effects to another with weaker ones.

Combine drugs only for specific indications Generally, drug combinations should be avoided (see Drug interactions, above). However, some drug combinations are of proven value for specific purposes; for example, benzodiazepines and antipsychotics to control acute symptoms of schizophrenia (see p. 130), and lithium and antidepressant for drug-resistant depressive disorder (see p. 111). Usually, drug combinations are initiated by a specialist because the adverse effects of such combinations can be more hazardous than those of a single drug. However, general practitioners may be asked to continue prescribing.

Adjust dosage carefully Dose ranges for some commonly used drugs are indicated later in this chapter; others will be found in the manufacturers' data sheets, or a work of reference. Within these ranges, the correct dose for an individual patient is decided from the severity of the symptoms, the patient's age and weight, and any factors that may affect drug metabolism or excretion.

Plan the interval between doses Less frequent administration has the advantage that patients are more likely to be reliable in taking drugs. The duration of action of most psychotropic drugs is such that they can be taken once or twice a day while maintaining a therapeutic plasma concentration between doses.

Decide the duration of treatment The duration depends on the risk of dependency and the nature of the disorder. In general, anxiolytic and hypnotic drugs should be given for a short time—a few days to 2 or 3 weeks—because of the risk of dependency. Antidepressants and antipsychotics are given for a long time—several months—because of the risk of relapse.

Advise patients Before giving a first prescription for a drug, the doctor should explain and give advice on the following points:

1. The likely *initial effects* of the drug (e.g. drowsiness or dry mouth).

2. The *delay* before therapeutic effects appear (about 2 weeks with antidepressants).

3. The likely *first signs of improvement* (e.g. improved sleep after starting an antidepressant).

4. *Common side effects* (e.g. fine tremor with lithium).

5. Any *serious effects* that should be reported immediately by the patient (e.g. coarse tremor after taking lithium).

6. Any *restrictions* while the drug is taken (e.g. not driving or operating machinery if the drugs reduce alertness).

7. *How long* the patient will need to take the drug: for anxiolytics, the patient is discouraged from taking them for too long; for antidepressants or antipsychotics, the patient is encouraged to continue after symptoms have been controlled.

Prescribing for special groups There are various groups of patients who need particular consideration when choosing the right drugs to prescribe (Box 17.1).

Adherence to treatment

Many patients do not take the drugs prescribed for them. Their unused drugs are a danger to children and a potential source of deliberate self-poisoning. Other patients take more than the prescribed dose, especially of hypnotic or anxiolytic drugs. It is important to check that repeat prescriptions are not being requested before the correct day. (Adherence to prescribed treatment was previously referred to as **compliance** and the agreement between the doctor and patient on a course of treatment is sometimes called **concordance**.)

There are three main points the patient must have accepted in order successfully to adhere to prescribed treatment:

1. The patient must *appreciate the need to take the drug*. Schizophrenic or seriously depressed patients may not be convinced that they are ill, or may not wish to recover. Some patients—including those with delusions—may distrust their doctors.

2. The patient should *have concerns* about its dangers. Some patients fear that antidepressant drugs will cause addiction; some fear unpleasant or dangerous side effects.

3. The patient needs to be *able to remember* to take it. Patients with memory impairment may forget to take medication, or take the dose twice.

Time spent at the start of treatment in discussing reasons for the drug treatment and the patient's concerns, and in explaining the beneficial and likely adverse effects of the drugs, increases adherence. Adherence should be checked at subsequent visits and, if necessary, the discussion should be repeated and extended to include any fresh concerns of the patient.

What to do if there is no therapeutic response

The first step is to find out whether the patient has taken the drug in the correct dose. If not, the points described above should be considered. If the prescribed dose has been taken, the diagnosis should be reviewed: if is confirmed, an increase of dosage should be considered. Only when these steps have been gone through should the original drug be changed.

Review of drugs used in psychiatry

Psychotropic drugs are those that have effects mainly on mental symptoms; they are divided into six groups according to their principal actions. Several have secondary actions used for other purposes. For example, antidepressants are sometimes used to treat anxiety (Table 17.1).

1. **Anxiolytic drugs** reduce anxiety. Because they have a general calming effect, they are sometimes called

BOX 17.1 **PRESCRIBING FOR SPECIAL GROUPS**

Children

Most childhood psychiatric disorders are treated without medication. Many drugs that are licensed for use in adults have not been adequately studied in children. The indications for drug treatment are considered in Chapter 20. When drugs are required, care must be taken in selecting the appropriate dose. Usually, medication will have been started by a specialist who will advise about continuing treatment.

Elderly patients

These patients are often sensitive to drug side effects and may have impaired renal or hepatic function, so it is important to start with low doses and increase to about half the adult dose in appropriate cases.

Pregnant women

Psychotropic drugs should be avoided if possible during the first trimester of pregnancy because of the risk of teratogenesis. If medication is needed for a woman who could become pregnant, advice is given about contraception. If the patient is already pregnant and medication is essential the manufacturer's advice should be followed and the risks discussed with the patient. If the patient becomes pregnant while taking a psychotropic drug the risk of relapse should be weighed against the reported teratogenic risk of the drug. In general, it is safer to use long-established drugs for which there has been ample time to accumulate experience about safety. The following points concern the classes of psychotropic drugs.

- **Anxiolytics** are seldom essential in early pregnancy since psychological treatment is usually an effective alternative.

- If **antidepressants** are required, amitriptyline and imipramine have been in long use, without convincing evidence of teratogenic effects.

- **Antipsychotic drugs**. It is important to discuss contraception with schizophrenic women, and to re-evaluate the need for antipsychotics if the patient becomes pregnant.

- **Lithium carbonate** should be avoided if possible in pregnancy because its use is associated with an increased rate of cardiac abnormality in the fetus (see p. 249). Contraception is especially important for women who may become manic and it is prudent to leave a month between the last dose of lithium and the ending of contraceptive measures. If a patient conceives when taking lithium, there is no indication for termination but the risks should be explained, specialist advice obtained, and the fetus examined by ultrasound. Mothers who are taking lithium at term should if possible stop gradually, well before delivery. The drug should not be taken during labour. Serum lithium concentration should be measured frequently during labour and the use of diuretics avoided.

- **Valproate** should be used cautiously in women of childbearing potential, and should not be started in pregnancy, because of its teratogenic potential.

Mothers who are breast-feeding

Psychotropic drugs should be prescribed cautiously to women who are breast-feeding because they pass into breast milk and the possibility is not ruled out that they may affect brain development. Some authorities recommend that women receiving psychotropic medication should not breast-feed. Others continue treatment cautiously with careful monitoring of the baby. Benzodiazepines pass readily into breast milk, causing sedation. Most neuroleptics and antidepressants pass rather less readily into the milk; sulpiride, doxepin, and dothiepin are secreted in larger amounts and should be avoided. Lithium carbonate enters milk freely and breast-feeding should be avoided. The advice of a specialist should be obtained.

BOX 17.1 **PRESCRIBING FOR SPECIAL GROUPS** (continued)

Patients with concurrent medical illness

Special care is needed in prescribing for patients with medical illness, especially liver and kidney disorders, which may interfere with metabolism and excretion of drugs. Conversely, medical disorders may be exacerbated by the side effects of some psychotropic drugs. For example, cardiac disorder and epilepsy may be affected adversely by some antidepressant drugs (see p. 243); while drugs with anticholingergic side effects exacerbate glaucoma and may provoke retention of urine.

TABLE 17.1	The main groups of psychotropic drugs	
Type	Indications	Classes of drug
Anxiolytic	Acute anxiety	Benzodiazepines
		Azapirones
Hypnotic	Insomnia	Benzodiazepines
		Cyclopyrrolones
		Zopiclone
Antipsychotic*	Delusion and hallucinations	Phenothiazines (conventional)
	Mania	Butyrophenones
	To prevent relapse in schizophrenia	Substituted benzamides (atypical)
Antidepressant	Depressive disorders	Tricyclics
	Chronic anxiety	MAOIs
	Obsessive-compulsive disorder	SSRIs
	Nocturnal enuresis	SNRIs
Mood stabilizer	To prevent recurrent mood disorder	Lithium
		Carbamazepine
		Valproate
		Lamotrigine
Stimulants	Narcolepsy	Amphetamine
	Hyperkinetic disorder in children	
Cognitive enhancers	Dementia	Donepezil
		Rivastigmine
		Galantamine

MAOI, monoamine oxidase inhibitor; SNRI, serotonin and noradrenaline reuptake inhibitor; SSRI, specific serotonin reuptake inhibitor.

*Antiparkinsonian drugs are used to control the side effects of antipsychotics.

minor tranquillizers (major tranquillizer is an alternative name for antipsychotic drugs, see below). In larger doses these drugs produce drowsiness and for this reason are sometimes called *sedatives*.

2. **Hypnotics** promote sleep; many hypnotics are of the same type as the drugs used as anxiolytics.

3. **Antipsychotic drugs** control delusions, hallucinations, and psychomotor excitement in psychoses. Sometimes they are called *major tranquillizers* because of their calming effect; or *neuroleptics* because of their parkinsonian and other neurological side effects. (Antiparkinsonian agents are sometimes employed to control parkinsonian side effects.)

4. **Antidepressants** relieve the symptoms of depressive disorders but do not elevate the mood of healthy people. Antidepressant drugs are also used to treat chronic anxiety disorders, obsessive-compulsive disorder, and, occasionally, nocturnal enuresis.

5. **Mood-stabilizing drugs** are given to prevent recurrence of recurrent affective disorders.

6. **Psychostimulants** elevate mood but are not used for this purpose because they can cause dependence. Their principal use in psychiatry is in the treatment of hyperactivity syndromes in children (see Chapter 20).

7. Cognition-enhancing drugs are used in dementia to delay deterioration.

The main groups of drugs will be reviewed in turn. For each group, an account will be given of important points concerning therapeutic effects, the compounds in most frequent use, side effects, toxic effects, and contraindications. General advice will also be given about the use of each group of drugs, but *specific applications to the treatment of individual disorders will be found in the chapters dealing with these conditions*. Drugs with a use limited to the treatment of a single disorder (e.g. disulfiram for alcohol problems), are discussed solely in the chapters dealing with the relevant clinical syndromes.

Anxiolytic drugs

Anxiolytic drugs reduce anxiety, and in larger doses produce drowsiness (they are **sedatives**) and sleep (they are also **hypnotics**, discussed on p. 238). These drugs are prescribed widely, and sometimes unnecessarily, for patients who would improve without them. Anxiolytics are used most appropriately to reduce severe anxiety. They should be prescribed for a short time—usually a few days, and seldom for more than

TABLE 17.2   Drugs used to treat anxiety
Primary anxiolytics
◆ Benzodiazepines
◆ Buspirone
Other drugs with anxiolytic properties
◆ Some antidepressants
◆ Phenothiazines
◆ Beta-adrenergic antagonists

2–3 weeks. Longer courses of treatment may lead to tolerance and dependence.

Buspirone (see below) seems to be an exception to the general rule that anxiolytics produce dependency, but its anxiolytic effect develops more slowly and is less intense than that of the benzodiazepines. The drugs called anxiolytics are not the only ones that reduce anxiety; antidepressant and antipsychotic drugs also have anxiolytic properties (Table 17.2). Since they do not induce dependence, they are sometimes used to treat chronic anxiety. Beta-adrenergic agonists are used to control some of the somatic symptoms of anxiety.

Benzodiazepines

Benzodiazepines act on specific receptor sites, linked with gamma-aminobutyric acid (GABA) receptors. They enhance GABA neurotransmission and affect indirectly 5-HT (serotonin or 5-hydroxytrypamine) and noradrenaline systems. As well as anxiolytic, sedative, and hypnotic effects, benzodiazepines have muscle-relaxant and anticonvulsant properties. Benzodiazepines are rapidly absorbed and metabolized into a large number of compounds, many of which have their own therapeutic effects.

Compounds in frequent use The many benzodiazepines are divided into short- and long-acting drugs. Short-acting drugs are useful for their brief clinical effect, free from hangover. Their disadvantage is that they are more likely than long-acting drugs to cause dependence. Examples of commonly used drugs of each group are shown for reference in Box 17.2.

Adverse effects The side effects are mainly *drowsiness*, with ataxia at larger doses (especially in the elderly). These effects, which may *impair driving skills* and the operation of machinery, are potentiated by alcohol. Patients should be warned about both these potential hazards. Like alcohol, benzodiazepines can *release aggression* by reducing inhibitions in people with a

BOX 17.2 GROUPING OF BENZODIAZEPINES

Group	Approximate duration of action	Examples
Short-acting	< 12 hours	Lorazepam
		Temazepam
		Oxazepam
		Triazolam
Long-acting	> 24 hours	Diazepam
		Nitrazepam
		Flurazepam
		Chlordiazepoxide
		Clobazam
		Chlorazepate
		Alprazolam

tendency to this kind of behaviour. This should be remembered, for example, when prescribing for women judged to be at risk of child abuse, or anyone with a history of impulsive aggressive behaviour.

Toxic effects are few, and most patients recover even from large overdoses.

Teratogenesis There is no convincing evidence of teratogenic effects; nevertheless, these drugs should be avoided in the first trimester of pregnancy unless there is a strong indication for their use.

Withdrawal effects occur after benzodiazepines have been prescribed for more than a few weeks; they have been reported in up to half the patients taking the drugs for more than 6 months. The frequency depends on the dose and type of drug. The symptoms of the withdrawal syndrome is shown in Table 17.3. Seizures

TABLE 17.3 Clinical features of the benzodiazepine withdrawal syndrome

- Apprehension and anxiety
- Insomnia
- Tremor
- Heightened sensitivity to stimuli
- Muscle twitching
- Seizures (rarely)

occur infrequently after rapid withdrawal from large doses. The obvious similarity between benzodiazepine withdrawal symptoms and those of an anxiety disorder makes it difficult, in practice, to decide whether they arise from withdrawal of the drug or the continuous presence of the anxiety disorder for which the treatment was initiated. A helpful point is that withdrawal symptoms generally begin 2–3 days after withdrawing a short-acting drug, or 7 days after stopping a long-acting one, and diminish again after 3–10 days. Anxiety symptoms often start sooner and persist for longer. Withdrawal symptoms are less likely if the drug is withdrawn gradually over several weeks. (For the treatment of benzodiazepine dependence, see p. 201.)

Buspirone

This anxiolytic, which is an azapirone, has no affinity for benzodiazepine receptors but stimulates $5-HT_{1A}$ receptors and reduces 5-HT transmission. It does not cause sedation but has side effects of headache, nervousness, and light-headedness. It does not appear to lead to tolerance and dependence. Its action is slower than that of benzodiazepines and less powerful. It cannot be used to treat benzodiazepine withdrawal.

Beta-adrenergic antagonists

These drugs do not have general anxiolytic effects but can relieve palpitation and tremor. They are used occasionally when these are the main symptoms of a chronic anxiety disorder. An appropriate drug is **propranolol** in a starting dose of 40 mg daily, increased gradually to 40 mg three times a day.

Contraindications The several contraindications limit the use of these drugs. These are: *asthma*, a history of *bronchiospasm*, or *obstructive airways disease*; incipient *cardiac failure* or *heart block*; *systolic blood pressure below 90 mm* mercury; a *pulse rate less than 60 per minute*; metabolic acidosis, for example in *diabetes*; and after prolonged fasting as in *anorexia nervosa*. Other contraindications and precautions are listed in the manufacturer's literature.

Drug interactions There are interactions with some drugs that increase the adverse effects of beta-blockers. Before prescribing these drugs, it is important to find out what other drugs the patient is taking, and consult a work of reference about possible interactions.

General advice about the use of anxiolytics

1. *Use sparingly.* Usually, attention to life problems, an opportunity to talk about feelings, and reassurance are enough to reduce anxiety to tolerable levels.

2. *Brief treatment.* Benzodiazepines should seldom be given for more than 3 weeks.

3. *Withdraw drugs gradually* to reduce withdrawal effects. When the drug is stopped, patients should be warned that they may feel more tense for a few days.

4. *Short- or long-acting drugs.* If anxiety is intermittent, a short-acting compound is used; if anxiety lasts throughout the day a long-acting drug is appropriate.

5. *Consider an alternative.* As explained in the section on anxiety disorders (see p. 81) some antidepressant and antipsychotic drugs have secondary anxiolytic effects and are useful alternatives to benzodiazepines.

Hypnotic drugs

An ideal hypnotic would increase the length and quality of sleep without changing sleep structure, leave no residual effects the next day, and cause no dependence and no withdrawal syndrome. No hypnotic drug meets these criteria, and most alter the structure of sleep: rapid eye movement sleep is suppressed while they are being taken and resumes once they have been stopped.

Benzodiazepines are the most frequently used hypnotic drugs. A short-acting drug such as temazepam is suitable for cases of initial insomnia and is less likely to cause effects the next day then long-acting compounds such as nitrazepam. These hangover effects can be hazardous for people who drive motor vehicles or operate machines.

Non-benzodiazepine drugs acting on GABA receptors

These drugs include **zopiclone**, **zolpidem**, and **zaleplon**, which bind selectively to omega-1 benzodiazepine sites on GABA receptors but not to the omega-2 sites involved in cognitive functions including memory. They are short-acting and have theoretical advantages over benzodiazepines. They have not been clearly shown to be clinically superior in patients with insomnia.

Chloral hydrate is commonly used and is an effective hypnotic, but it should only be used as a short-term treatment because it may lead to tolerance and addiction. It may also affect hepatic enzymes and should be avoided in people with severe renal, hepatic, or cardiac disease.

Patients should be warned that **alcohol potentiates** the effects of hypnotic drugs, sometimes causing dangerous respiratory depression. This effect is particularly likely to occur with chlormethiazole and barbiturates, which should not be prescribed to people taking excessive amounts of alcohol except under careful supervision in the management of withdrawal (see p. 193).

Hypnotic drugs tend to be prescribed too frequently and for too long. Some patients are started on long periods of dependency on hypnotics by the prescribing of night sedation in hospital. These drugs should be prescribed only when there is a real need, and should be stopped before the patient goes home. The management of insomnia is discussed in Chapter 12.

Prescribing for special groups

For **children**, the prescription of hypnotics is not justified except occasionally for the treatment of night terrors or somnambulism. For the **elderly**, hypnotics should be prescribed with particular care since they may become confused and thereby risk injury.

Antipsychotic drugs

Antipsychotic drugs reduce psychomotor excitement, hallucinations, and delusions occurring in schizophrenia, mania, and organic psychoses. Antipsychotic drugs block dopamine-2 receptors to varying degrees. The degree to which they do so may account for their therapeutic effects, and certainly explains the propensity of individual drugs to cause extrapyramidal side effects. Several drugs, particularly the newer 'atypical' antipsychotics, are also serotonin-2A receptor antagonists and this may explain their different clinical effects. Antipsychotic drugs also block noradrenergic and cholinergic receptors to varying degrees and these actions account for some of their many side effects.

Antipsychotic drugs are well absorbed and partly metabolized in the liver into numerous metabolites, some of which have antipsychotic properties of their own. Measurements of plasma concentrations of the parent drug are therefore not helpful for the children.

Types of antipsychotic drugs

There are many antipsychotic drugs available, with different chemical structures. For non-specialists, the following simplified grouping is sufficient.

1. **Conventional** (also known as '**typical**' or '**first generation**') **antipsychotic drugs** bind strongly to postsynaptic dopamine D_2 receptors. This action seems to account for their therapeutic effect, but also their propensity to cause movement disorders.

2. **Atypical** (also known as '**second generation**') **antipsychotic drugs** vary in the extent to which they bind to dopamine D_2/D_4, 5-HT$_2$, alpha$_1$-adrenergic, and muscarinic receptors. It is thought that the

balance between the D_2 and 5-HT$_2$ antagonism may account for their therapeutic actions. They are less likely to cause movement disorders than the typical antipsychotics and do not cause hyperprolacti-naemia. This group of drugs includes **clozapine**, **olanzapine**, **risperidone**, **quetiapine**, **sertindole**, **zotepine**, and **ziprasidone**.

Clozapine was the first atypical drug. It binds only weakly to D_2 receptors and has a higher affinity for D_4 receptors. It also binds to histamine H$_1$, 5-HT$_2$, alpha$_1$-adrenergic, and muscarinic receptors. At the time of writing, clozapine is the only antipsychotic that has been demonstrated to be effective in patients who are unresponsive to conventional antipsychotics. Clozapine does not cause extrapyramidal side effects, but it causes neutropenia in 2–3 per cent of patients, which progresses to agranulocytosis in 0.3 per cent of patients. For this reason, it is used only when other drugs have failed and then with regular blood tests, and an explanation of the risks and benefits.

Dopamine system stabilizers The current target for new drug development is the production of molecules that 'stabilize' the dopaminergic system. These drugs are partial agonists and can increase dopamine transmission in D_2 receptors when it is low and decrease transmission when it is high. Thus, it may be possible to achieve the relief of psychotic symptoms without inducing parkinsonism. **Aripiprazole** is the prototype of this class of drugs, although older drugs such as sulpiride and amisulpiride may have some of the same characteristics.

Slow-release depot preparations are given by injection to patients who improve with drugs but cannot be relied on to take them regularly by mouth. These preparations are esters of the antipsychotic drug, usually in an oily medium. Examples include fluphenazine decanoate, flupenthixol decanoate, and risperidone. Their action is much longer than that of the parent drug, usually 2–4 weeks after a single intramuscular dose. Because their action is prolonged, a small test dose is given before the full dose is used.

Adverse effects

The numerous adverse effects of antipsychotic drugs are related mainly to the antidopaminergic, anti-adrenergic, and anticholinergic effects of the drugs (Table 17.4). They are common even at therapeutic doses and so are described in some detail. When prescribing, the general account given here should be supplemented with that found in the manufacturer's literature, or in a standard pharmacological work of reference.

Antidopaminergic effects give rise to four kinds of *extrapyramidal* symptoms and signs (Table 17.5). These effects often appear at therapeutic doses and are most frequent with conventional antipsychotic drugs.

1. *Acute dystonia* occurs soon after the treatment begins. It is most frequent with butyrophenones and phenothiazines with a piperazine side chain. The clinical features are shown in Table 17.6. The term *oculogyric crisis* denotes the combination of ocular muscle spasm and opisthotonus. The clinical picture is dramatic and sometimes mistaken for histrionic behaviour. Acute dystonia can be controlled by an anticholinergic drug such as biperiden given carefully by intramuscular injection following the manufacturer's advice about dosage.

2. *Akathisia* is an unpleasant feeling of physical restlessness and a need to move, leading to inability to keep still. It starts usually in the first 2 weeks of treatment but can be delayed for several months. The symptoms are not controlled reliably by antiparkinsonian drugs but generally disappear if the dose is reduced.

3. *Parkinsonian effects* are the most frequent of the extrapyramidal side effects (Table 17.7). The syndrome often takes a few weeks to appear. Parkinsonism can sometimes be controlled by lowering the dose. If this cannot be done without losing the therapeutic effect, an antiparkinsonian drug can be prescribed. With continued treatment, parkinsonian effects may diminish even though the dose of the antipsychotic stays the same. It is appropriate to check at intervals that the antiparkinsonian drug is still required since these compounds may increase the risk of tardive dyskinesia.

4. *Tardive dyskinesia* is so called because it is a late complication of antipsychotic treatment. The clinical features are shown in Table 17.8. The condition may be due to supersensitivity of dopamine receptors resulting from prolonged dopamine blockade. Tardive dyskinesia occurs in about 15 per cent of patients on long-term treatment. Since it does not always recover when the antipsychotic drugs are stopped, and responds poorly to treatment, prevention is important. This is attempted by keeping the dose and duration of dosage of antipsychotic drugs to the effective minimum and by limiting the use of antiparkinsonian drugs (see above). Usually, the best treatment for tardive dyskinesia is to stop the antipsychotic drug when the state of the mental illness allows this. At first the dyskinesia may worsen, but often it improves after several drug-free months. If the

TABLE 17.4 Unwanted effects of typical antipsychotic drugs

Effect	Comments
Antidopaminergic effects	
◆ Acute dystonia	See text
◆ Akathisia	
◆ Parkinsonism	
◆ Tardive dyskinesia	
Antiadrenergic effects	
◆ Postural hypotension	Hypotension particularly likely after intramuscular injection and in the elderly
◆ Nasal congestion	
◆ Inhibition of ejaculation	Anticholinergic effects especially important in the elderly
◆ Dry mouth	
◆ Reduced sweating	
◆ Urinary hesitancy and retention	
◆ Constipation	
◆ Blurred vision	
◆ Precipitation of glaucoma	
Other effects	
◆ Cardiac arrhythmias	
◆ Hypothermia	Especially important in the elderly
◆ Weight gain	
◆ Amenorrhoea	
◆ Galactorrhoea	Chlorpromazine and some other drugs
◆ Worsening of epilepsy (some)	
◆ Photosensitivity (some)	
◆ Accumulation of pigment in the skin, cornea, and lens (some)	
Neuroleptic malignant syndrome	See Table 17.9 and text

TABLE 17.5 Extrapyramidal effects of antipsychotic drugs

Effect	Usual interval from starting treatment
Acute dystonia	Days
Akathisia	Days to weeks
Parkinsonism	A few weeks
Tardive dyskinesia	Many years

TABLE 17.6 Clinical features of acute dystonia

- ◆ Torticollis
- ◆ Tongue protrusion
- ◆ Grimacing
- ◆ Spasm of ocular muscles
- ◆ Opisthotonus

condition does not improve, or if the antipsychotic drug cannot be stopped, an additional drug can be prescribed in an attempt to reduce the dyskinesia. No one drug is uniformly successful and specialist advice should be obtained. (The specialist may try a dopamine receptor antagonist such as sulpiride or a dopamine-depleting agent such as tetrabenazine.)

Depression Antipsychotic drugs may cause depression but this symptom is part of the clinical picture of

TABLE 17.7	Clinical features of parkinsonism

- Akinesia
- Expressionless face
- Lack of associated movements when walking
- Stooped posture
- Rigidity of muscles
- Coarse tremor
- Festinant gait (in severe cases)

TABLE 17.8	Clinical features of tardive dyskinesia

- Chewing and sucking movements
- Grimacing
- Choreoathetoid movements
- Akathisia

TABLE 17.9	Clinical features of the neuroleptic malignant syndrome

Principal features

- Fluctuating level of consciousness
- Hyperthermia
- Muscular rigidity
- Autonomic disturbance

Associated symptoms

Mental symptoms

- fluctuating consciousness
- stupor

Motor symptoms

- increased muscle tone
- dysphagia
- dyspnoea

Autonomic symptoms

- hyperpyrexia
- unstable blood pressure
- tachycardia
- excessive sweating
- salivation
- urinary incontinence

Laboratory findings

- raised white cell count
- raised creatinine phosphokinase (CPK)

Consequent problems

- pneumonia
- cardiovascular collapse
- thromboembolism
- renal failure

chronic schizophrenia, and it is not certain whether antipsychotic drugs have an independent effect.

Neuroleptic malignant syndrome This is a rare but extremely serious effect of neuroleptic treatment, especially with high potency compounds. The cause is unknown. The symptoms, which begin suddenly, usually within the first 10 days of treatment, are summarized in Table 17.9. Treatment is symptomatic. The drug is stopped, the patient is cooled, fluid balance is maintained, and any infection is treated. There is no drug of proven effectiveness. The condition is serious and about one-fifth of patients die. If a patient has had this condition in the past, specialist advice should be obtained before any further antipsychotic treatment is prescribed.

Weight gain Both conventional and atypical drugs, but particularly clozapine and olanzapine, can cause substantial weight gain and this can limit their acceptability to patients. It is important to inform the patient about the possibility of weight gain and to monitor their weight while taking the drugs.

Hyperglycaemia There is evidence that several of the atypical drugs, including olanzapine and risperidone, can induce hyperglycaemia and *diabetes*. They should therefore be used with caution in patients at risk of developing diabetes, and blood sugar should be routinely monitored in such patients. It should be noted that many patients with schizophrenia have other risk factors for developing diabetes.

Specific adverse effects of clozapine About 2–3 per cent of patients taking clozapine develop *leucopenia*, and this can progress to agranulocytosis. With regular monitoring leucopenia can be detected early and the drug stopped; usually the white cell count returns to normal. (Monitoring is usually weekly for 18 weeks and twice weekly thereafter.) Clozapine may also cause excessive salivation, postural hypotension, weight gain, and hyperthermia; and, in high doses, seizures. Clozapine is sedating and respiratory depression has been reported when it has been combined with benzodiazepines.

Teratogenesis

Although the drugs have not been shown to be teratogenic, they should be used with caution in early pregnancy.

Contraindications

There are few contraindications to the use of antipsychotic drugs. They include myasthenia gravis, Addison's disease, glaucoma, and past or present bone marrow depression. Caution is required when there is liver disease (chlorpromazine should be avoided), renal disease, cardiovascular disorder, parkinsonism, epilepsy, or serious infection. The manufacturer's literature should be consulted for further contraindications to the use of specific drugs.

Choice of drug

Of the many compounds available, the following are among the appropriate choices:

* a more sedating drug: olanzapine, chlorpromazine;

* a less sedating drug: trifluoperazine or haloperidol;

* a drug with fewer extrapyramidal side effects: sulpiride or risperidone;

* an intramuscular preparation for rapid calming: chlorpromazine or haloperidol;

* a depot preparation: fluphenazine decanoate or risperidone;

* for patients resistant to other antipsychotics: clozapine (to be initiated by a specialist).

Antiparkinsonian drugs

Although these drugs have no direct therapeutic use in psychiatry, they are used to control the extrapyramidal side effects of antipsychotic drugs. For this purpose, the anticholinergic compounds used most commonly are benzhexol, benztropine mesylate, procyclidine, and orphenadrine. An injectable preparation of biperiden is useful for the treatment of acute dystonia.

Although these drugs are used in psychiatry to reduce the side effects of antipsychotic drugs, they have side effects of their own. Their anticholinergic side effects can add to those of the antipsychotic drug to increase constipation, and precipitate glaucoma or retention of urine. Also, they may increase the likelihood of tardive dyskinesia (see p. 239). Benzhexol and procyclidine have euphoriant effects, and are sometimes abused to obtain this action.

Antidepressant drugs

Antidepressant drugs have therapeutic effects in depressive illness, but do not elevate mood in healthy people (contrast the effects of stimulants like amphetamine). Drugs with antidepressant properties are divided conveniently into: tricyclic antidepressants; modified tricyclics and related drugs; selective serotonin reuptake inhibitors (SSRIs); serotonin and noradrenaline reuptake inhibitors (SNRIs); selective noradrenaline uptake inhibitors; and monoamine oxidase inhibitors (MAOIs). These drugs have not been shown to differ substantially in efficacy or speed of action but only in their adverse effects.

Antidepressant drugs increase 5-HT and/or noradrenaline function. The development of specific 5-HT reuptake inhibitors suggested that the antidepressant effects result from increased 5-HT function. However, specific noradrenaline reuptake inhibitors have been developed and they too are antidepressants. Thus, the mechanism of antidepressant action remains uncertain.

Antidepressants have a long half-life and most can be given once a day. Antidepressants should be withdrawn slowly, because sudden cessation may lead to restlessness, insomnia, anxiety, and nausea. Antidepressant action appears usually 10–14 days after the drug was first taken. The reason for this delay is not known—it could be due to the delay in achieving steady plasma levels or because of the requirement for an adaptive response by the neurons before therapeutic activity commences.

Tricyclic antidepressants

These drugs are so named because their chemical structure has three benzene rings. They have many adverse effects (see below) and toxic effects on the cardiovascu-

TABLE 17.10	Side effects of tricyclic antidepressants
Anticholinergic effects	Dry mouth
	Constipation
	Impaired visual accommodation
	Difficulty in micturition
	Worsening of glaucoma
	Confusion (especially in elderly)
Alpha-adrenoceptor blocking effects	Drowsiness
	Postural hypotension
	Sexual dysfunction
Cardiovascular effects	Tachycardia
	Hypotension
	Cardiac conduction deficits
	Cardiac arrhythmia
Other effects	Seizures
	Weight gain

lar system. Because of these effects, tricyclics are being replaced for many purposes by drugs without these side effects. However, they are still important because they are of proven effectiveness in severely depressed patients. Also, they are generally less expensive than other antidepressant drugs.

Adverse effects Tricyclic antidepressants have many side effects, which can be divided into the groups shown in Table 17.10. Most of the effects are common and those that are infrequent are important, so the list should be known before prescribing. The following points should be noted:

- Difficulty in micturition may lead to the retention of urine in patients with prostatic hypertrophy.

- Cardiac conduction deficits are more frequent in patients with pre-existing heart disease. If it is necessary to prescribe a tricyclic drug to such a patient, a cardiologist's opinion should be sought (it is often possible to choose a drug of another group without this side effect, see below).

- Seizures are infrequent but important. Antidepressant drugs should be avoided if possible in patients with epilepsy. If their use is essential, the dose of anticonvulsant should be adjusted—usually with the advice of the neurologist treating the case.

Toxic effects In overdosage, tricyclic antidepressants can produce serious effects requiring urgent medical treatment. These effects include: ventricular fibrillation, conduction disturbances, and low blood pressure; respiratory depression; agitation, twitching, and convulsions; hallucinations, delirium, and coma; retention of urine, and pyrexia.

Teratogenic effects have not been proved but antidepressants should be used cautiously in the first trimester of pregnancy and the manufacturer's literature consulted.

Drug interactions These should be studied before prescribing. They are summarized in Box 17.3.

Contraindications include *agranulocytosis*, severe *liver damage*, *glaucoma*, and *prostatic hypertrophy*. The drugs should be used cautiously in epileptic patients because they are epileptogenic, in the elderly because they cause hypotension, and after myocardial infarction because of their effects on the heart.

Modified tricyclics and related drugs

The chemical structure of the tricyclics has been modified in various ways to produce drugs with fewer side effects. Of the many drugs, only two will be mentioned here.

BOX 17.3 PRINCIPAL INTERACTIONS BETWEEN TRICYCLIC ANTIDEPRESSANTS AND OTHER DRUGS

With antihypertensives Tricyclic antidepressants interact with adrenergic neuron blockers such as bethanidine, debrisoquine, and guanethidine, and with clonidine. (They do not interfere with beta-adrenoreceptor antagonists or thiazide diuretics.) They can *increase* the hypotensive effect of angiotensin-converting enzyme (ACE) inhibitors such as captopril.

With monoamine oxidase inhibitors These important interactions are described on p. 246.

With phenytoin Because they share a metabolic pathway, tricyclic antidepressants may increase concentrations of phenytoin.

With pressor amines Tricyclic antidepressants potentiate the pressor effects of *adrenaline* and *noradrenaline*, so that there is a potential hazard when a local anaesthetic is used with a pressor amine (e.g. in dentistry).

---

1. **Lofepramine** has less strong anticholinergic side effects than amitriptyline and is less sedating; however, it may cause anxiety and insomnia. In overdose it is less cardiotoxic than conventional tricyclics.

2. **Trazodone** also has few anticholinergic effects, but has strong sedating properties.

Selective serotonin reuptake inhibitors

These drugs selectively inhibit the reuptake of serotonin (5-HT) into presynaptic neurons. Examples are fluoxetine, fluvoxamine, paroxetine, and sertraline. Their antidepressant effect is comparable to that of the

TABLE 17.11	Side effects of SSRIs
Gastrointestinal	Nausea
	Flatulence
	Diarrhoea
Central nervous system	Insomnia
	Restlessness
	Irritability
	Agitation
	Tremor
	Headache
	(Acute dystonia, rarely)
Sexual	Ejaculatory delay
	Anorgasmia

TABLE 17.12   Indications for SSRI treatment for depressive disorder*

- Concomittant cardiac disease
- Intolerance to anticholinergic side effects
- Significant risk of deliberate overdose
- Excessive weight gain with previous tricyclic treatment
- Sedation undesirable
- Obsessive-compulsive disorder with depression

* SSRIs are safer than tricyclics but caution is required.

tricyclic antidepressant drugs, and because they lack anticholinergic side effects they are safer for patients with prostatism or glaucoma, and when taken in overdose. They are not sedating. Their side effects are listed in Table 17.11 and indications for their use in Table 17.12. Recently, there has been concern that SSRIs may induce suicidal actions in some patients and this has led, in the UK, to all SSRIs apart from fluoxetine being banned in children and adolescents. Whether or not SSRIs do induce suicidal thinking remains unclear but they can certainly cause severe restlessness, which in some patients might increase any suicidal thinking. It is important to monitor all patients who start antidepressant drugs of any kind for the emergence of suicidal thoughts.

Drug interactions The combination of SSRIs with *MAOIs* should be avoided since the combination may produce a 5-HT toxicity syndrome with hyperpyrexia, rigidity, myoclonus, coma, and death. *Lithium* and *tryptophan* also increase 5-HT function when given with SSRIs. Combinations of lithium and SSRIs are sometimes used cautiously by specialists for depressive disorders resistant to other treatment. Other interactions are listed in the manufacturer's literature.

Toxic effects Overdosage leads to vomiting, tremor, and irritability.

Serotonin and noradrenaline reuptake inhibitors

Venlafaxine blocks 5-HT and noradrenaline reuptake but does not have the anticholinergic effects that characterize tricyclic antidepressants and is not sedative. The side effects resemble those of SSRIs; in full doses it may cause hypotension. Venlafaxine appears to be slightly more effective than SSRIs in comparative trials.

Selective noradrenaline reuptake inhibitors

Several tricyclic antidepressants are relatively specific noradrenaline reuptake inhibitors (e.g. desimiprimanine and lofepramine). Recently, a non-tricyclic drug,

reboxetine, has been developed with a specific action on noradrenaline reuptake. Clinical trials show that it has antidepressant effects greater than placebo and is comparable to other antidepressants. At the time of writing reboxetine has not been evaluated fully. (See p. 48 for advice on searching for evidence about the effectiveness of new drugs.)

Choice of antidepressant

The clinician should become familiar with the use of one drug from each of the following groups:

1. An SSRI with few anticholinergic effects.

2. A sedating tricyclic: for example, amitriptyline or trazodone.

3. A less sedating tricyclic: for example, imipramine or lofepramine.

4. A drug of optimal efficacy with few anticholinergic effects: for example, venlafaxine.

In general, however, since there is very little difference between antidepressants in efficacy or speed of action, the choice depends on an assessment for each patient of the likely importance of side effects, toxic effects, and interactions with other drugs. Finally, cost should be taken into account.

Side effects Sedating side effects are useful when depression is accompanied by anxiety and insomnia, but may be troublesome for drivers of motor vehicles or other forms of transport, and for operators of machinery. Anticholinergic side effects need to be avoided for patients with prostatism or glaucoma.

Toxic effects Cardiotoxic effects should be considered, especially when there is an increased risk that the patient may take a deliberate overdose or there is cardiac disease.

Epilepsy All antidepressants have the potential of provoking seizures; as a consequence the dose of antiepileptic drugs may have to be increased in patients with epilepsy.

Drug interaction A work of reference should be consulted if the patient is taking or is likely to commence medication for another condition, and a choice made to prevent unwanted drug interactions.

Cost It is appropriate to choose the least expensive drug within the group that is clinically appropriate.

Advice to patients

Before prescribing, the following points should be explained and discussed with the patient:

1. *Delayed response*. The therapeutic effect is likely to be delayed for up to 2 or 3 weeks but side effects will appear sooner.

2. *Adverse effects*. The common effects should be described, including drowsiness, and a warning given of the dangers of driving a motor vehicle or using machinery even when only slightly drowsy. With tricyclics, dry mouth and accommodation difficulties are common side effects. Patients taking 5-HT reuptake blockers may feel irritable or restless.

3. Effects of alcohol. The effects of alcohol are increased when antidepressants are taken.

4. *Older patients* should be warned about the effects of postural hypotension and told how to minimize these (e.g. by rising slowly from bed). The effects of tricyclics on bladder function should be explained. Reassurance can be given that most of these effects are likely to decrease with time.

Starting treatment

When tricyclics are prescribed, the starting dose should be moderate; for example, amitriptyline 75–100 mg per day increasing after 3–7 days to 125–150 mg per day according to the urgency. The dose may be increased further if there is no response, after the extent of the side effects has been observed.

Drugs with sedative side effects can be given in a single dose at night, so that sedative effects help the patient to sleep and the peak of other side effects occurs during sleep. SSRIs and other drugs that cause insomnia should be given in the first half of the day, usually in a single dose.

Doses should be reduced for elderly patients, those with cardiac disease, prostatism, or other conditions that may be exacerbated by the drugs, and those with disease of the liver or kidneys. If agitation, as a symptom of depressive disorder, is not controlled by a sedative antidepressant, a phenothiazine can be added.

Since patients feel the side effects of the drug before experiencing its benefits, they should be seen again after a week, or earlier if the disorder is severe. At this interview, the severity of the depression is reassessed, side effects are discussed, and encouragement is given to continue taking the medication until the therapeutic response occurs.

Non-response

The management of depressed patients who fail to respond to antidepressant medication is discussed on pp. 113–14.

Monamine oxidase inhibitors

MAOIs are seldom used as the first antidepressant treatment because of their side effects and hazardous interactions with other drugs and foodstuffs (described below). They are usually started by a specialist, but since general practitioners and hospital doctors may treat patients who are taking MAOIs, their hazardous interactions should be known.

MAOIs inactivate enzymes that metabolize noradrenaline and 5-HT and this action probably accounts for their therapeutic effects. They also interfere with the metabolism of tyramine, and certain other pressor amines taken medicinally. MAOIs also interfere with the metabolism in the liver of barbiturates, tricyclic antidepressants, phenytoin, and antiparkinsonian drugs. When the drug is stopped, these inhibitory effects on enzymes disappear slowly, usually over about 2 weeks, so that the potential for food and drug interactions outlasts the taking of the MAOI. Recently, MAOIs with more rapidly reversible actions have been produced. Reversible MAOIs are less likely to give rise to serious interactions with foodstuffs and drugs. The various MAOIs differ little in their therapeutic effects.

Commonly used drugs include phenelzine, isocarboxazid, and tranylcypromine. The latter has an amphetamine-like stimulating effect in addition to its property of inhibiting monoamine oxidase. This additional effect improves mood in the short term but can cause dependency. Moclobemide is a *reversible* MAOI.

Adverse effects The common adverse effects of MAOIs are listed in Table 17.13.

Interactions with tyramine in food and drinks Some food and drinks contain tyramine, a substance that is normally inactivated in the body by monoamine oxidases. When these enzymes are inhibited by MAOIs,

TABLE 17.13	Side effects of MAOIs	
Autonomic	Dry mouth	
	Dizziness	
	Constipation	
	Difficulty in micturition	
	Postural hypotension	
Central nervous system	Headache	
	Tremor	
	Paraesthesia	
Other	Ankle oedema	
	Hepatotoxicity (hydrazines)	

BOX 17.4 INTERACTIONS OF MAOIS WITH DRUGS AND FOOD

Due to inactivation of monoamine oxidase

Foods and drinks with high tyramine content

* Most cheeses
* Extracts of meat and yeast
* Smoked or pickled fish
* Hung poultry or game
* Some red wines

Drugs with pressor effects

* Adrenaline, noradrenaline
* Amphetamine, ephedrine
* Fenfluramine
* Phenylpropanolamine
* L-Dopa, dopamine

Due to effects on other enzymes

* Morphine, pethidine
* Procaine, cocaine
* Alcohol
* Barbiturates
* Insulin and oral hypoglycaemics

Drugs that promote brain 5-HT function

* Selective serotonin reuptake inhibitors (SSRIs)
* Clomipramine
* Imipramine
* Fenfluramine
* L-Tryptophan
* Buspirone

tyramine is not broken down and exerts its effect of releasing noradrenaline, with a consequent pressor effect. (As noted above, with most MAOIs the inhibition lasts for about 2 weeks after the drug has been stopped. With the reversible MAOI, meclobemide, inhibition lasts for a shorter time, usually about 24 hours.) If large amounts of tyramine are ingested, the blood pressure rises substantially with a so-called *hypertensive crisis* and, occasionally, a cerebral haemorrhage. An important early symptom of such a crisis is a severe, usually throbbing, headache.

The main tyramine-containing food and drinks to be avoided are listed for reference in Box 17.4. About four-fifths of reported interactions between foodstuffs and MAOIs, and nearly all deaths, have followed the consumption of *cheese*. It is important to consult this list and the manufacturer's literature before prescribing MAOIs. Patients should be given a list of foodstuffs and other substances to be avoided (available usually from the manufacturer).

Drug interactions Patients taking monoamine oxidase inhibitors should not be given drugs metabolized by enzymes inhibited by MAOIs or those that enhance 5-HT functions (Box 17.4). The former fall into three groups:

1. *Drugs metabolized by amine oxidases with pressor effects*. Of these, ephedrine is a constituent of some 'cold cures' and adrenaline is used with local anaesthetics.

2. *Drugs metabolized by other enzymes affected by MAOIs*. The most important of these drugs are listed in Box 17.4. Sensitivity to oral antidiabetic drugs is increased leading to the risk of hypoglycaemia.

3. *Drugs that potentiate brain 5-HT function*. Combinations of these drugs with MAOI may produce a *5-HT syndrome* with:

   * hyperpyrexia;
   * restlessness, muscle twitching, and rigidity;
   * convulsions and coma.

Combinations of MAOIs and tricyclics in specialist practice Combinations of MAOIs and tricyclic antidepressants are sometimes used for resistant depression. Other doctors are unlikely to start this treatment but they may treat patients already taking the combination. Key points about the combined treatment are summarized in Box 17.5.

Treatment of hypertensive crises Hypertensive crises are treated by parenteral administration of phentolamine to block alpha-adrenoceptors, or if this drug is not available, by intramuscular chlorpromazine. Blood pressure should be followed carefully.

Treatment of the 5-HT syndrome All medication should be stopped and supportive measures given. Drugs with 5-HT antagonists properties may be tried but their benefits have not been proved—propranolol and cypropeptadine are possible choices.

Contraindications These include liver disease, phaeochromocytoma, congestive cardiac failure, and conditions that require the patient to take any of the drugs that react with MAOIs.

BOX 17.5 COMBINATIONS OF MAOIS AND TRICYCLICS

◆ To avoid a 5-HT syndrome, combinations of MAOI with imipramine or clomipramine should be avoided. Also, MAOIs and SSRIs should not be combined, see p. 244.

◆ When a MAOI and a suitable tricyclic are combined they should be started together, both at low dosage; or MAOI is added to a previously prescribed tricyclic. *Tricyclics should not be added to a MAOI since this sequence is more likely to provoke a 5-HT syndrome.*

◆ Since the effects of MAOIs (except moclobemide) continue for at least 2 weeks after the drugs have been stopped, tricyclics should not be given for this period after stopping an MAOI. (If tricyclics are given first no drug-free interval is required.)

◆ The value of this combined therapy has not been evaluated fully and generally it should be started by a specialist.

Management Because the drugs have so many interactions, MAOIs should not be prescribed as the first drug for the treatment of depressive disorders, and specialist advice should usually be obtained when they appear to be indicated.

Information for patients The dangers of interactions with foods and other drugs should be explained carefully, and a warning card provided (Box 17.6). Patients should be told to show this card to any doctor or dentist who is treating them. They should be warned not to buy any proprietary drugs except from a qualified pharmacist, to whom the card should always be shown.

Choice of drug Phenelzine is a suitable choice, starting with 15 mg twice daily and increasing cautiously to 15 mg four times a day. Tranylcypromine, which has amphetamine-like effects as well as MAOI properties, is often effective but as noted above some patients become dependent on its stimulant action.

Changing drugs As noted above, if an MAOI is not effective, *at least 2 weeks* must pass between ceasing the MAOI and starting another kind of antidepressant. As MAOIs should be discontinued slowly, the time for

BOX 17.6 A SAMPLE MAOI TREATMENT CARD

Treatment card

Carry this card with you at all times. Show it to any doctor who may treat you other than the doctor who prescribed this medicine, and to your dentist if you require dental treatment.

Instructions to patients

Please read carefully.
While taking this medicine and for 14 days after your treatment finishes you must observe the following simple instructions:

1. Do not eat CHEESE, PICKLED HERRING, or BROAD BEAN PODS.

2. Do not eat or drink BOVRIL, OXO, MARMITE, or ANY SIMILAR MEAT or YEAST EXTRACT.

3. EAT ONLY FRESH foods and avoid food that you suspect could be stale or 'going off'. This is especially important with meat, fish, poultry, or offal. Avoid game.

4. Do not take any other MEDICINES (including tablets, capsules, nose drops, inhalations, or suppositories) whether purchased by you or previously prescribed by your doctor, without first consulting your doctor or your pharmacist. NB Treatment for coughs and colds, pain relievers, tonics, and laxatives are medicines.

5. Drink ALCOHOL only in moderation and avoid CHIANTI WINE completely.

Keep a careful note of any food or drink that disagrees with you, avoid it, and tell your doctor.
Report any severe symptoms to your doctor and follow any other advice given by him.

(Prepared by the Royal Pharmaceutical Society and the British Medical Association on behalf of the Health Departments of the United Kingdom (revised September 1998). Reproduced from the *British National Formulary* (copyright BNF).)

changeover is even longer. These periods are shorter for the reversible MAOI, moclobemide (see above).

Mood-stabilizing drugs

Drugs that prevent the recurrence of bipolar disorder are often called mood stabilizers. The term is simply descriptive and does not denote a pharmacological class. The main mood stabilizers are lithium and a number of antiepileptic drugs including sodium valproate, carbamazepine, and lamotrigine. Mood stabilizers may also be effective at treating acute mood episodes. For example, lithium and sodium valproate are used to treat acute mania, and lithium and lamotrigine are used in depressive disorders—especially those occurring in bipolar disorder.

Lithium

Pharmacology It is not known which of lithium's many pharmacological actions explains its therapeutic effects, but its effect in increasing brain 5-HT function may be relevant. Lithium is absorbed and excreted by the kidneys where, like sodium, it is filtered and partly reabsorbed. Lithium concentrations rise, sometimes to dangerous levels in three circumstances:

1. *Dehydration*: when the proximal tubule absorbs more water, more lithium is reabsorbed.

2. *Sodium depletion*: lithium is carried by the mechanism that carries sodium, and more lithium is transported when there is less sodium.

3. *Thiazide therapy*: thiazide diuretics increase the excretion of sodium but not of lithium, and plasma lithium rises.

Dosage and plasma concentrations General practitioners are often asked to supervise continuing treatment with lithium started by specialists, and hospital doctors treat these patients for other conditions. Because the therapeutic and toxic doses are close together, it is essential to measure the plasma concentrations of lithium regularly during treatment. Measurement is made first after 4–7 days; then weekly for 3 weeks; and then, provided that a satisfactory steady state has been achieved, once every 6 weeks.

The *timing of the measurement* is important. After an oral dose, plasma lithium levels rise by a factor of two or three within about 4 hours and then fall to the steady-state level. Since the steady-state level is important in therapeutics, concentrations are normally measured *12 hours after the last dose*, usually just before the morning dose, which can be delayed if necessary for an hour or two. It is the steady-state level 12 hours after the last dose, not the 'peak', which is the level referred to when discussing the concentrations aimed at in treatment and prophylaxis. If an unexpectedly high concentration is found the first step is to find out whether the patient has inadvertently taken the morning dose before the blood sample was taken.

The required plasma concentrations are:

♦ for *prophylaxis*: 0.5–1.0 mmol/litre (increased occasionally to a maximum of 1.2 mmol/litre);

♦ for *treatment of acute mania*: 0.8–1.5 mmol/litre.

Toxic effects begin to appear over 1.5 mmol/litre and may be serious over 2.0 mmol/litre.

Although the therapeutic effects is related to the steady-state concentration of lithium, any renal effects caused by the drug (see below) may relate to the peak concentrations. For this reason, the drug is often given twice a day. Delayed-release tablets have been introduced for the same reason but the time course of plasma levels resulting from these tablets is not substantially different from that of standard preparations.

Adverse effects These effects are listed in Table 17.14, and the following points should be noted:

TABLE 17.14	Side effects of lithium
Early effects	Polyuria
	Tremor
	Dry mouth
	Metallic taste
	Weakness and fatigue
Later effects	Fine tremor*
	Polyuria and polydipsia
	Hair loss
	Thyroid enlargement
	Hypothyroidism
	Impaired concentration
	Weight gain
	Gastrointestinal distress
	Sedation
	Acne
	Impaired memory (see text)
	ECG changes†
Long-term effects on the kidney (see text)	

*Coarse tremor is a sign of toxicity.
† T-wave flattening; QRS widening (reversible when drug is stopped).

- *Polyuria* can lead to dehydration with the risk of lithium intoxication. Patients should be advised to drink enough water to compensate for the fluid loss.

- *Tremor.* Fine tremor occurs frequently. Most patients adapt to this; for those who do not, propranolol 10 mg three times daily often reduces the symptom. *Coarse tremor is a sign of toxicity.*

- *Enlargement of the thyroid* occurs in about 5 per cent of patients taking lithium. The thyroid shrinks again if thyroxine is given while lithium is continued; and it returns to normal a month or two after lithium has been stopped.

- *Hypothyroidism* occurs commonly (up to 20 per cent of female patients) with a compensatory rise in thyroid-stimulating hormone. Tests of thyroid function should be performed every 6 months, and a continuous watch kept for suggestive clinical signs, particularly lethargy and substantial weight gain. If hypothyroidism develops and lithium treatment is still necessary, thyroxine treatment should be added.

- *Impaired memory.* This usually takes the form of everyday lapses such as forgetting well-known names. The cause is not known.

- *Long-term effects on the kidney.* Ten per cent of patients develop a persistent impairment of concentrating ability. A few patients develop nephrogenic diabetes insipidus due to interference with the effect of antidiuretic hormone. This syndrome does not respond to antidiuretic treatments but usually recovers when the drug is stopped. Provided doses are kept below 1.2 mmol/litre, renal damage is rare in patients whose renal function is normal at the start. Nevertheless, it is usual to test renal function every 6 months.

TABLE 17.15 Toxic effects of lithium

- Nausea, vomiting
- Diarrhoea
- Coarse tremor
- Ataxia, dysarthria
- Muscle twitching, hyperreflexia
- Confusion, coma
- Convulsions
- Renal failure
- Cardiovascular collapse

Toxic effects The toxic effects of lithium (Table 17.15) constitute a serious medical emergency as they can progress through coma and fits to death. If these symptoms appear, lithium should be stopped at once and a high intake of fluid provided, with extra sodium chloride to stimulate an osmotic diuresis. Lithium is cleared rapidly if renal function is normal but in severe cases renal dialysis may be needed. Most patients recover completely, some die, and a few survive with permanent neurological damage.

Teratogenesis Lithium crosses the placenta and, there are reports of increased rates of fetal abnormalities, most affecting the heart. Therefore, the drug should be avoided in the first trimester of pregnancy. If possible, lithium should be stopped a week before delivery or otherwise reduced by half and stopped during labour to be restarted afterwards. However, lithium is *secreted into breast milk* to the extent that plasma lithium concentrations of breast-fed infants can be half or more of that in the maternal blood. Therefore, bottle-feeding is usually advisable.

Drug interactions There are several important interactions between lithium and other drugs. The manufacturer's literature or a book of reference should be consulted whenever lithium treatment is started and a second drug is prescribed for a patient taking lithium. The principal interactions are listed for reference in Box 17.7.

Contraindications These include *renal failure* or *recent renal disease*, *cardiac failure* or *recent myocardial infarction*, and *chronic diarrhoea* sufficient to alter electrolytes. It is advisable not to use lithium for *children* or, as explained above, in *early pregnancy*. The precautions needed during delivery and lactation are referred to on p. 234. Lithium should not be prescribed if the patient is judged unlikely to observe the precautions required for its safe use.

Management Lithium is usually continued for at least 2 years, and often for much longer. The need for the drug should be reviewed once a year, taking into account any persistence of mild mood fluctuations that suggest the possibility of relapse if treatment is stopped (Box 17.8). Continuing medication is more likely to be needed if the patient has previously had several episodes of affective disorder within a short time, or if previous affective disorders were so severe that even a small risk of recurrence should be avoided. There should be compelling reasons for continuing treatment for more than 5 years, although patients have taken lithium safely for longer periods.

BOX 17.7 PRINCIPAL INTERACTIONS BETWEEN LITHIUM AND OTHER DRUGS

Lithium concentrations may be increased by several drugs

- Haloperidol
- Thiazide diuretics (potassium sparing and loop diuretics seem less likely to increase lithium levels but should be used cautiously)
- Muscle relaxants: when a patient on lithium is to have an operation the anaesthetist should be informed in advance because the effect of muscle relaxants may be potentiated. If possible, lithium should be stopped 48–72 hours before the operation
- Non-steroidal anti-inflammatory agents (NSAIDs)
- Some antibiotics (e.g. metronidazole and spectinomycin)
- Some antihypertensives (e.g. angiotensin-converting enzyme inhibitors and methyldopa)

Interaction with antipsychotics

- Potentiation of extrapyramidal symptoms
- Occasionally, confusion and delirium

Interaction with specific serotonin reuptake inhibitors (SSRIs)

- 5-HT syndrome (see p. 246)

Later action with ECT may cause a reaction similar to a 5-HT syndrome

Withdrawal effects Lithium should be withdrawn gradually over a few weeks; sudden withdrawal may cause irritability, emotional lability, and, occasionally, relapse (more often into mania than depression).

Carbamazepine

Pharmacology Carbamazepine was introduced as an anticonvulsant. Later it was found to prevent the recurrence of affective disorder. It is effective in some patients unresponsive to lithium, and for some with rapidly recurring bipolar disorder. Both the effect in acute mania and the long-term efficacy of carbamazepine are less certain than those of lithium, but it is used successfully both as monotherapy and in combination with lithium in some patients.

Dosage and plasma concentration Carbamazepine is usually started at 400 mg daily in outpatients but may be increased up to 800–1000 mg or higher in inpa-

tients. The doses used for long-term treatment depend on tolerability and can range from 200 to 1600 mg daily. Monitoring of blood levels is less important than continued clinical vigilance for the emergence of adverse effects.

Adverse effects may be troublesome if plasma levels are high and include drowsiness, dizziness, nausea, double vision, and skin rash. A rare but serious side effect is agranulocytosis. A full blood count and liver function tests should be done before commencing treatment.

Drug interactions Carbamazepine can accelerate the metabolism of some other drugs and of the hormones in the contraceptive pill, reducing its effectiveness. It is advisable therefore to consider another form of contraception. Drug interactions should be checked in a reference source before prescribing other drugs to a patient taking carbamazepine.

Teratogenesis Carbamazepine seems to be one of the safest mood stabilizers for a pregnant patient.

Sodium valproate

Pharmacology Like carbamazepine, sodium valproate was introduced as an anticonvulsant. Later it was found to control acute mania. The evidence that it prevents the recurrence of bipolar disorder is less strong, but it is increasingly used and, in the USA, is used more commonly than lithium. There are several formulations of valproate that vary in terms of pharmacokinetics. Most trials have investigated valproate semisodium, but this is currently more expensive than other formulations.

Dosage and plasma concentration The doses depend on the formulation. Here we refer to valproate semisodium—the equivalent doses for other formulations may need to be 30 per cent higher. For most outpatients valproate should be started at 250–500 mg in divided doses or as a single dose at night. The dose can be titrated upward by 250–500 mg/day every few days, depending on adverse effects. The usual maintenance dose is between 750 and 1250 mg/day.

Adverse effects Common adverse effects include sedation, tiredness, tremor, and gastrointestinal disturbance. Reversible hair loss may occur in 10 per cent of patients. Sodium valproate may cause thrombocytopenia and has other unwanted effects that should be studied in a reference source before a patient is treated.

Drug interactions Valproate displaces highly protein-bound drugs such as other antiepileptic drugs from their protein-binding sites and may therefore

BOX 17.8 THE MANAGEMENT OF PATIENTS ON LITHIUM

Treatment with lithium is usually started by a specialist, but general practitioners are often involved in continued treatment. Careful management is essential because of the potential effects of therapeutic doses of lithium on the thyroid and, possibly, the kidneys; and the toxic effects of excessive dosage.

Before starting lithium

Before starting lithium a note should be made of any other medication taken by the patient and a **physical examination**, including weight, should be done. Thyroid function tests, electrolytes and urea, and blood creatinine levels should be checked (and a creatinine clearance test done if indicated). Haemoglobin, erythrocyte sedimentation rate (ESR), and a full blood count are often done as well. If indicated, an electrocardiograph (ECG) and pregnancy tests, should be done.

Advice to the patient

The doctor should explain:

- common side effects;
- early toxic effects that might indicate an unduly high blood level of lithium;
- the need to keep strictly to the dosage prescribed;
- arrangements for monitoring blood levels of lithium;
- circumstances in which unduly high levels are most likely to arise—low salt diet, unaccustomed severe exercise, gastroenteritis, renal infection, or dehydration secondary to fever;
- the need to stop the drug and seek medical advice if these conditions arise.

If the patient consents, it is usually appropriate to include another member of the family in these discussions. An explanatory leaflet should be provided, repeating the same points for reference.

Starting lithium prophylaxis

Lithium carbonate is usually given in a single night-time dose. The commonest dose for adults is 800 mg per day, tapered as indicated. The dose is adjusted until a lithium level of 0.5–1.0 mmol/litre is achieved in a sample taken 12 hours after the last dose. The optimal level is usually the highest level within this range tolerated without significant adverse effects. Levels between 1.0 and 1.5 mmol/litre may be used in the treatment of acute mania, but vigilance is required for adverse effects. Steady-state levels are usually achieved 5 days after a dose adjustment.

Continuing treatment

As treatment continues lithium estimations should be carried out every 3–6 months or whenever the clinical status of the patient changes. Thyroid and renal function tests should be checked every 12 months. It is important to have a way of reminding the doctor about repeat investigations. If two consecutive thyroid function tests 1 month apart show hypothyroidism, lithium should be stopped or L-thyroxine prescribed. Mild but troublesome polyuria is a reason for attempting a reduction in dose, whereas severe persistent polyuria is an indication for specialist renal investigation. A persistent leucocytosis is not uncommon and is apparently harmless; it reverses soon after the drug is stopped.

While lithium is continued, the doctor must keep in mind the possibility of interactions if new drugs are required by the patient.

increase plasma levels. Valproate inhibits the metabolism of lamotrigine, which must be used at about 50 per cent of the usual dose when prescribed in combination.

Teratogenesis Valproate is teratogenetic and so must be avoided if possible in pregnant women and used with caution in women of childbearing potential.

Lamotrigine
Pharmacology Lamotrigine also is primarily an anticonvulsant. It may be effective in bipolar depression, possibly without inducing mania, and it also prevents depressive (but not manic) relapse in bipolar disorder.

Dosage and plasma concentration Lamotrigine must be initiated very gradually: initially 25 mg daily for 2 weeks, then 50 mg daily for 2 weeks, then further gradual increase. The usual dose in bipolar disorder is 100–300 mg/day.

Adverse effects A rash may occur in 3–5 per cent of patients—the risk can be reduced by using gradual dosing (see above). Other side effects include nausea, headache, tremor, and dizziness.

Drug interactions Lamotrigine levels are increased by valproate. The combination of lamotrigine and carbamazepine may cause neurotoxicity.

Teratogenesis Lamotrigine does not appear to be teratogenetic.

Central nervous system stimulant drugs

Central nervous system stimulant drugs are used in the treatment of attention deficit disorder (see p. 287). The most commonly used drug is *methylphenidate* which acts mainly by releasing dopamine from presynaptic dopamine terminals. The mode of action is unclear, but methylphenidate improves attention and reduces overactivity and impulsiveness.

Adverse effects The main adverse effects are nervousness and insomnia.

These drugs should be started after full assessment by a specialist (p. 287). Monitoring of continued therapy is essential. Methylphenidate is also increasingly used in adults with ADHD.

Cognition-enhancing drugs
Anticholinesterase inhibitors
These drugs, including donepezil, rivastigmine, and galantamine, have been recently introduced for the treatment of mild to moderate Alzheimer's disease.

These drugs increase the function of acetylcholine, which can improve cognitive functioning. They have a modest beneficial effect in some patients that might persist for a number of months. Anticholinesterase inhibitors are used following assessment in a specialist clinic, including tests of cognitive, global, and behavioural functioning and the assessment of activities of daily living.

Adverse effects The main adverse effects of anticholinesterase inhibitors include anorexia, nausea, vomiting, and diarrhoea.

Other physical treatments
Electroconvulsive therapy (ECT)
ECT is given by psychiatrists. The general reader requires only a general knowledge of its use; those requiring further information should consult *The Shorter Oxford Textbook of Psychiatry* or another specialist text.

In ECT, an electric current is applied to the skull of an anaesthetized patient to produce seizure activity while the consequent motor effects are prevented with a muscle relaxant. The electrodes that deliver the current can be placed with one on each side of the head (bilateral ECT) or with both on the same side (unilateral ECT). Unilateral placement on the *non-dominant side* results in less memory impairment but may be less effective than bilateral ECT. Bilateral placement is therefore preferred when a rapid response is essential, or when unilateral ECT has not been effective.

The beneficial effect, which depends on the cerebral seizure, not on the motor component, is thought to result from neurotransmitter changes probably involving 5-HT and noradrenaline transmission. ECT acts more quickly than antidepressant drugs, although the outcome after 3 months is similar.

Indications
The are a number of main indications for ECT.

1. The *need for an urgent response*:
   - when life is threatened in a severe depressive disorder by refusal to drink or eat or very intense suicidal ideation;
   - in puerperal psychiatric disorders when it is important that the mother should resume the care of her baby as quickly as possible.

2. For a *resistant depressive disorder*, following failure to respond to thorough treatment with antidepressant medication.

3. For two uncommon syndromes:

- **catatonic schizophrenia** (see p. 122);
- **depressive stupor** (see p. 101).

Adverse effects

ECT has a number of adverse effects. Patients often have a brief period of headache after the treatment. A degree of cognitive impairment after treatment is relatively common although this clears rapidly in most patients. The more effective forms of ECT (e.g. higher dose, bilateral) appear to be more likely to cause cognitive problems. Some patients report a persistent loss of autobiographical memories but this has been difficult to show objectively in research studies. Depressive disorder can also lead to cognitive impairment including memory problems and it is therefore possible that the disorder itself is responsible. It is probably best to inform the patient that they may experience some short-term problems and that some patients report longer term problems but that these appear to be uncommon. There are occasional effects from the anaesthetic procedure: the teeth, tongue, or lips may be injured while the airway is introduced and, rarely, muscle relaxants cause prolonged apnoea.

Mortality of ECT

The death rate from ECT is about 4 per 100 000 treatments, closely similar to that of an anaesthetic given for any minor procedure to a similar group of patients. Mortality is greater in patients with cardiovascular disease, and due usually to ventricular fibrillation or myocardial infarction

Contraindications

The contraindications are those for any anaesthetic procedure and any condition made worse by the changes in blood pressure and cardiac rhythm that occur even in a well-modified fit: serious heart disease, cerebral aneurysm, and raised intracranial pressure. Extra care is required with diabetic patients who take insulin and for patients with the sickle cell trait. Although risks rise somewhat in old age, so do the risks of untreated depressive disorder and of drug treatment.

Consent to ECT

Before ECT, a full explanation is given of the procedure and its risks and benefits, before asking for consent. If a patient refuses consent or is unable to give it (for example, because he is in a stupor), and if the procedure is essential, the psychiatrist should seek a second opinion and discuss the situation with relatives (although they cannot consent on behalf of the patient). In the UK and many other countries there are procedures for authorizing an ECT when the patient refuses but it is essential (these are set out in the Mental Health Act or corresponding legislation). Patients treated under these provisions seldom question the need for treatment once they have recovered.

ECT technique

ECT is administered by a psychiatrist, who applies the current, and an anaesthetist and a nurse. The procedure is described in specialist textbooks. ECT is usually given twice a week with a total of 6–12 treatments, according to progress. Response begins usually after two or three treatments; if there has been no response after 6–8 treatments, it is unlikely that more ECT will produce useful change.

As some patients relapse after ECT, antidepressants are usually started towards the end of the course to reduce the risk of relapse.

Treatment with bright light

There is some evidence that bright light treatment is effective in seasonal affective disorder (SAD) (see p. 104). When a therapeutic effect appears it is rapid, but relapse is common. Light is administered usually at about 6–8 a.m. using a commercially available light box. The intensity of the light is usually about that of a bright spring day. The mode of action is uncertain; the light may correct circadian rhythms, which seem to be phase-delayed in seasonal affective disorder.

Psychosurgery

Psychosurgery refers to the use of neurological procedures to modify the symptoms of psychiatric illness by operating either on the nuclei of the brain or on the white matter. The treatment had a period of wide use after its introduction in 1936 until the development of effective psychotropic drugs in the 1960s. Nowadays, it is used rarely and then only in a few special centres, mainly for a very small minority of patients with obsessional or prolonged depressive disorders that have failed to respond to vigorous and prolonged pharmacological and behavioural treatment.

Modern surgery involves small lesions placed by stereotaxic methods, usually to interrupt the fronto-limbic connections. With these restricted lesions, side effects are unusual; when they occur they include apathy, weight gain, disinhibition, and epilepsy.

There have been no randomized controlled trials to test the value of the operation, and its use is diminishing even further as pharmacological and behavioural treatments continue to improve.

Further reading

Stahl, S. M. (2000). *Essential Psychopharmacology*. Cambridge University Press, Cambridge.

A comprehensive and very well illustrated review of psychopharmacology.

CHAPTER 18

Psychological treatment

Chapter contents

Basic procedures *256*

Supportive treatment *257*

Problem-solving techniques *257*

Cognitive behaviour therapies *258*

Dynamic psychotherapy *262*

Treatment in groups *264*

Psychotherapy for couples and families *266*

There are many kinds of psychological treatment but only a few are of direct concern to non-specialists. All doctors need to be able to employ basic psychological procedures in their everyday practice. They also need to know enough about the commonly used special methods of psychological treatment to be able to decide when to refer patients appropriately. In this chapter, psychological treatments will be described under the following headings:

1. **Basic procedures** common to every form of therapy and relevant also to all interactions between the doctor and patient.

2. **Supportive treatment**, which is a part of all clinical practice.

3. **Problem-solving techniques** useful for patients with adjustment disorders and similar conditions.

4. **Behavioural and cognitive treatments** used to alter patterns of behaviour and thinking that prevent recovery from certain psychiatric disorders.

5. **Psychodynamic methods** that enable patients to recognize unconscious determinants of their behaviour and thereby gain more control over it.

6. **Treatment in groups**.

7. **Treatment of couples and families**.

Terminology

Two terms may cause confusion because they are used with more than one meaning.

Psychotherapy is sometimes used to mean all forms of psychological treatment, often with an additional qualifying term; for example, behavioural psychotherapy. Sometimes, however, the term refers solely to psychodynamic methods.

Counselling refers to a wide range of the less technically complicated psychological treatments ranging from the giving of advice, through sympathetic listening, to structured ways of encouraging problem solving. By itself, the term does not have a precise meaning and it should be qualified to indicate either the procedures that are employed (e.g. problem-solving counselling) or the problem that is being addressed (e.g. bereavement counselling).

Basic procedures

Certain basic procedures are involved in all forms of psychological treatment whatever additional techniques may be employed (Table 18.1). These basic procedures are also involved in every therapeutic relationship, including prescribing drugs and supporting patients for whom there is no effective specific treatment.

Develop a therapeutic relationship to gain patients' confidence, improve their adherence to more specific methods, and sustain them through periods of distress. Although helpful in these ways, a therapeutic relationship can become too intense so that it impedes progress (see below). In an appropriate therapeutic relationship, patients should feel that the therapist is concerned about them but understand that the relationship is professional, clearly distinct from a friendship, and one that the therapist maintains with other patients.

Listen to patients' concerns Patients feel helped when they describe their problems to a sympathetic person, and many complain that doctors do not listen for long enough before they offer advice. To be effective, listening requires adequate time, and patients should feel that they have the doctor's undivided attention and have been understood. Non-verbal signs of attention and occasional rephrasing of what has been said can help to achieve this.

Provide information, explanation, and advice All three need to be accurate, clear, free from jargon, and relevant to the patient's physical and mental condition. They should correct any misunderstandings about the nature of the condition or the likely outcome. Explanations of the cause of symptoms should be positive. It is not enough to say that no physical disease has been found for the symptoms—an accurate and convincing explanation should be given of the psychosocial causes.

Allow the release of emotion It is everyday experience that the expression of strong emotion is followed by a sense of relief. Some patients feel ashamed to reveal their feelings to others and need to be assured that to do this is not a sign of weakness. Sometimes further emotional release is needed on a second occasion, but frequently repeated outpourings of emotion are seldom helpful.

Improve morale Patients who have prolonged or recurrent medical or social problems may give up hope of improvement. Low morale, caused in this or other ways, undermines further treatment and rehabilitation. Even if there is no hope of recovery, it is usually possible to improve morale; for example, by describing how pain and distress can be minimized.

Review and develop assets Diagnosis focuses on what is wrong but treatment needs to take into account what abilities and social supports are intact, and help patients to develop them.

Encourage self-help Patients should be helped to achieve an appropriate balance between collaboration with treatment and a determination to be self-sufficient. It is usually possible to achieve this important aim even with the most handicapped patients provided a dependent relationship is not allowed to develop.

Problem of dependency

It is important that patients do not become dependent on their therapists. This problem is most likely to arise during psychological treatment but it can occur in the course of any treatment. Signs that the relationship is becoming too intense include:

TABLE 18.1 Basic procedures of supportive psychological treatment

- Develop a therapeutic relationship
- Listen to patients' concerns
- Provide information, explanation, and advice
- Allow the expression of emotion
- Improve morale
- Review and develop assets
- Encourage self-help

- asking questions about the doctor's personal life;

- efforts to prolong interviews beyond the agreed time;

- attempts to contact the doctor for unwarranted reasons.

Dependent patients do not make appropriate efforts to help themselves. They demand increased attention and if the therapist does not respond, they may become anxious or angry, or make increasingly unreasonable demands. If such signs appear, the doctor should discuss them with the patient without delay, and explain why too intense a relationship is unhelpful.

Transference

In the practice of psychotherapy, an intense relationship between the patient and doctor is called a transference. The term originates from Freud's theory that in such a relationship, the patient transfers to the doctor feelings and thoughts that originated in a close relationship during childhood—usually with one or other parent. When the current feelings are positive, there is said to be a **positive transference**; when the current feelings are negative, there is said to be a **negative transference**.

Countertransference

Not only may patients transfer to their therapists feelings that properly belong elsewhere, therapists may do the same with their patients. Thus therapists may develop strong positive or negative feelings because a particular patient reminds them, consciously or unconsciously, of a parent or another close figure in their lives. Such feelings toward the patient are called countertransference. If countertransference is not recognized in its early stages and corrected, it may impair the doctor's ability to maintain an appropriate professional relationship and to provide impartial advice.

Supportive treatment

Supportive therapy uses the general therapeutic factors described above to:

- reduce distress during a short episode of self-limiting illness or personal misfortune;

- tide the patient over until a specific treatment has a beneficial effect (e.g. while waiting for the therapeutic effects of an antidepressant drug);

- sustain patients whose medical or psychiatric condition cannot be treated, or whose stressful life problems cannot be resolved (e.g. the problems of caring for a handicapped child).

Before choosing supportive therapy, the question should always be asked whether a more active form of psychological or other treatment could bring about change. Sessions generally last for about 15 minutes, though the first session of treatment is often longer. Sessions are often weekly at first but may become less frequent. The length, frequency, and number of sessions should be agreed with the patient at the start.

Problem-solving techniques

The aim of these treatments is to help patients to solve stressful problems and to make changes in their lives. Problem solving is used as the main treatment for acute reactions to stress and for adjustment disorders; and as an addition to other treatments for psychiatric disorders in which associated life problems need to be resolved.

Problem solving is used for problems requiring:

- a **decision**; for example, whether a pregnancy is to be terminated, or an unhappy marriage brought to an end;

- **adjustment** to new circumstances such as bereavement or the discovery of terminal illness, or a move to an unfamiliar environment (e.g. by a student starting university life);

- **change** from an unsatisfactory way of life to a healthier one; for example, as part of treatment for dependence on alcohol or drugs.

Problem-solving counselling includes the basic processes described above together with some extra techniques (Table 18.2).

1. A *list of problems* is drawn up by the patient with help from the therapist, who helps to define and separate the various aspects of a complex set of problems.

2. The patient *chooses one of the problems* to work on.

TABLE 18.2 Basic procedures of problem-solving counselling

Basic techniques of supportive therapy, plus:
1. Define and list the problems
2. Choose a problem for action
3. List alternative courses of action
4. Evaluate the courses of action and choose the best
5. Try the chosen course of action
6. Evaluate the results
7. Repeat until all the important problems have been resolved

3. The therapist helps the patient to *list alternative courses of action* that could solve or reduce the problem. A written list of problems and possible actions helps a patient to identify a plan of action that is specific, practical, and likely to succeed. The listed problems and actions are considered one by one to determine what should be done, and how success will be judged.

4. The patient *considers the pros and cons* of each plan of action and *chooses the most promising.*

5. The patient *attempts the chosen course of action* for the first problem.

6. The *results are evaluated.* If successful, the next problem is acted upon. If the plan for the first has not succeeded, the attempt is reviewed constructively by the patient and therapist to decide how to increase the chance of success on the next occasion. Lack of success is not viewed as a personal failure but as an opportunity to learn more.

7. The *sequence is repeated* until all the selected problems have been resolved.

Throughout treatment, patients are encouraged to take the lead in identifying problems and solutions so that they learn not only a way of resolving the present difficulties but also a strategy for dealing with future problems. Sessions of treatment last for about 30 minutes. Four to eight sessions are usual according to the complexity of the problems.

Crisis intervention

When patients are overwhelmed by stressful events or adverse circumstances they are said to be in crisis and help for them is called crisis intervention. People in crisis include those who have harmed themselves, victims of physical or sexual assault, and people involved in man-made or natural disasters. Such patients are highly aroused and usually require some additional help to reduce this arousal before they can concentrate effectively on problem solving.

Crisis intervention uses the techniques of problem solving with a special focus on the following:

♦ **Reducing anxiety and promoting sleep** by giving support and encouraging the expression of distress. When distress is severe, an anxiolytic or hypnotic drug (usually a benzodiazepine) may be needed for a few days to calm the patient and ensure sleep.

♦ **Recall of traumatic events.** Some clinicians think that avoiding the recall of the traumatic experience prolongs the stress reaction. For this reason patients in crisis are often encouraged to relive the expe-

rience, and express the associated feelings. Although this release of emotion may produce immediate relief, it has not been shown to have lasting benefit unless at the same time the memories are discussed in a way that integates them with the rest of the patient's experience (see Debriefing, p. 65).

Cognitive behaviour therapies

Behaviour therapy is used to treat symptoms and abnormal behaviours that persist because of certain actions of the patient or other people that produce immediate relief of distress but nevertheless prolong the disorder. An example of such an action by the patient is the avoidance of situations that provoke anxiety. An example of an action by another person that has the same effect is paying more attention to patients when they behave abnormally than when they behave normally.

Cognitive therapy is used to treat symptoms and abnormal behaviours that persist because of the way that patients think about them. An example of such a way of thinking is the conviction that palpitations, occurring as part of an anxiety response, are evidence of an impending heart attack.

Cognitive behaviour therapy Because thoughts and actions of these kinds often occur together, behavioural and cognitive techniques are often used together. The combination is called cognitive behaviour therapy.

Most cognitive behaviour therapies require special training and generalists need know only the principles of the treatments and the main reasons for referral. There are, however, some simpler procedures that can be used by non-specialist, namely **relaxation**, **exposure**, and **anxiety management**. These procedures will be described after the principles of treatment have been outlined.

Principles of cognitive behaviour therapy

The *general approach* to cognitive behaviour therapy is that the therapist helps patients first to become aware of, and then to modify, their maladaptive thinking and behaviour. Because patients have to practise new ways of thinking and behaving between the sessions of treatment it is particularly important that they understand the procedures clearly and are well motivated to carry them out. Written instructions are often used to supplement the explanations given by the therapist during treatment sessions.

Behavioural analysis Symptoms, cognitions, and behaviour are monitored by recording them in a diary in which are noted the occurrence of: (i) symptoms;

TABLE 18.3 Two examples of behaviour diaries

A. A diary to record anxiety

Date/Time	The situation in which you felt anxious	Symptoms	Rating of anxiety (0–10)	What you were thinking	What you did
12/6/98 4pm	In a queue at the supermarket	Palpitations and dizziness	8	I am going to die	Ran away from the queue
13/6/98 10am	In town centre	Palpitations and sweting	5	I must relax	Stood still. Tried to relax

B. A diary to record an eating disorder

Date/Time	The problem	The situation at the time	What you were thinking	What you did
18/7/98 7pm	Ate a whole loaf of bread with butter and jam	Feeling despondent after being criticized at work	Everything I do goes wrong	Made myself vomit
19/7/98 1pm	Bought 3 bars of chocolate and a cake	Angry with my friend	No one respects me	Sat alone and ate it all

(ii) thoughts and events that precede and possibly provoke the symptoms; and (iii) thoughts and events that follow and possibly reinforce the symptoms (Table 18.3). This detailed examination of thoughts, behaviour, and provoking events is called behavioural analysis.

Graduated approach Treatment takes the form of a graduated series of tasks and activities such that patients gain confidence in dealing with less severe problems before attempting more severe ones.

Experimental format Tasks and activities are presented as experiments in which the achievement of a goal is a success, while non-achievement is not a failure but an opportunity to learn more by analysing constructively what went wrong. This format helps to avoid discouragement and maintain motivation.

Commonly used techniques of behaviour therapy (Table 18.4)

Relaxation training

This treatment is used to reduce anxiety by lowering muscle tone and autonomic arousal. Relaxation training is useful in the treatment of some physical conditions that are made worse by stressful events (e.g. some cases of mild hypertension). Used alone, relaxation is not effective for severe anxiety disorders but it is a component of anxiety management training (see below), which is often effective in these conditions.

The essential procedures are:

- **relaxing** muscle groups one by one;
- **breathing** slowly as in sleep;

TABLE 18.4 Some techniques of behaviour therapy

- ◆ Relaxation training
- ◆ Exposure
- ◆ Response prevention
- ◆ Thought stopping
- ◆ Assertiveness training
- ◆ Self-control
- ◆ Contingency management
- ◆ (Aversion therapy)

- ◆ **clearing the mind** of worrying thoughts by concentrating on a calming image; for example, a tranquil scene.

These techniques can be combined in a variety of ways but the results of all methods appear to be similar. One typical form of relaxation training has the following steps:

- ◆ *Distinguish between tension and relaxation* by first tensing a group of muscles and then letting go.
- ◆ *Breathe slowly* and regularly.
- ◆ *Imagine* a *restful scene* such as a quiet beach on a warm cloudless day.
- ◆ *Relax one muscle group* (e.g. the muscles of the left forearm). Follow this by relaxing other groups one by one, for example the left upper arm, right forearm, right upper arm, neck and shoulders, face, abdomen, back, left thigh, left calf, right thigh, and right calf.

◆ *Relax larger muscle groups* (e.g. all the muscles of a limb together) so that complete relaxation is achieved more rapidly.

◆ *Resume activity gradually* as in waking from sleep.

The first relaxation session usually lasts for about 30 minutes and each subsequent session usually lasts about 15 minutes. Throughout the sessions the person continues to breathe slowly and imagine restful scenes. After about six sessions, most people can relax rapidly. It is useful to provide a tape recording of the instructions for relaxation to be used at home in quiet surroundings at a time when disturbance is unlikely.

Exposure

Exposure is used mainly for phobic disorders. The basic procedure is to persuade patients to enter, repeatedly, situations that they have avoided previously or, if this is not practicable, to imagine doing so. When re-entry to feared situations is gradual the term **desensitization** is used. When the re-entry to feared situations is rapid, the term **flooding** is used.

The *stages of treatment* are:

1. Determine in detail which *situations* are *avoided*.

2. Arrange these situations in order of the amount of anxiety that each provokes (the resulting list is called a **hierarchy**). Check whether the difference in the amount of anxiety induced by each item in the hierarchy and the next is about the same throughout the list. If it is not, add or remove items until this aim has been achieved A hierarchy might include items such as the local shop when there are no other customers; the local shop when it is crowded; a supermarket when there are no queues at the checkouts; a supermarket with long queues.

3. *Teach relaxation training* (see above) so that it can be used subsequently to reduce anxiety during exposure.

4. Persuade the patient *to enter a situation* at the bottom of the hierarchy and stay until anxiety has declined. It is important that anxiety should have subsided before the patient leaves the situation otherwise no benefit will follow. The procedure is repeated until the situation can be experienced without anxiety.

5. Repeat with the next situation on the hierarchy and so on until the top of the hierarchy is reached.

Patients should practise exposure for about an hour every day. To ensure this it is often helpful to enlist a relative or friend who can encourage practice, praise success, and sustain motivation. If repeated and adequately prolonged exposure does not reduce anxiety, another situation is chosen lower on the hierarchy.

Other behaviour therapy methods

Response prevention

Response prevention is used to treat obsessional rituals. It is based on the observation that rituals become less frequent and intense when patients make prolonged and repeated efforts to suppress them. To be effective, the ritual must be suppressed until the associated anxiety has waned, and this may take up to an hour. Since the immediate effect of response prevention is to increase anxiety, patients require much support if they are to suppress the rituals for the required time. When this stage has been achieved, the procedure is repeated in the presence of any factors that tend to provoke the rituals (e.g. someone with a washing ritual would suppress it while the hands are dirty). Usually, any associated obsessional thoughts decline as the rituals improve.

Thought stopping

Thought stopping is used to treat obsessional thoughts occurring without obsessional rituals (and therefore not treatable by response prevention). A sudden, intrusive stimulus is used to interrupt the thoughts; for example, the mildly painful effect of snapping an elastic band worn around the wrist. When treatment is successful, patients become able to interrupt the thoughts without the aid of the distracting stimulus.

Assertiveness training

This method is for people who are abnormally shy or socially awkward. Socially acceptable expression of thoughts and feelings is encouraged as follows:

◆ *analyse the problem* in terms of facial expression, eye contact, posture, and tone of voice, and what is said;

◆ *exchange of roles* to help the patient understand the viewpoint of the other person in the situation;

◆ *demonstrate* appropriate social behaviour;

◆ *practise* appropriate behaviour within the sessions;

◆ *practise* appropriate social behaviour in everyday life;

◆ *record* the outcome of this practice.

Self-control

Self-control techniques are used to increase control over behaviours such as excessive eating or smoking. The treatment may be used alone or as part of a wider treatment as in cognitive behaviour therapy for bulimia nervosa (see p. 262). The treatment has two stages.

Self-monitoring is the keeping of daily records of the problem behaviour and of the circumstances in which it occurs. For example, a patient who overeats would record what is eaten, when it is eaten, and any associations between eating and stressful events or moods. The keeping of such records is itself a powerful aid to self-control, because many patients have previously avoided facing the true extent of their problems.

Self-reinforcement is the rewarding of oneself when a goal has been achieved successfully. For example, a woman who has reached a target might buy herself a new pair of shoes. Rewards of this kind help to maintain motivation.

Contingency management

Contingency management is used to control abnormal behaviour that is being reinforced unwittingly by other people; for example, by parents who attend more to a child during temper tantrums than at other times. The *treatment* has two aims: first, to identify and reduce the reinforcers of the abnormal behaviour; and second, to find ways of rewarding desirable behaviour. Praise and encouragement are the usual rewards but they may be added to with material rewards such as points or stars that will earn a child a desired toy or treat. Contingency management has four stages:

1. The *behaviour to be changed is recorded* by the patient or another person (e.g. a parent might count the frequency of a child's temper tantrums).

2. Events that immediately follow the behaviour and appear to be *reinforcers are identified*; usually these events involve extra attention given to the child when behaving badly.

3. The *undesirable behaviour is ignored* as far as this is practicable.

4. *Appropriate behaviour is rewarded* (e.g. the parent would attend to the child when behaving well).

Parents or others *monitor progress* by recording the frequency of the relevant behaviour. Attention is also given to events that precede and seem to provoke the behaviour. For example, the child's temper tantrums may occur after the mother pays attention to a younger sibling. The approach may seem mechanistic, but in practice the procedures can be carried out in a caring way.

Aversion therapy

This method, which is now used rarely, is mentioned for completeness. Undesirable behaviour is linked to a stimulus such as a very mild electric shock that acts as a negative reinforcement. There are ethical problems concerned with giving even mildly painful stimuli as treatment. Also, although the treatment has the immediate effect of reducing behaviour, it has not been proved to have lasting benefits.

Outline of cognitive therapy

Cognitive therapy proceeds through four stages:

1. *Identify maladaptive thinking* by asking patients to keep a daily record of the thoughts that precede and accompany their symptoms or abnormal behaviour. The thoughts are recorded as soon as possible after they have occurred.

2. *Challenge* the maladaptive thinking by correcting misunderstandings with accurate information, and pointing out illogical ways of reasoning.

3. *Devise alternatives* to the maladaptive ways of thinking.

4. *Test* these alternatives.

Until maladaptive thinking has changed, *distraction* is used to control the thoughts. It is achieved by *focusing attention* on some external object (e.g. patients may count blue cars in the street or look intently at an object in the room) and by using *mental exercises*, such as mental arithmetic, that require full attention.

Commonly used cognitive behavioural techniques

Anxiety management

The components of anxiety management are relaxation, techniques for changing anxiety-provoking cognitions, and exposure. Treatment is preceded by assessment (Box 18.1).

Anxiety-provoking cognitions are reduced in the following ways. The therapist explains the nature of the normal anxiety response and that the symptoms

---

BOX 18.1 ANXIETY MANAGEMENT

- Organize *a diary record of the behaviour* (see Table 18.3) to assess:

    the nature and severity of symptoms;

    situations in which anxiety occurs;

    avoidance.

- Give *information* to correct misunderstanding about the cause of symptoms.

- *Explain* the vicious circle of anxiety ('fear of fear') and the effects of avoidance.

- Teach *relaxation* (see p. 259).

- Teach *exposure* (see p. 259).

- Teach *distraction* from anxious thoughts (see above).

(For further information see Kennerley, H. (1995). *Managing Anxiety*, 2nd edn. Oxford University Press, Oxford.)

are harmless. This information is discussed in relation to the principal symptoms and concerns of the patient; for example, that dizziness will lead to fainting. The therapist explains how fearful concerns about the symptoms ('fear of fear') can produce a vicious circle of anxiety (see p. 74). Anxious cognitions and symptoms usually improve somewhat after this explanation. **Distraction** (see above) is used to reduce the anxiety-producing effect of any remaining thoughts.

Most anxious patients avoid situations that provoke anxiety and this avoidance maintains anxiety (see Chapter 6). **Exposure** (see p. 259) is therefore an important component of anxiety management.

Cognitive therapy for panic disorder

Patients with panic disorder are convinced that some of the physical symptoms are not caused by anxiety but are the first indications of a serious physical illness (often that palpitations signal an impending heart attack). This conviction causes further anxiety so that a cycle of mounting anxiety is set up. The treatment includes the general components listed above with the following additional features:

◆ The *therapist explains* that physical symptoms are part of the normal response to stress, and that fear of these symptoms sets up a vicious circle of anxiety.

◆ *Patients record* the fearful thoughts that precede and accompany their panic attacks. Patients who cannot identify their thoughts during naturally occurring panic attacks can often do so if panic-like symptoms are induced by voluntary hyperventilation.

◆ The *therapist demonstrates* that fearful cognitions can induce anxiety, by asking patients to remember and dwell on these cognitions and observe the effect.

◆ *Patients attempt to think in the new way* when they experience symptoms, and they observe the effect of this change on the severity of the panic attacks. By repeating this sequence many times they gradually gain control of the panic attacks.

Cognitive therapy for depressive disorder

The cognitive disorder found in depressive disorder is more complex than that in the anxiety disorders, and cognitive treatment is correspondingly more elaborate. The three kinds of cognitive abnormality in depressive disorder (see p. 106) are dealt with as follows.

1. **Intrusive thoughts**, usually of a self-depreciating kind (e.g. 'I am a failure'). When they are weak such thoughts can be counteracted by distraction, using the methods described above, but when they are strong they are difficult to control.

2. **Logical errors** distort the way in which experiences are interpreted, and maintain the intrusive thoughts (Box 18.2). The therapist helps the patient recognize these irrational ways of thinking and change them.

3. **Maladaptive assumptions** are often about social acceptability; for example, the assumption that only good looking and successful people are liked by others. The patient is helped to examine how ideas of this kind influence the ways in which they think about themselves and other people.

As well as helping patients to change their ways of thinking, the therapist also suggests activities to overcome depressed patients' tendencies to withdraw and to be inactive. This last procedure, **activity scheduling**, is especially important for severely depressed patients.

Cognitive behaviour therapy for bulimia nervosa

This treatment begins with self-control methods (see p. 260), which are used to re-establish normal patterns of eating (three meals a day and no snacks between meals). Patients keep records of what and when they eat, and of the events and thoughts and feelings that precede a binge. They also record vomiting and laxative abuse. Self-control procedures usually reduce bingeing, vomiting, and laxative abuse but without cognitive procedures, relapse is common. The four basic stages of cognitive therapy are used: (i) abnormal cognitions are identified using daily records; (ii) the logical basis of these cognitions is challenged; (iii) alternative views are formulated; and (iv) the effect of thinking in new ways is tested. These procedures can also be carried out as a self-help programme (Box 18.3).

BOX 18.2 LOGICAL ERRORS IN DEPRESSIVE DISORDERS

◆ **Exaggeration**: magnifying small mistakes and thinking of them as major failures.

◆ **Catastrophizing**: expecting serious consequences of minor problems (e.g. thinking that a relative who is late home has been involved in an accident).

◆ **Overgeneralizing**: thinking that the bad outcome of one event will be repeated in every similar event in the future (e.g. that having lost one partner, the person will never find a lasting relationship).

◆ **Ignoring the positive**: dwelling on personal shortcomings or on the unfavourable aspects of a situation while overlooking favourable aspects.

BOX 18.3 SELF-HELP FOR BULIMIA NERVOSA

Monitoring:

- a daily record of eating, binges, and vomiting
- weighing once a week

Regular planned meals:

- three normal-sized meals a day with three small between-meal snacks

Stop binges:

- eat only the planned amount
- keep other food out of sight
- keep limited stocks
- take just enough money when buying food

Control vomiting:

- urge to vomit declines as binges stop

Control purging:

- reduce laxatives/diuretics, if necessary, in stages

Find alternatives to binge eating:

- list distracting activities
- try them

Reduce life problems

- problem-solving counselling (Table 18.2)

(For further information see Fairburn, C. G. (1995). *Overcoming Binge Eating*. Guilford Press, New York and London.)

BOX 18.4 ETHICAL ISSUES OF IMPOSING VALUES IN DYNAMIC PSYCHOTHERAPY

Therapists should always respect their patients' values and never impose their own. This rule applies to all therapeutic situations, for example when counselling about a possible termination of pregnancy. It is especially important in dynamic psychotherapy in which value judgements are often involved, for example in deciding what relationship changes would be desirable. Therapists may impose their own values:

- directly by expressing their values or challenging those of the patient;
- indirectly, for example by giving more attention to arguments against a course of action than to arguments for it.

The problem arises also in couple therapy and family therapy in which therapists should not support, directly or indirectly, the values and approach of one member of the couple or family against those of the others.

The cognitive approach in everyday practice

Although cognitive therapies are complex procedures requiring special training, three features of the cognitive approach are useful in everyday clinical practice:

1. *Recording thoughts* occuring when symptoms are experienced.

2. *Recording abnormal behaviours and events* that precede and follow them.

3. *Asking patients to evaluate* their progress both as a way of judging the success of treatment and as a way of increasing their collaboration with treatment.

Dynamic psychotherapy

Brief psychodynamic therapy

In this treatment, patients are helped to obtain a greater understanding of aspects of their problems and of themselves, with the expectation that this will help them to overcome these problems. The focus of treatment is on aspects of the problems and of the self of which the person was previously unaware (unconscious aspects). The treatment may be brief and focused on a small number of specific problems (**focal psychotherapy**) or long term and dealing with a broader range of problems. Dynamic psychotherapy is a specialist treatment requiring lengthy training. Those who are not specialists need to understand the indications for referral and broad principles of treatment.

The main *indications* for brief dynamic therapy are problems of low self-esteem and difficulties in making relationships, either of which may be accompanied by emotional disorders, eating disorders, or sexual disorders. Because treatment is so much concerned with self-concept and relationships, which involve judgements about the kind of change that is desirable and good, it highlights some ethical problems concerned with values (Box 18.4).

Patients referred for dynamic psychotherapy need to be insightful and willing to consider links between their present difficulties and events at earlier stages of their lives. The principal steps of treatment (Table 18.5) are:

1. The patient and therapist *agree on the problems* that will be the focus of treatment.

2. Patients *discuss recent and past experiences* of the problem. To encourage the necessary self-revelation, the

TABLE 18.5 Some techniques of brief psychodynamic therapy
◆ Agree problems to be discussed
◆ Discuss recent and past experiences of the problem
◆ Review patients' part in problems they ascribe to others
◆ Identify common themes
◆ Link present with past behaviour (interpretations)
◆ (Sometimes) comment on the relationship with the therapist (transference interpretations)
◆ Consider alternative ways of thinking and relating

TABLE 18.6 Some techniques of long-term dynamic therapy
◆ Free association
◆ Recall of dreams
◆ Interpret transference
◆ Control countertransference

therapist speaks infrequently and responds more to the emotional than the factual content of what is said. For example, instead of asking for more factual detail he may say 'you seemed angry when you spoke about that experience'.

3. Patients are encouraged to *review their own part in problems* that they ascribe to other people.

4. Patients are helped to *identify common themes* in what they are describing; for example, fear of being rejected by other people.

5. Patients are helped to *recall similar problems* at an earlier stage of life. They are encouraged to consider whether the present maladaptive behaviour may have originated as a way of coping that was adaptive at that time but is now self-defeating. For example, failure to trust others following the experience of sexual abuse in childhood.

6. The *therapist makes interpretations* to help patients discover connections between past and present behaviour, or between different aspects of their present behaviour. Interpretations should be presented as hypotheses to be considered by the patient, rather than truths to be accepted.

7. The patient is encouraged to consider *alternative ways of thinking and relating* and to try these out first with the therapist and then in everyday life.

Dynamic psychiotherapy tends to give rise to intense emotional relationships between the patient and therapist (transference, see p. 257). In some forms of brief psychotherapy, the transference is examined to throw light on the patient's relationship with his parents, as in long-term therapy (see below). Whether or not transference is used in this way, it is important to reduce its intensity before the planned end of treatment, otherwise patients are left in a dependent state, which makes it difficult to terminate the therapy.

Long-term dynamic psychotherapy

This treatment, which originates from Freud's original methods of psychoanalysis, aims to change longstanding patterns of thinking and behaviour that contribute to personal and relationship problems and may be associated with psychiatric disorder. Patients are seen three or more times a week, for at least a year. As well as the basic procedures of psychotherapy, the following special techniques are used (Table 18.6):

1. **Free association**, i.e. encouraging patients to allow their thoughts to wander freely and illogically from a starting point of relevance to the problem. This technique and the next are used to encourage the recall of previously repressed memories.

2. **Recall of dreams** and discussion of their meaning.

3. **Transference interpretation**. Intense transference (see p. 257) develops readily in this form of treatment because the therapist sees the patient frequently and over a long period but reveals little of himself. Transference is used as a tool of treatment on the assumption that it reflects patients' relationships with their parents in earlier life. (In psychodynamic theory these early relationships are important in aetiology.) The therapist comments on the significance of the transference reactions (he makes transference interpretations) and helps the patient to practice controlling the strong emotions that are part of the transference—and similar to emotions experienced outside the therapy sessions.

3. **Control of countertransference**. The factors that encourage transference in the patient also provoke countertransference (see p. 257) on the part of the therapist. It is for this reason that therapists are required to understand their emotional reactions better by undergoing dynamic psychotherapy themselves before using these intensive methods with patients.

The problems of dependency, noted above under brief dynamic therapy, are even greater with long-term therapy and termination should be anticipated and discussed long before the planned end of treatment.

TABLE 18.7 Additional therapeutic influences in group therapy
◆ Group support
◆ Learning from others
◆ Testing opinions, etc. against those of others
◆ Practising social behaviour

No randomized controlled trials have demonstrated that this long and intensive form of psychotherapy is more effective than brief dynamic treatment or cognitive behaviour therapies. For this reason, these methods are seldom used in everyday practice.

Treatment in groups

Small group therapy

A small group usually has about eight patients. When several patients are treated together, certain psychological processes develop which do not occur in individual therapy (Table 18.7). These processes are useful both in psychiatric treatment and in the general practice of medicine where groups can be used to support patients or their relatives. These additional factors are:

1. **Group support**, which can help the members through difficult periods in their treatment or in their lives.

2. **Learning from others**, for example how others in the group have overcome problems similar to the patient's own.

3. **Testing beliefs, opinions, and attitudes** against those of other people. This experience is often more effective in bringing about change than is advice from a professional.

4. **Practising adaptive social behaviour**, especially by those who are shy or socially awkward.

In group therapy, close relationships develop between patients as well as between each patient and the therapist. The therapist should ensure that these relationships do not become too intense, and particularly that members do not form relationships outside the group meetings. Each member of a group discusses personal problems with other group members, and this requirement can lead to ethical problems concerning confidentiality (Box 18.5).

Types of small group therapy

Group therapy can be used for any of the purposes for which individual therapy is used, that is for *support*, *problem solving*, *behavioural treatment*, and *dynamic psycho-*

BOX 18.5 **ETHICAL ISSUES OF CONFIDENTIALITY IN GROUP THERAPY**

In individial psychotherapy, patients have a confidential relationship with the therapist. Members of a group reveal their problems not only to the therapist but also to each other. Two consequences follow this:

1. **Patients** need to agree: (i) that they will speak about personal matters in the group; and (ii) that they will treat as confidential the revelations of other group members.

2. **Therapists** need to ensure that anything that they have learned in a one-to-one interview (e.g. as part of an assessment for group therapy) is not revealed to the group. If such information is important for the group process, the therapist must wait until the patient reveals it.

therapy. The length of treatment, its intensity, and the techniques vary according to the purpose, as they do with individual therapy.

Special forms of small group therapy

There are several special kinds of group treatment, of which only two will be mentioned. In **psychodrama** problems are enacted (as in a play) rather than merely talked about. In **encounter groups** a confrontational style of questioning and interpretation is used in the hope that it will hasten change. There is no research evidence that confrontational methods produce additional benefit and some evidence that they may increase the symptoms of some patients. For these reasons confrontational methods should be used only after special training and only with patients selected to have enough psychological strength to tolerate the methods.

Large group treatment

In some psychiatric wards, patients meet regularly in a group containing 20 or more people. The usual purpose is supportive, enabling patients to talk about the problems of living together in the ward, and thereby to prevent an increase in these problems.

A **therapeutic community** uses group methods not just for support but also to modify personality. Patients reside in the community for many months, living and working together, and attending small and large groups in which they discuss problems in relationships and try to help each other to recognize and resolve their problems. This kind of treatment has been used mainly for patients with personality disorders characterized by antisocial or aggressive behaviour. The value of the methods is uncertain and the approach is available in only a few special centres.

Self-help groups

These groups are organized by people who have a problem in common, for example obesity, alcoholism, postnatal depression, or the rearing of a child with a congenital disorder. The group is often led by a person who has coped successfully with the problem. The members usually meet without a professional therapist although the leader may have a professional adviser. Alcoholics Anonymous (see p. 194) is an example of such a group, Weight Watchers is another. When well run by informed persons these groups are valuable sources of support.

Psychotherapy for couples and families

Couple therapy

Couple therapy (or **marital therapy**) is used to help couples who have problems in their relationships. In medical practice this therapy is used when relationship problems are maintaining a psychiatric disorder (e.g. a depressive disorder) in one or both partners. Treatment focuses on the ways in which the couple interact rather than on their individual problems. The aim is to promote concern by each partner for the welfare of the other, tolerance of differences, and an agreed balance of decision making and dominance. To avoid imposing the therapist's own values, the couple first identify the difficulties that they wish to put right. The therapist does not to take sides with either partner but helps the couple understand each other's point of view. Problems of communication are pointed out. Common problems of this kind include failure to express wishes directly, failure to listen to the other's point of view, 'mind reading' (A knows better than B what is in B's mind), and following positive comments with criticism (the sting in the tail).

Marital therapy can be carried out in several ways using a number of approaches.

1. *Problem-solving methods* like those described on p. 257.

2. *Behavioural approaches* that focus on the ways that each person reinforces, or fails to reinforce, the behaviour of the other.

3. *Transactional methods* in which attention is given to the private rules that govern the couple's behaviour towards each other; and to the question of who makes these rules (e.g. whose work takes priority and who decides this).

4. *Dynamic methods* intended to uncover hitherto unconscious aspects of the couple's interaction; for example, the possibility that a husband repeatedly criticizes his wife because she fails to show the self-reliance that he lacks himself.

Depending on the nature of the marital problem, and on the couple's capacity for psychological insight, each approach can be of value. There is, however, insufficient evidence from clinical trials on which to evaluate these treatments.

Family therapy

Family therapy is usually employed when a child or adolescent has an emotional or conduct disorder. In addition to the young person, the parents are involved together with any other family members (such as siblings or grandparents) who are involved closely with the young person. The aim of treatment is to reduce the problem rather than to produce some ideal state of family life.

Problems-solving methods, *transactional methods*, and *dynamic approaches* can be used as in marital therapy. Specific forms of family therapy have been devised to deal with factors thought to lead to relapse in eating disorders and schizophrenia.

Further reading

Bloch, S. (ed.) (2003). *An Introduction to the Psychotherapies*, 4th edn. Oxford University Press, Oxford.
Although nearly 20 years old the book still contains one of the best introductions to the subject.
Hawton, K., Salkovskis, P. M., Kirk, J. & Clark, D. M. (1989). *Cognitive Behaviour Therapy for Psychiatric Problems: a Practical Guide*. Oxford University Press, Oxford.
Although somewhat dated, this book contains a particularly clear and practical account of the basic procedures used in this group of treatments.

CHAPTER 19

Mental health care for the community

Chapter contents

Psychiatric disorder in the community 267

Provision of mental health services 269

This chapter is concerned with the provision and organization of services for people with psychiatric disorder. It is not concerned with the treatment of individuals, but with the provision of mental health services for a population. It deals mainly with the services needed for people between the ages of 18 and 65 (services for children are discussed in Chapter 20, and services for the elderly in Chapter 16). It does not deal with services for people with learning disability (these services are described in Chapter 21). Mental health services are organized in different ways from country to country. This chapter describes mainly the provision of services in the UK, but the principles apply much more widely.

The chapter begins by describing the overall epidemiology of mental disorder. This gives a measure of the need for services. It then goes on to describe the principles of providing services and current models of service provision. Ethical issues are discussed in Box 19.1.

Psychiatric disorder in the community

Prevalence

To understand the range of psychiatric services that are required for a specific community it is necessary to know:

1. The frequency of mental disorders in the population.

2. How patients with these disorders come into contact with the health services.

The local prevalence of mental disorders will vary from place to place, but approximate estimates can be

---

BOX 19.1 ETHICAL ISSUES OF COMMUNITY CARE

Confidentiality

The doctor–patient relationship usually includes a high level of confidentiality in which the doctor only releases information to a third party without the patient's consent if there is an overwhelming need to do so for the purposes of the health or safety of the patient or a third party.

In community care, this level of confidentiality is difficult to guarantee for several reasons:

1. Effective multidisciplinary community care requires good communication between team members. However, the various professional groups may not have exactly the same practices in relation to confidentiality and the sharing of information.

2. Neighbours and other members of the community may become aware of visits to patients by members of the community team.

3. Assertive outreach programmes may need to make enquiries concerned with the whereabouts of patients who need to be seen, but are not present when visited. In emergencies, the right to confidentiality and privacy needs to be balanced with the risks of harm to the patient and/or others.

Many of these potential problems can be predicted and avoided if they are discussed with the patient and professionals at a care planning meeting. For example, by agreeing with patients when they well, the actions that the team might need to take to help them should they relapse.

Resource allocation

In the planning of health services, it is usual for the demands for services to outstrip available resources. Allocation of resources across services therefore requires an ethical framework to:

- decide on the relative needs of people with different disorders;
- assess the relative costs and benefits of different treatments;
- make acceptable decisions in the absence of complete information.

---

obtained from national surveys. Table 19.1 shows prevalence estimates from a large population survey in the UK. From this table it can be seen that mental disorders are common. From this and other studies, it appears that between 1 in 4 and 1 in 5 of the population at risk experience such disorders in the course of a year.

Higher rates of neurotic disorder are found in people who are:

- divorced/separated;
- single parents;
- unemployed;
- city or town dwellers.

Higher rates of psychotic illness are found in:

- homeless people;
- inner cities.

Psychiatric disorders in different health care settings

The prevalence of psychiatric disorder also varies in different health care settings. This information can be used as an estimate of *need* for mental health services as well as describing where the majority of mental disorders are treated.

Relationship between primary and secondary care

A commonly used model of the proportion of mental illness that is seen at different levels of service is that of Goldberg and Huxley, who described a **pathway to psychiatric care** (Box 19.2).

Anxiety and moderately severe depressive disorders are very common in primary care. It has been estimated that about 5 per cent of general practice attenders suffer from a significant depressive disorder. Specialist psychiatric care focuses on the

TABLE 19.1 Approximate prevalence of psychiatric disorder in the community (1-week prevalence per 1000 population; age 16–65 years)		
	Women	Men
Any non-psychotic mental disorder	200	125
Non-specific neurotic disorder	100	50
Generalized anxiety disorder	50	40
Depressive episode	30	20
Obsessive-compulsive disorder	20	10
Panic disorder	10	10
Functional psychosis*	5	5
Alcohol dependence*	20	75
Drug dependence*	15	30

* One-year prevalence per 1000 population.

From Jenkins, R., Lewis, G., Bebbington, P., Brugha, T., Farrell, M., Gill, B. & Meltzer, H. (1997). The National Psychiatric Morbidity Surveys of Great Britain—initial findings from the Household Survey. *Psychological Medicine* **27**, 775–89.

(NB These figures differ from those in Chapter 6, illustrating the effect of differing survey methods and definitions of disorder.)

BOX 19.2 PATHWAY TO PSYCHIATRIC CARE AND THE APPROXIMATE PREVALENCE OF MENTAL DISORDERS IN THE POPULATION AND HEALTH CARE SETTINGS

Level 1. Mental disorder in the community
200 per 1000 population aged 16–65
Filter 1. The decision to consult a doctor

Level 2. Mental disorders in all primary care patients
180–200 per 1000 population aged 16–65
Filter 2. The detection of mental disorder in primary care

Level 3. Mental disorders diagnosed in primary care patients
100 per 1000 population aged 16–65
Filter 3. Referral to secondary mental health services

Level 4. All mental disorders in secondary care patients
20 per 1000 population aged 16–65
Filter 4. Admission to psychiatric hospitals

Level 5. Patients in psychiatric hospital
< 5 per 1000 population aged 16–65

(From Goldberg, D. & Huxley, P. (1980). *Mental Illness in the Community.* Tavistock, London.)

---

needs of patients with schizophrenia, bipolar disorder, and severe and treatment-resistant depressive disorders.

Psychiatric disorders in general hospital settings

The prevalence of depressive, anxiety, and substance abuse disorders is high in general hospitals, both in patients with physical illness and in patients with somatoform disorders. This subject is dealt with fully in Chapter 11.

Provision of mental health services

In this section, we describe the different kinds of services available for people suffering from psychiatric disorders. The basic principles of the provision of mental health services are the same as for any other health service. They should be:

- accessible to those who require them;
- appropriate to the needs of the whole community;
- effective;
- equitable (fair);
- acceptable to patients;
- efficient and economical.

What makes mentally ill people seek help?

Not everyone with a psychiatric disorder seeks medical advice. Some people with minor emotional reactions to stress obtain help from their family, friends, the Church, or non-medical counselling agencies (see Chapter 6). Many people with problems of substance abuse do not seek help of any kind. Nevertheless, in Britain, about 9 in 10 of people with mental disorder attend a general practitioner, although many do not complain directly of psychological symptoms (see below). Whether a person with *clinically significant psychiatric disorder* consults a general practitioner depends on several factors (Table 19.2). Mental disorders are stigmatized and there is much misunderstanding about them among the general population. For example, most people believe that depression is wholly due to adverse life events, the best treatment is counselling, and that antidepressants are addictive. There have been recent efforts to improve the general population's knowledge

TABLE 19.2 Factors influencing a person's decision to seek medical advice

- Severity and duration of the disorder

- The person's attitude to psychiatric disorder—some people feel ashamed of the disorder and embarrassed to ask for help

- Attitudes and knowledge of family and friends—if these people are unsympathetic the affected person may be less likely to admit the problem or seek help for it

- The person's knowledge about possible help—if he does not know that help can be provided, or if he has false expectations about the likely treatment he may not seek help

- The person's perception of the doctor's attitude to psychiatric disorder—if the doctor is viewed as unsympathetic, the person is less likely to ask for help

although the effectiveness of such campaigns is unknown.

It is commonly believed that people with mental health problems are more likely to make use of, and to benefit from, services that take fully into account the views of those who use them. For this reason, patients are encouraged to be involved in all stages of service development.

Psychiatric disorder in primary care

Detection of psychiatric disorder

Most people with psychiatric disorder who seek help from a general practitioner have symptoms of anxiety or depression. Not all these patients tell the doctor about these psychiatric symptoms; many describe physical symptoms instead. These physical symptoms may be of an associated minor physical illness, or may be somatic symptoms of anxiety (e.g. palpitations) or of depression (e.g. tiredness). Patients present physical rather than psychological symptoms for two reasons. Some patients are aware of the emotional symptoms as well as the physical ones but are uncertain whether the doctor will respond sympathetically to a request for help with psychological symptoms; they hope he will discover them for himself. Other patients are unaware that their physical symptoms may have a psychological cause. Up to a third of people with a psychiatric disorder who consult a general practitioner present in the above two ways. General practitioners vary in their ability to detect these undeclared psychiatric disorders; two factors will help:

1. The doctor should always consider the *possibility of mental disorder* in consultations.

2. The doctor needs good *interviewing skills*. The key skills are the ability to gain the patient's confidence (and so

enable him to disclose any psychiatric symptoms) and the ability to identify any psychological factors that are contributing to physical symptoms.

General practitioners can improve their ability to detect common psychiatric disorders, such as depression, by using screening questions or questionnaires and by improving their interviewing skills (see pp. 16–20).

Treatment of psychiatric disorder

The majority of identified psychiatric disorder is treated by general practitioners themselves. They deal with nearly all adjustment disorders, the majority of the anxiety and depressive disorders, and many problems of alcohol abuse. They refer to psychiatrists about 5–10 per cent of the patients identified as having psychiatric disorders, selecting particularly those with severe depressive disorders, schizophrenia, dementia, and other disorders when severe and persistent.

For depressive disorders, drug treatment is usually indicated. There is evidence that depressive disorders are undertreated in primary care—both in terms of dose and duration of treatment. It has been shown that if depressive disorders in primary care are optimally treated, the outcome is much improved. Some depressive disorders go untreated because they have not been recognized; some that are recognized are treated inadequately, often because of an erroneous belief that antidepressants are ineffective when depressive mood is understandably related to adverse life events. Some patients do not wish to take antidepressants and, provided the depressive disorder is not severe, many can be helped with problem-solving therapy (see p. 111). For most adjustment and anxiety disorders, brief psychological treatments are more appropriate than drug therapy (see p. 78). However, most general practitioners lack the time to provide psychological treatments for all who need it. Some primary care teams include a counsellor or another professional who can provide brief psychological treatment. Without one of these ways of providing psychological treatment, it may be necessary to prescribe anxiolytic drugs to suppress symptoms, or to refer the patient for secondary care.

Patients who do not respond to treatment, have severe illnesses, or need treatments not available in primary care need to be referred to the specialist psychiatric services. The decision to refer to a psychiatrist is determined by several factors (Table 19.3).

Links between the specialist mental health services and primary care

Most patients with a psychiatric disorder are treated in primary care and it is important to develop good links

TABLE 19.3 Factors influencing a general practitioner's decision to refer to the specialist psychiatric services

♦ Uncertainty about diagnosis

♦ Severity of the condition—the most severely ill patients may need admission to hospital

♦ Serious suicidal ideas

♦ Need for treatment that is unavailable in primary care

♦ Willingness of the patient to see a psychiatrist

♦ Accessibility of psychiatric services, how far the patient has to travel, and how promptly patients are seen by the psychiatrist

between general practitioners and the specialist mental health services. In the past, this collaboration was in two ways: (i) a **consultation-liaison** arrangement in which the psychiatrist advised on the management of patients whom the general practitioner continued to treat; and (ii) by psychiatrists **transferring outpatient clinics** from the hospital to primary care. The balance of these arrangements depended on local factors, including the needs of the general practitioners and their patients, the accessibility of outpatient clinics to patients, and the number of psychiatrists available to provide services for the population. A substantial difficulty with this approach was the small number of consultant psychiatrists relative to the need for services. More recently, with the expansion of community mental health teams, much of the liaison with primary care is done by members of the team other than psychiatrists. This arrangement allows the consultant psychiatrists to focus on patients who need their particular expertise. One difficulty of making specialist mental health services more accessible to primary care is that it can result in the referral of an increasing number of milder cases. Therefore, the criteria for referral need to be agreed between the general practitioner and the psychiatric team and managed carefully.

For patients with chronic and enduring mental health problems, the most appropriate form of management is often **shared care** in which both the primary care and specialist mental health teams have an agreed and coordinated role.

Specialist mental health services

Patients reaching the psychiatric services are a selected group of the population of people with psychiatric disorder. The number and type of patients referred depends on the general practitioners' confidence, ability, and willingness to treat psychiatric problems, and on the resources at their disposal. The principles that apply to the provision of psychiatric services are:

♦ to treat patients outside hospital whenever feasible;

♦ to provide services close to patients' homes;

♦ to prevent, as far as possible, the occurrence and recurrence of psychiatric disorder;

♦ to involve families and voluntary organizations in the planning and provision of care.

All psychiatric services must provide for patients with serious disorders such as severe and chronic anxiety disorders, severe mood disorder, schizophrenia, dementia, and people who are suicidal or dangerous to others by reason of mental disorder. Specialist adult psychiatric services provide these services in several ways including:

♦ community mental health teams (CMHTs);

♦ outpatient clinics;

♦ day services;

♦ inpatient facilities;

♦ rehabilitation resources.

Community mental health teams

These have been developed in order to avoid unnecessary admission to hospital, to provide services as close as possible to a patient's home, and to provide continuity of care for patients with chronic psychiatric disorders. They are usually *multidisciplinary*, including several other clinical disciplines as well as psychiatry (Table 19.4). In a well-functioning CMHT, the members work flexibly as well as performing task specific to their profession.

There are two main models of community care. In the first, **case management**, a *key worker* is identified. The key worker is often a community mental health nurse and is reponsible for making sure that the patient's needs and clinical status are regularly assessed. This assessment often takes place at a multidisciplinary meeting. In this model, other members of the team are involved as required to carry out specific tasks. For example, if the patient's clinical state deteriorates, a psychiatrist will reassess the problem, while if the patient needs help with housing, the social worker will be involved. In the second model, **assertive community treatment**, care is focused on the most severely ill patients with the aim of improving adherence with treatment and avoiding the need for hospital admission. In this second model, unlike case management, clinical responsibility for each patient is shared by the team, and each member is involved with each patient. In the UK, case management is the model used most often.

TABLE 19.4 Mental health professionals in a community mental health team (CMHTs)	
Profession	Role
Psychiatrist	The clinical leader of the team and responsible for psychiatric assessments. Initiates and supervises drug treatments and provides brief psychological interventions. Supervises outpatients, inpatients, and day patients
Community mental health nurse	The core members of the team who usually work exclusively in the CMHT. Act as key workers for patients with chronic mental disorders, monitor medication and side effects, and provide some psychological treatments
Clinical psychologist	Performs psychological assessments and provides a full range of psychological treatments
Occupational therapist	Performs functional assessments, provides social skills training, some psychological treatments, and assists the patient in finding occupation
Social worker	Performs social and Mental Health Act assessments and assists the patient in meeting accommodation and financial needs. May also provide some psychological treatments

Whichever model of community care is used, several elements are required to ensure that a CMHT can work effectively with patients suffering from severe mental illness, such as schizophrenia.

Regular and systematic reassessment of the patient's clinical status and needs It may be necessary to arrange a *multidisciplinary needs assessment* in which CMHT members with specific skills (Table 19.4) assess various aspects of the patient's functioning and decide which interventions are likely to help.

Effective collaboration between all those involved in care Team members should meet regularly and between meetings should communicate effectively with each other and with the patients, relatives, or carers, and any others involved in the patient's care such as social services and the general practitioner. A written *care plan* should be made for each patient and circulated to everyone who needs to know about the arrangements. It is important to start care planning meetings *before* a patient is discharged from hospital.

Adequate support for carers *Family and friends* are the main carers of most patients living outside hospital. For the most handicapped patients they encourage suitable behaviours such as getting up and eating at appropriate times; maintaining personal hygiene; and using time constructively. They provide psychological support and encourage adherence with treatment. They have to tolerate unusual behaviour or social withdrawal. Prolonged involvement in care can be stressful and carers may need counselling as well as periods of respite. *Voluntary carers* play a significant part in community care. Trained volunteers may provide psychological and practical support for patients and families. Some charitable organizations provide professional carers and hos-

tel staff. Voluntary carers need training, supervision, and adequate access to mental health professionals.

Provision of suitable accommodation Many patients live with their families, and some can care for themselves in rented accommodation. Others need more help, which can be provided in two main ways:

1. *Group homes.* Some patients are able to live in group homes, which are houses in which four or five patients live together. These houses are often owned by a charitable organization. Patients perform all the essential tasks of running the house together, even though separately they could do only some of them. They receive support and supervision, usually from a community nurse who ensures that the arrangements are continuing to work well.

2. *Staffed hostels.* Patients with greater handicaps can live in hostels where members of staff are present throughout the day and often at night, ensuring greater supervision and assistance than in a group home.

Difficulties finding suitable accommodation can often delay a patient's discharge from hospital.

Provision of appropriate occupation Some patients with chronic psychiatric disorder can undertake normal employment or, if beyond retirement age, can take part in the same activities as healthy people of similar age. Other patients require *sheltered work*, in which they can work productively, but more slowly than would be possible elsewhere. Often such work includes the making of craft items or horticulture. Patients who are too handicapped to undertake sheltered work, need *occupational therapy* to avoid boredom, understimulation, and lack of social contacts.

Arrangements to ensure the patient's collaboration with treatment This is one of the main challenges of community care. Several methods have been tried, ranging from providing the patient with good quality information about their treatment to using compulsory treatment orders (see p. 321). The most promising approaches are currently the use of family interventions (see p. 131) and 'compliance therapy', a hybrid of cognitive therapy and motivational interviewing.

Outpatient clinics

Outpatient clinics are an efficient way of providing psychiatric assessment and treatment. Most of the treatment could be provided in general practice or the community by a visiting psychiatrist or other mental health clinician, but central clinics have three advantages:

1. They employ the time of the professional staff effectively because they do not spend time traveling.

2. They ensure that a senior person is available immediately to give advice to less experienced staff.

3. They provide facilities for physical examination and investigations which may not be so readily available in the community.

Their disadvantages are that patients may have to travel long distances and that it may be more difficult for family members to attend when this is necessary.

Day services

There are two main types of day service, with different functions.

Day hospitals provide assessment and treatment for patients who need intensive treatment but can sleep safely at home or in a hostel. Day hospitals provide supervised drug treatment, occupational therapy and rehabilitation, and a range of psychological treatments. Such hospitals are suitable for patients with moderately severe depressive disorder, chronic schizophrenia, and severe and chronic neuroses. Day hospitals can shorten the length of inpatient stay and avoid admission altogether for some patients.

Day centres provide long-term support for patients suffering from chronic mental illness, but do not offer an alternative to hospital admission. Occupational therapy and rehabilitation may be provided, but medical and nursing services are not. Voluntary organizations often provide day centres or 'drop-in centres'.

Inpatient facilities

Every specialist psychiatric service requires an inpatient unit, capable of treating patients with severe mental disorders, and able to admit patients promptly in an emergency. Admission to hospital is needed when patients:

♦ need a level of assessment that cannot be provided elsewhere;

♦ need a treatment that cannot be provided in any other setting;

♦ have insufficient social support;

♦ might put themselves or other people at risk;

♦ when arrangements for care outside hospital break down and a comprehensive care plan needs to be put in place.

Psychiatric inpatient units serving a large area used to be grouped together in a single psychiatric hospital; now they are often smaller, dispersed, and accommodated in general hospitals serving smaller areas. Units in specialist hospitals have the advantage that a wider range of treatments can be made available (e.g. specialized occupational and rehabilitation facilities); units in a general hospital have the advantages of reduced stigma, early liaison with other specialties, and, usually, closeness to the patient's home.

In the past, patients often remained in inpatient units long after the acute stage of illness had passed; when recovery was incomplete some patients remained for many years. Now patients with residual problems are usually discharged from hospital and are given continuing treatment. The advantage of remaining in hospital ('asylum') is easier provision of accommodation, treatment, rehabilitation, and protection; the disadvantage of a prolonged stay in hospital can be institutionalism that adds to the handicap produced by the disorder. This institutionalism is the result of lack of social stimulation, idleness, boredom, and a monotonous routine with a lack of responsibility for personal decisions. If community care can meet patients' needs it is generally better than prolonged inpatient care and is preferred by patients and their carers. However, when patients are discharged from hospital without adequate provision for their needs for accommodation and treatment, community care can be worse for the patient than long-term care in hospital.

A range of specialist residential provision is required to provide adequate services for a population. Approximate estimates of the number of places required in each type of accommodation for a population are shown in Table 19.5. The actual provision required will depend on local factors such as the amount of social deprivation and unemployment (high rates of social deprivation increase the need for residential services).

TABLE 19.5 Estimated need for specialist residential provision per 250 000 population

Type of accommodation	Estimate (range)
Acute and crisis care	100 (50–150)
Intensive care unit	10 (5–15)
Secure unit	4 (1–10)
Hostel wards	50 (25–75)
24-hour staffed hostels	75 (40–110)
Day-staffed hostels	50 (25–75)
Group homes (visited)	45 (20–70)

From Wing, J. (1992). Epidemiologically based needs assessment. In: Steven, A. & Raftery, J. *Epidemiologically Based Needs Assessment*. NHS Executive, London.

Further reading

Goldberg, D. & Huxley, P. (1992). *Common Mental Disorders: a Bio-social Approach*. Routledge, London.
Describes the reasons that lead people with psychiatric disorders to present to doctors, and the factors which lead to referral to the specialist psychiatric services.

CHAPTER 20

Child and adolescent psychiatry

Chapter contents

General issues 276

Problems of pre-school children 281

Disorders of older children 282

Disorders of development 291

Psychological disorders of physically ill children 294

Disorders of adolescence 295

Disorders of parent–child relationships 296

Some ethical problems in child psychiatry 299

Appendix: A comprehensive scheme for history taking and examination in child psychiatry 300

Emotional and behavioural problems are common among children of all ages, and doctors are often asked for advice about them by parents. It is estimated that about 1 in 5 children have a significant problem in any one year. Many of these children come to the notice of general practitioners but only about 1 in 10 needs the help of a specialist. To help these children and their families requires a basic knowledge of normal child development and of the behaviour disorders of this time of life, together with the skills needed to interview the child, assess the problem, and use basic forms of management. Problems vary with age:

1. Among **pre-school children** the most common problems concern sleeping, eating, elimination, and rebelliousness.

2. Among **school-age children** most problems are of anxiety or disordered conduct.

3. Among **adolescents** mood disorders, eating disorders, and conduct disorders are common.

Help is also sought for problems in the development of specific skills, especially speech and reading.

Generally the problems are reported by parents but at times parents conceal a problem from professionals, usually a problem of child abuse or neglect. Problems of these last two kinds are considered at the end of the chapter.

The plan of this chapter is shown in Table 20.1. It starts with a brief account of some relevant aspects of normal development.

TABLE 20.1	Organization of this chapter
General issues	Normal development
	Assessment of a psychiatric problem in childhood
	Types of psychiatric disorder in childhood
	General causes of childhood psychiatric disorder
	Principal methods of treatment
Problems of pre-school children	See Table 20.6
Disorders of older children	Emotional disorders (see Table 20.8)
	Sleep disorders
	Disorders of elimination
	Hyperkinetic disorder
	Conduct disorder
	Other problem behaviours
Disorders of development	Specific developmental disorders
	Childhood autism
	Other disorders affecting speech
	Gender identity disorders
Psychological disorders of physically ill children	See p. 294
Disorders of adolescence	See pp. 294–6
Disorders of parent–child relationships	Physical abuse
	Sexual abuse
	Emotional abuse
	Neglect
	Munchausen syndrome by proxy
Some ethical problems in child psychiatry	Conflicts of interest
	Confidentiality
	Consent
A comprehensive scheme for history taking and examination in child psychiatry	See Appendix pp. 300–1

General issues

Normal development

Detailed accounts of child development are provided in textbooks of paediatrics. The following account summarizes points that are particularly relevant to the study of childhood emotional and behavioural disorders. *It is important to remember that there are wide variations in the speed of development of healthy children.*

First year

This is a period of rapid intellectual and motor development. The child learns about the basic attributes of common objects, spatial relationships, and simple links between cause and effect. By about 7 months most children can sit without support, and by about 14 months most can take a few steps unaided. In the first year, the child develops a regular pattern of feeding and sleeping. The child forms a strong, secure emotional bond, especially with the mother but also with the father, siblings, and others closely involved. By about 8 months the child shows signs of distress when separated from the mother, and in the presence of strangers.

Second year

The child begins to walk, explores the environment, and learns that this exploration will be limited at times by the parents (e.g. to avoid danger). The parents demand more of the child as they encourage bowel and bladder training. For a time, the child resists these constraints and demands, and shows frustration, sometimes with displays of temper. Although these tantrums may at first be alarming to the parents, provided they are dealt with consistently and lovingly they gradually resolve, although displays of temper may continue infrequently into the next year.

Language develops during the second year and by the age of 20 months most children have learnt the words 'dada', 'mama', and three others. As speech and language comprehension increase, it becomes easier for the parents to understand their child's wishes and feelings and to respond to them appropriately.

Age 2–5 years

In this period there is rapid development of language and intellectual functions and children ask many questions. Attention span increases, motor skills are refined, and continence is achieved. Children become less self-centred and more sociable and they learn to share in the life of the family. Gender roles become established, the parents' values are absorbed, and a sense of conscience develops. During this period children are capable of vivid fantasy, expressed in imaginative games. Play helps children learn how to relate to other children and adults, explore objects, and increase their motor skills.

Later childhood

When children start school, they learn about social relationships with other children and with adults other than the parents. Skills and knowledge increase. Ideas of right and wrong develop further at this age as the influence of school is added to that of the family.

Children develop a feeling of self-worth, while learning that they are less successful in some activities than their peers are. A loving family and good teachers help with these developments.

Adolescence

Considerable changes—physical, psychosexual, and social—take place in adolescence and they are usually accompanied by some emotional turmoil. Generally, the latter does not last long and it may go unnoticed by adults. Among older adolescents rebellious behaviour is common, especially during the last years of compulsory attendance at school. Other common problems are in relationships, sexual difficulties, delinquent behaviour, excessive drinking of alcohol, and abuse of drugs and solvents. These behaviours and the associated emotional turmoil may be difficult to distinguish from psychiatric disorder.

Assessment of a psychiatric problem in childhood

Four special points should be kept in mind when assessing the emotional or behavioural problems of a child or adolescent.

1. It is usually the *parents*, and not the child, who *seek help*. For this reason, whether such a disorder becomes known to the family doctor depends not only on its nature and severity but also on the attitudes and tolerance of the parents. Some healthy children are brought to the doctor by overanxious parents for advice about behaviour that is normal for the child's age; other parents do not seek help for serious problems.

2. Psychiatric disturbance in a child may *result from problems in other members of the family*, usually the parents. For example, the child may be distressed because the parents quarrel frequently. For this reason assessments in child psychiatry are, even more than in adult psychiatry, concerned with the whole family and not just with the patient.

3. Whether a behaviour is abnormal depends in part on the *child's stage of development*. For example, repeated bed-wetting is clearly normal in a child aged 18 months but clearly abnormal in a child aged 7 years. Between these ages its significance has to be assessed carefully.

4. *Environmental factors* are important both in the neighbourhood and the school.

Aims of assessment

The aims of assessment are to:

- obtain a clear account of the presenting problems and make a diagnosis;
- relate these problems to the child's temperament, development, and physical condition;
- relate problems to the influences of the family, school, and wider social environment;
- make a management plan.

Differences between the assessment of children and adults

Although the psychiatric assessment of children resembles that of adults, there are two important differences.

1. When the child is young, the *parents supply most of the verbal information*. Despite this, the child should usually be seen without the parents at some stage. This arrangement is especially important when child abuse is suspected.

2. When interviewing a child it is often difficult to follow a set routine and a *flexible approach is required*. Nevertheless, whatever the order in which the data are collected, they should always be recorded in a standard order to assist others who may use the case record.

Interviewing the parents

The parents are usually seen together. The interviewer should put them ease and make them feel that the interview is intended to help not criticize, and that it does not undermine their confidence. They should feel that they are part of the solution to the child's difficulties rather than part of the problem. The interviewer uses the general interview techniques described in Chapter 2: for example, he should be alert to feelings and attitudes as well as to facts. Before asking systematic questions, the interviewer should encourage parents to talk spontaneously about the child's problem. The main items for assessment are shown in Table 20.2 (a more complete list is provided for reference in Appendix 20.1, pp. 300–1).

Home visits

In assessing more severe problems, it is often helpful for a member of the child psychiatry team to visit the home. This visit provides useful information, not only about the material circumstances of the home and the neighbourhood, but also about the relationships between family members and the pattern of their life together.

Interviewing and observing the child

Starting the interview Children are usually brought to the interview by their parents; few have chosen to

TABLE 20.2 Interviewing parents: the main items*

The presenting problem

- Nature, severity, and frequency
- Situations in which it occurs
- Factors that make it worse or better

Other current problems concerning

- Mood and energy level
- Activity, concentration
- Physical symptoms
- Eating, sleeping, elimination
- Relationships with parents and siblings
- Relationships with other children
- Antisocial behaviour
- School performance

Family history

- Family structure
- Current emotional state of parents and children
- Separations from and illness of parents
- Quality of relations with parents and siblings

Personal history of the child

- Problems in pregnancy, delivery, and neonatal life
- Previous and current levels of development
- Past illness and injury; hospital stays
- Attendance and attainments at school

* See Appendix 20.1 (p. 300) for details.

TABLE 20.3 Principal observations of a child's behaviour and emotional state

- Rapport with the interviewer
- Relationship with parents
- Stage of development
- Appearance
- Activity level
- Ability to concentrate
- Mood
- Habits, mannerisms
- Physical examination

come. It is important therefore to: (i) establish a friendly atmosphere and win the child's confidence before asking about the problems; and (ii) explain how the psychiatrist and other team members may be able to help. With younger children an indirect and gradual approach is needed; starting with general topics that may engage the child's interest such as pets, games, or birthdays, before asking about the problems. With older children and adolescents it may be possible to follow an approach similar to that for adults.

Continuing the interview Older children can usually talk about their problems and their circumstances directly but young children need to be helped, for example by asking about their likes and dislikes, and what they would ask for if given three wishes. The interview techniques recommended for adults (see Chapter 2), such as the use of open questions, apply equally to interviews with children. Children who have difficulty in expressing their problems and feelings in words, may be able to show them in other ways:

- during imaginative play;
- when asked to make a drawing or painting and then to talk about it;
- when asked whom they would like to accompany them to a desert island;
- when asked what they would ask for if given three magic wishes.

Observing behaviour While trying to engage a child in these ways, the interviewer should observe how the child interacts with them, and with the parents when they are present. Specific items of the child's behaviour and mental state should be recorded. The main points are listed in Table 20.3 and a more complete list is given in the appendix to this chapter (see p. 300). A general assessment should be made of the child's development relative to other children of the same age.

Physical examination Any relevant physical examination should be performed with particular attention to the central nervous system.

Interviewing other informants

The most important additional informants, other than members of the family, are the child's *teachers*. They can describe classroom behaviour, educational achievements, and relationships with other children. They may also have useful information about the family and their circumstances.

Types of psychiatric disorder in childhood

The psychiatric problems of childhood can be divided into four groups:

1. Behaviour problems of pre-school children.

2. Problems of behaviour and emotion among older children.

3. Disorders of development.

4. Abuse of children by parents or other adults.

The individual disorders within these groups are described in a later section. First, some general issues are discussed concerning the aetiology and treatment of childhood psychiatric disorders.

General causes of childhood psychiatric disorder

Although there are causes specific to each disorder, many others are general. As in adult psychiatry causes are multiple and fall into three interacting groups: **heredity**, **physical disease**, and **environment** (Table 20.4). Of these, environmental factors are particularly important.

Heredity

Hereditary factors in child psychiatry are polygenic and, as in the disorders of adult life, they interact with environmental factors. For many conditions genetic factors exert their effects indirectly through the control of temperament and intelligence, but in others the effect is more specific—for example in autism (see pp. 291–3).

Physical disease

In childhood any serious physical disease can lead to psychological problems, but brain disorders are particularly likely to have this effect. Serious damage to the brain (usually from birth injury) predisposes to psychiatric disorder. It has been suggested that minor damage to the brain may be a cause of some otherwise unexplained psychiatric disorders such as conduct disorder. However, evidence for this latter idea is not convincing.

Environmental factors

Factors within the family and in the wider environment are important in most of the psychiatric disorders of childhood.

The family

To progress successfully from complete dependence on the parents to independence, children need a stable and secure family environment in which they are loved, accepted, and provided with consistent discipline. Lack of any of these elements can predispose to psychiatric disorder.

Prolonged absence or loss of a parent can predispose to both emotional and conduct disorders in the child. How children react to separation depends on:

- their *age* at the time of separation;

- their previous *relationship with the parents*;

- the *reason for the separation*—for example, separation due to divorce of the parents may follow a long period of quarrelling, which itself affects the child;

- *how the separation is managed* by those remaining with the child. When separation leads to institutional care, this experience may itself predispose to psychiatric disorder.

Other family factors associated with psychiatric disorder in the child include: discordant family relationships, illness of a parent, personality deviance of a parent, large family size, child abuse, neglect, and rejection.

Social factors outside the family

Wider social influences become increasingly significant as the child grows older, spends more time outside the family, and is influenced by the attitudes and behaviour of other children, teachers, and older people in the neighbourhood. Such influences are particularly important in the aetiology of conduct disorder.

The importance of social factors is reflected in the finding that rates of childhood psychiatric disorder are higher in areas of social disadvantage, such as deprived inner city areas with overcrowded living conditions, lack of play space for younger children, inadequate social amenities for teenagers, and lack of community involvement.

TABLE 20.4 Causes of childhood psychiatric disorder
◆ Heredity
◆ Physical disease
◆ Environment
◆ Family factors:
separation
illness of a parent
parental discord
personality deviance of parent
large family size
child abuse and neglect
◆ Social and cultural factors:
influences at school
peer group behaviours
poor social amenities and overcrowding
lack of community involvement

TABLE 20.5 Basic treatment plan for childhood psychiatric problems

- Engage and reassure the child
- Discuss problems with parents:
  nature
  causes
  probable outcome
- Reduce stressors on the child:
  at home
  at school
  elsewhere
- Assess and if necessary change the response to the problem of parents or others
- Avoid medication except for specific indications (see text)
- With the parents' agreement, involve the child's teachers

Principal methods of treatment

General issues

Although treatment differs in important ways according to the type of disorder, there are many common features. For most childhood disorders, treatment need not be complex. The basic plan, which can often be carried out by the general practitioner, is shown in Table 20.5. It is often enough to:

- *discuss the problem* with the parents and the child;
- *discuss the concerns* of the parents and the child;
- *correct any misconceptions* by giving information about the nature, causes, and likely outcome of the disorder;
- *reduce any stressors*, if possible, acting on the child or help him to cope better with them. To achieve this, it may be necessary to talk with other family members or teachers;
- *consider simple behavioural approaches*—for example reducing the parents' inadvertent reinforcement of problem behaviour (see p. 260);
- *decide whether to involve the child's teachers*. Sometimes the problems are related to conditions at school, including bullying, and the teachers need to be aware of this. Sometimes the causes are outside the school but conduct and work in school are affected and teachers need advice about how to respond to the child. Occasionally, remedial teaching is needed, or a change in the child's school timetable or, very occasionally, a change of school.

The role of specialist services In most cases, the primary care team can treat the child. A child psychiatry clinic has the additional resource of a *team* usually consisting of a psychiatrist, social worker, psychologist, and nurses. Usually one of these people is chosen as the '*key worker*' to whom the child relates, while the other team members take on specific tasks, such as liaison with parents or teachers, or cognitive behaviour treatment. The family is involved closely in treatment, and so is any agency concerned with the child and his family such as the social or educational psychology services. Nearly all children referred for specialist psychiatric treatment are treated as outpatients although in some places there are facilities for day patients.

Inpatient care is seldom necessary. It is chosen for one of three reasons:

1. *To treat a severe behaviour disorder* that cannot be managed in another way (e.g. some cases of anorexia nervosa).
2. *For observation* when the diagnosis is uncertain (e.g. to decide whether an epileptic child's behaviour problems are related to the epilepsy, or to emotional and social factors).
3. *To separate the child* temporarily from home to assess behaviour in a different environment (e.g. when abuse is suspected as a cause).

In some special units, the *mother is admitted* to hospital with the child to allow observation and modification of the ways in which she responds to the child, most often in cases of child abuse. Sometimes other family members are admitted as well as the mother.

Specific techniques of treatment

Problem-solving counselling (see p. 257) for the parents and child may form part of the treatment of any of the problems considered in this chapter.

Family therapy Families are always involved in some way in the treatment of children. Family therapy refers to a specific psychological treatment in which the child's symptoms are considered as an expression of difficulties in the functioning of the family. Members of the family meet to discuss their difficulties that appear related to the child's disorder, while the therapist helps them to find ways of overcoming the problems. (See also p. 266.)

Behaviour therapy Behavioural principles (see p. 258) are used in the management of many kinds of childhood psychiatric problem. The aim is often to reduce the attention given to a child when a problem behaviour occurs, and increase the attention given to more appropriate behaviour. As well as these general approaches, specific techniques of behaviour therapy are available for phobias (see p. 259) and enuresis (see p. 286). *Cognitive therapy* (see p. 261) is sometimes used with older children.

Dynamic psychotherapy is usually employed after simpler measures have been tried. Since younger children cannot communicate their problems and feelings effectively in words, play, drama, drawing, and painting may be used as an alternative means of expression.

Drug treatment Medication is considered last because it has only a limited place in the treatment of childhood psychiatric disorders. Although *anxiolytic* and *hypnotic drugs* are sometimes prescribed occasionally, most anxiety and sleeping problems can be treated better in other ways (see pp. 283 and 282). *Antidepressant drugs* are indicated for the more severe depressive disorders of childhood and adolescence, usually when psychological and social measures have failed. They are used also for the rare obsessive-compulsive disorders of older children, and they have a limited place in the treatment of enuresis (p. 286). *Stimulant drugs* have a beneficial effect in attention deficit hyperactivity disorder (see p. 288). *Antipsychotic drugs* are of use in schizophrenia starting in adolescence.

Other forms of help for the child

Special education Some children benefit from special education designed to: (i) remedy associated problems of difficulties in writing, reading, or arithmetic that often accompany psychiatric disorders, especially conduct disorder and hyperkinetic disorder; and (ii) receive help from teachers skilled in working with children with emotional or behavioral problems.

Substitute care This term refers to the placement of a child in a foster home, a children's home, or a special residential school. Such placements are sometimes necessary when the family is very unstable, but should be considered only after every practicable effort has been made to improve the home environment.

Problems of pre-school children

Common problems at this age are attention-seeking, disobedience, temper tantrums, aggression, impaired attention, and problems of sleeping and feeding (Table 20.6). Other problems include excessive and indiscriminate attachment, sometimes seen among children raised in institutions, and inhibited attach-

TABLE 20.6 Disorders of pre-school children

- Temper tantrums
- Breath-holding
- Sleep problems:
  insomnia
  nightmares and night terrors
- Feeding problems:
  food fads and food refusal
  pica

ment to the carer, sometimes seen in children who have been abused (see p. 297). Most problems are short lived and whether they are reported to doctors depends on the attitudes of the parents as well as on the severity of the problem.

Aetiology

Psychological problems at this age are related to the child's stage of development, to temperament, and to influences in the family.

Development As noted earlier, there are wide individual variations in rates of development, seen most obviously in relation to sphincter control and language acquisition.

Temperament Differences in temperament are evident from soon after birth when some babies are more active and responsive than others. Such early characteristics may affect the parents' response to the child (e.g. how often they pick up the child) and these parental responses may affect the child's subsequent development.

Family problems Many behaviour problems at this age are associated with factors within the family such as inadequate parenting skills, maternal depression, marital disharmony, and rivalry between siblings.

Assessment

In assessing the problems of pre-school children, the interviewer has to rely mainly on information from the parents. The assessment should decide whether:

- the child's behaviour is abnormal, or the problem is the parents' inappropriate concerns about behaviour within the normal range;
- the behavioural problem is part of a wider delay in development suggesting learning disability (see Chapter 21) or a pervasive developmental disorder (see p. 291);

◆ the child's behaviour is caused by other problems in the family.

Common problems

Temper tantrums

Most toddlers have occasional mild temper tantrums, and only frequent or severe tantrums are abnormal. Tantrums are often provoked by inconsistent discipline and reinforced unintentionally by excessive attention to the child when they take place. Parents should be informed about the nature and causes of the problem. Temper tantrums usually improve when the parents set consistent limits to the child's behaviour, enforce these limits kindly but firmly, and pay less attention to the child during the tantrums. It is important to discover why the parents have been unable to achieve consistent discipline (e.g. there may be marital problems), and to give common-sense advice on setting and enforcing limits.

Breath-holding

Periods of breath-holding are not uncommon in pre-school children. Like temper tantrums, they are often caused by frustration leading to rage. The behaviour can be alarming for parents, especially if the child becomes cyanosed before breathing resumes. The nature of the attacks should be explained to the parents, and they should be helped to respond calmly, and to avoid reinforcing the behaviour with excessive attention. Managed in this way, the behaviour disappears with time.

Insomnia

One-fifth of children aged between 1 and 2 years of age take at least an hour to fall asleep or are repeatedly wakeful for long periods during the night, thus disturbing their parents. Most of these problems resolve within a few months. When the insomnia is not severe and there are no other problems, the only requirement is to reassure parents that it will pass and to help them not to overreact to it. If the sleep problem is more severe or persistent, the parents' response to the problem should be studied. Often, they are inadvertently maintaining the problem by responding as soon as the child cries, spending long periods at the child's bedside, allowing the child to return to the living room, or taking the child into their own bed. The condition usually improves if the parents:

◆ understand the causes;

◆ establish a regular bedtime routine;

◆ do not reinforce the problem behaviour;

◆ make the child's bedroom a pleasant place.

Hypnotic medication should be used seldom and then only briefly in conjunction with the above measures. At first, it may be difficult to persuade the parents to keep to the new rules, and continued support may be needed. When this simple approach fails, there may be a wider problem in the child or the family and specialist assessment may be required.

Nightmares and night terrors

These problems (described further on p. 285) are quite common among healthy toddlers but seldom persist for long. Usually all that is needed is to advise the parents to calm the child on waking and help him to return to sleep. If this is not successful, there may be a wider problem, requiring specialist assessment.

Feeding problems

Food fads and food refusal are common in pre-school children. In a minority, the behaviour is severe or persistent. When this happens it is often because the parents are unintentionally reinforcing behaviour that would otherwise be transient. Some parents offer alternative (and sometimes unsuitable) food, or take other steps to persuade the child to eat. Parents should be helped to understand the causes of the problem and then advised how to manage it differently. They are encouraged to ignore the feeding problem as far as possible, to refrain from offering the child alternatives when he does not eat what is first offered, and to stop using other special ways to persuade him to eat.

Pica is the eating of items that are not foods (e.g. soil, paint, and paper). Pica is often associated with other behaviour problems, and sometimes with learning disability. Parents should be reassured that the problem is a recognized disorder that usually improves. They should take common-sense measures to keep the child away from the abnormal items of diet. Any stressful circumstances should be modified if possible. With this approach the problem usually disappears; if it does not there may be a wider problem requiring specialist assessment. Even in these more severe cases, the problem usually diminishes as the child grows older.

Disorders of older children

These disorders generally occur between about 5 years of age and the transition to adolescence. This section includes, in addition to the groups of disorders shown in Table 20.7, an account of school refusal—a pattern of behaviour which is not itself a psychiatric disorder but is commonly associated with psychiatric disorder.

TABLE 20.7 Approxiamate frequency of some disorders of school age children

Emotional disorders
Generalized anxiety: unknown
Phobic anxiety: 2%
Separation anxiety: 2–4%
Major depression: 0.5–1%
Obsessive-compulsive disorder: up to 1.0%
Hyperkinetic disorder: 3 –5%

Estimates vary considerably (see text) and the figures are provided mainly to show the relative frequencies of the various disorders.

TABLE 20.8 Emotional disorders of children

- Anxiety disorder
- Phobic disorder
- Separation anxiety disorder
- Social anxiety disorder
- Unexplained physical symptoms (somatization)
- Depressive disorder
- Repetitive behaviours and obsessive-compulsive disorder

TABLE 20.9 Symptoms of childhood anxiety disorder

- Fearfulness and phobia
- Timidity
- Excessive worrying
- Poor concentration
- Poor sleep
- Physical symptoms:
  headache
  nausea, vomiting
  abdominal pain
  bowel disturbance
- Overdependence
- Separation anxiety

TABLE 20.10 Treatment of childhood anxiety disorder

- Explain the nature of the problem to the parents and child
- Help the child to talk about his worries
- Reduce or avoid stressors
- Help the parents to support the child
- Use anxiolytics rarely

Emotional disorders

The term emotional disorder refers to childhood disorders characterized by anxiety or depression, or by physical symptoms that are an expression of anxiety or depression ('**somatization**'), or by repetitive or compulsive behaviours (Table 20.8). Emotional disorders are common (only conduct disorders are more frequent) but most improve with time leaving no residual symptoms. When these disorders continue into adult life, it is usually as an anxiety or mood disorder.

Anxiety disorder

The symptoms of childhood anxiety disorder are listed in Table 20.9. Anxiety is common in childhood. Anxiety disorder is diagnosed when the anxiety is severe enough to cause significant problems in social functioning.

The focus of *normal childhood anxieties* changes with age:

- *infants* pass through a stage of fear of strangers;
- *pre-school children* fear separation from their parents, and often fear animals and darkness;
- *older children* fear certain social situations.

Anxiety disorders in childhood follow the same sequence: separation anxiety and phobic disorder usually start in pre-school years, while social anxiety starts later.

Aetiology Anxiety disorders are thought to be caused by the interaction of anxious temperament and environmental factors, but the exact nature of these factors is unknown.

Treatment The stages of treatment are summarized in Table 20.10. It is important to discover the child's worries and to discuss them in ways appropriate to their age. The parents need advice on how to help the child to gain confidence and overcome the fears. Anxiolytic drugs should be used only when anxiety is extremely severe, and then only for a few days.

Phobic disorder

Phobic symptoms are common in childhood. Most concern animals, insects, darkness, or death. Some children fear going to school so that phobic disorder is a cause of school refusal (see p. 290). Most childhood phobias improve without treatment provided that the parents adopt a firm but reassuring approach. When phobias do not improve with these simple measures, behavioural treatment is usually effective. The child is helped to return gradually to the feared situations following the procedures used for similar phobic disorders in adults (see p. 80).

Separation anxiety disorder

Children with separation anxiety cling to their parents and are extremely distressed when parted from them. They may worry that an accident or illness will befall their parents. The condition may be initiated by a frightening experience such as admission to hospital, or by insecurity in the family; for example, when the parents are contemplating divorce. Separation anxiety is often maintained by overprotective attitudes of the parents and treatment is directed to changing these attitudes and reassuring the child (see also school refusal, p. 290).

Social anxiety disorder

Younger children with this disorder are abnormally anxious in the presence of strangers, and avoid them. The fears of older children resemble those of adults with social phobia (see p. 80).

Somatic symptoms of emotional disorder

Children often communicate distress by complaining repeatedly of physical symptoms for which no physical cause can be found. The term **functional symptoms** is sometimes used, and the process is called **somatization**. The symptoms are usually associated with stressful circumstances or with parental anxiety. Common complaints are of abdominal pain, headache, limb pains, and sickness. Of these, abdominal pain is particularly frequent.

Treatment The steps in treatment are summarized in Table 20.11. The doctor explains to the child and parents that the physical symptoms are undoubtedly real, and are treatable. The relationship to stress and anxiety is explained: the analogy with headache is often helpful. The child is helped to talk about the symptoms, the situations in which they are worse or better, and any other problems. Any stressful circumstances should be reduced or avoided as far as possible. When the symp-tom is pain, the parents are advised to convey sympathy but not to focus attention on the pain. The child and parents are helped to find ways of reducing the experience of pain without taking analgesics, for example by arranging distracting activities.

Depressive disorder

Most depression in childhood is a normal response to distressing circumstances such as the serious illness of a parent, the death of a close family member, or parental disharmony. The child is sad and tearful, and may eat poorly and sleep badly. As well as these normal responses to adversity, a few older children may develop depressive disorders. These disorders are related to the depressive disorders of adult life in that there is an increased rate of depressive disorder among first-degree adult relatives of affected children, and there are continuities between depressive disorder in childhood and adult life.

Clinical picture Depressive disorder in children is generally similar to that in adults with *low mood*, *loss of interest and pleasure* in usual activities, *self-blame*, *hopelessness*, and *disturbance of appetite and sleep*. Sometimes *physical symptoms* take the place of obvious low mood. Extreme guilt is less common among children than adults. *Bipolar disorder does not seem to occur before puberty*.

Treatment is similar to that for anxiety disorders in childhood (see Table 20.10). The parents are informed about the nature of the problem and helped to support the child. The problem is explained to the child in terms appropriate to their age and the child is helped to talk about the feelings of depression and his worries. Any stressful circumstances are reduced or avoided if possible. Medication should be reserved for older children with definite evidence of a severe depressive disorder. The choice of medication requires special knowledge and a child psychiatrist should be consulted before an antidepressant drug is prescribed.

Prognosis Although most children with depressive disorder improve with treatment, they have a high risk of recurrence. Poor outcome is related to the intensity of the initial depression and to family and social difficulties.

Suicide in childhood

Suicide in childhood is considered on p. 181.

Repetitive behaviours and obsessive-compulsive disorder

Many children engage in repetitive behaviours such as counting or repeatedly handling, touching, or avoiding

---

TABLE 20.11 Treatment of somatic symptoms of emotional disorder

- Explain that symptoms are real but have psychological causes
- Help the child to talk about the symptoms and his worries
- Reduce or avoid any stressors if possible
- Help parents to support the child
- Use distraction rather than analgesics (see text)

certain objects. These behaviours usually diminish with time. Although similar to compulsive symptoms in adults, these repetitive behaviours do not fulfil one of the important criteria for obsessive-compulsive disorder (see pp. 85–6): the child does not resist the urge to carry them out. Obsessional and compulsive disorder of the adult type is uncommon in childhood, and when these symptoms occur they are often secondary to an anxiety or depressive disorder. True obsessive-compulsive disorder in childhood is likely to recur in adolescence or adult life.

Treatment The child and parents can be reassured that repetitive behaviours usually disappear without treatment. When obsessional and compulsive symptoms are part of a primary anxiety or depressive disorder, the primary disorder should be treated. True obsessive-compulsive disorders are difficult to treat and specialist help should be sought. Treatment involves the reduction of any stressful circumstances, behaviour therapy similar to that used for adults (see p. 260), and, in some cases, medication (see p. 88).

Sleep disorders

The commonly encountered disorders of sleeping are **nightmares**, **night terrors**, and **sleep-walking** (sleep problems of younger children are considered on p. 282).

Nightmares

Nightmares occur during *REM (rapid eye movement) sleep*. The child wakens to full consciousness and recall of an unpleasant dream. Nightmares are common in childhood, especially around the ages of 5 or 6 years. Often, they are provoked by frightening experiences during the day. Frequent nightmares may be accompanied by daytime anxiety.

Treatment The parents should be informed about the nature of the disorder and reassured that it is likely to improve with time. The child is given information appropriate to his age and any stressful circumstances are discussed and reduced if possible.

Night terrors

Night terrors are less common than nightmares. A few hours after going to sleep the child sits up and appears terrified and confused and may scream. Night terrors occur during stages 3 and 4 of *non-REM sleep*. After a few minutes, the child settles slowly and returns to normal calm sleep.

Treatment There is no specific treatment. The parents should be informed about the nature of the problem. It is sometimes helpful to wake children shortly before the usual time of their night terror. Night terrors seldom persist into adult life.

Sleep-walking

In this condition children walk around while still asleep. The eyes are usually open and the child avoids familiar objects. Sleep-walking occurs during *deep non-REM sleep*, usually in the early part of the night. The child may appear agitated, does not respond to questions, and is often difficult to wake, although he can usually be led back to bed. Some children do not walk, but sit up and make repetitive movements. Episodes usually last for a few minutes, although rarely they may continue for as long as an hour. Sleep-walking is most common between the ages of 5 and 12 years, occurring at least once in 15 per cent of children in this age group. Occasionally, the disorder persists into adult life.

Treatment There is no specific treatment. Parents should be told what is known about the condition, and that it usually resolves. Meanwhile, as sleep-walkers occasionally harm themselves, they should protect the child from injury by fastening doors and windows securely, barring stairs, and removing dangerous objects.

Disorders of elimination

Functional enuresis

Functional enuresis is the repeated involuntary voiding of urine, occurring after an age at which continence is usual and in the absence of any identified physical disorder. The condition may be **nocturnal** (bed-wetting) or **diurnal** (occurring during waking hours), or both. Nocturnal enuresis is referred to as **primary** if there has been no preceding period of urinary continence for at least 1 year. It is called **secondary** if there has been a preceding period of urinary continence for this period. Nocturnal enuresis can cause great unhappiness and distress, particularly if the parents blame or punish the child, and if the condition restricts staying with friends or going on holiday.

Most children achieve regular daytime and night-time continence by 3 or 4 years of age, and *5 years is generally taken as the youngest age for the diagnosis*. Nocturnal enuresis occurs in about 10 per cent of children at 5 years of age, 4 per cent at 8 years, and 1 per cent at 14 years. The condition is more frequent in boys. Daytime enuresis has a lower prevalence and is more frequent in girls.

Aetiology *Primary nocturnal enuresis* seems usually to result from delay in the maturation of nervous control of the bladder. Rarely, there is an anatomical or functional abnormality of the bladder itself. Most children are free from psychiatric disorder (although psychiatric disorder is more frequent than among non-enuretic children). Factors that may contribute to aetiology in some cases include abnormal toilet training, whether unduly lax or unduly rigid, and anxiety due to stressful events. *Secondary cases* are often related to stressful events in the home or at school.

Assessment There are six stages of assessment:

1. *Exclude a primary physical cause*, particularly urinary infection, diabetes, or epilepsy.

2. *Exclude a primary psychiatric cause*: learning disability or psychiatric disorder.

3. *Identify any stressful circumstances* in the family, at school, or elsewhere.

4. *Identify the child's concerns* about the bed-wetting and any other problems.

5. *Identify the patents' attitudes* and other family members to the bed-wetting.

6. *Find out how the parents have tried to help* the child already.

Treatment (Table 20.12) If the condition is *secondary*, the causative physical or psychiatric disorder should be treated. Children with a serious psychiatric disorder should be referred to a child psychiatrist. Most *primary* cases can be treated successfully in general practice.

- The parents and the child are *reassured* that the condition is common and that the child is not to blame.

- The parents are told that *punishment and disapproval are inappropriate* and ineffective.

TABLE 20.12 Stages in the treatment of nocturnal enuresis

- Treat any primary physical disorder
- Treat any psychiatric disorder
- Advice to parents and child:
  avoid disapproval and punishment
  reward success (star charts)
- Modify any stressors if possible
- Restrict fluids before bedtime
- Wake during the night

For persistent cases

- Enuresis alarm (see text)
- Medication for temporary relief (see text)

- Parents are encouraged to *reward success* (e.g. with star charts), and *not to focus attention on failure*.

- If *stressors* have been found, they should be *reduced if possible*.

Many younger enuretic children improve spontaneously soon after advice of this kind, but those over 6 years of age are likely to need more than advice. The next steps are:

- *restrict fluid* intake before bedtime;

- *wake the child* to pass urine once during the night;

- use an *enuresis alarm* if the child is aged over 6 years (see below);

- *medication* (see below).

Enuresis alarms A sensor to detect urine is attached to the child's pyjama trousers and a miniature alarm is carried in the pocket or on the wrist. The child turns off the alarm and rises to complete emptying the bladder while the bed is remade if necessary. (In the past, before the necessary sensors were available, the passage of urine was detected by two metal plates separated by a cotton pad. When the pad became wet, the current flowed and an alarm bell rang. The term *pad and bell method* is still in use to describe this approach to treatment.) About 70 per cent of children improve within a month of this treatment, but a third relapse within a year. Children under 6 years of age seldom improve with this method.

Medication Treatment with the *tricyclic antidepressant* imipramine can reduce bed-wetting. The drug is given at a low dose, related to the child's age, in accordance with the manufacturer's instructions. Most bed-wetters improve partially on the drug, and about a third stop completely although most relapse when the drug is stopped. Because of this high relapse rate, the side effects of tricyclics, and the potential danger of accidental overdose, the use of antidepressant drugs is limited mainly to enabling the child to be dry over a short but important period, such as a school journey.

The *synthetic antidiuretic hormone* desmopressin leads to short-term improvement in about half the cases in which it is used though most children relapse when it is stopped.

Functional encopresis

Functional encopresis is an uncommon disorder in which the child passes faeces in inappropriate places, after the age at which bowel control is usual. The age at which control is reached varies, but at the age of

3–4 years 94 per cent of children have control with only occasional accidents. The disorder may be present continuously from the time when bowel control is normally acquired (**primary encopresis**), or it may start after a period of continence (**secondary encopresis**). The condition is more common in boys than girls.

Aetiology Encopresis is sometimes a consequence of chronic constipation due to conditions causing pain on defecation (e.g. anal fissure) or Hirschsprung's disease (*secondary encopresis*). Cases without a physical cause (*primary encopresis*) are sometimes associated with learning disability. In some cases the parents have adopted either an excessively strict, and in other cases an inconsistent, approach to bowel training. However, it is unlikely that either can be the sole cause of the condition because many other children reared in these ways do not develop encopresis. Sometimes soiling begins after an upsetting event, or during a period of rebellion against the parents, but again this cannot be the sole cause. Emotional disorders are common among children with encopresis, but they are as likely to be the result as the cause of the condition.

Assessment Most cases require assessment by a specialist. The assessment is similar to that for enuresis (see above):

* seek a primary physical or psychiatric cause;
* identify any stressful conditions;
* assess the attitudes of the parents and any siblings;
* explore the child's concerns about the problem;
* ask the parents how they have tried to help the child.

Treatment The plan of treatment resembles that for enuresis (see above and Table 20.12):

* Treat any primary physical or psychiatric disorder.
* Reassure the parents that the problem occurs in other children and will improve in time.
* Encourage normal bowel habits, starting by asking the child to sit on the toilet for 5 minutes after each meal.
* Encourage the parents to reward the child for opening his bowels in the appropriate place, and not to dwell on failure.
* Modify any stressful circumstances if possible.

Occasionally, admission to hospital is needed to establish a new routine. Untreated encopresis seldom persists beyond the middle teenage years. When treated it usually improves within a year.

Attention deficit hyperactivity disorder (hyperkinetic disorder)

About a third of children are described by their parents as overactive, and up to a fifth of schoolchildren are so described by their teachers. These reported cases of overactivity vary from little more than normal high spirits to a severe disruptive and persistent disorder—which in the more severe cases is accompanied by inattention. Because of this association, the term used in DSM for the abnormal condition is **attention deficit hyperactivity disorder**. Although this term is widely used, readers will also encounter the alternative term **hyperkinetic disorder** which is used in ICD (the international classification, see p. 13). The prevalence of these disorders is certainly less than that of the hyperactivity reported by parents and teachers, but the reported rates vary with the criteria for diagnosis: 5–10 per cent using DSM criteria, and 1–2 per cent with the more restrictive ICD criteria.

Clinical features (Table 20.13)

These children are restless, fidgety, and cannot sit still for long. They have difficulty in attending to one thing for long and in following instructions. Their school work is disorganized and contains many careless errors. They are boisterous, reckless, and accident prone. Their behaviour exhausts their parents and their teachers, alienates other children, and disrupts their school work. All these problems lead to low self-esteem and sometimes to disobedience, temper tantrums, aggression, and other antisocial behaviour. Depressive mood is common. These behaviours vary in severity between places—for example worse at school than at home—and from day to day.

TABLE 20.13 Clinical features of attention deficit hyperactivity disorder

* Extreme restlessness
* Sustained overactivity
* Poor attention
* Learning difficulty
* Impulsiveness
* Recklessness
* Accident proneness
* Disobedience
* Temper tantrums
* Aggression

Children with these symptoms often have another disorder ('co-morbidity') including conduct disorder, depressive disorder, and anxiety disorder.

Aetiology

Aetiology is multifactorial. Twin, adoption, and family studies all suggest *genetic predisposition*. Linkage has been reported with some of the genes involved in the dopamine system suggesting an abnormality of dopaminergic transmission. The restlessness and difficulty in concentration suggest an abnormality in the prefrontal cortex and related subcortical structures since these are involved in guiding and sustaining behaviour, and delaying responses. As these brain regions are rich in catecholamines, this observation appears to link with the genetic findings and with the observed therapeutic effect of stimulant drugs (see below). Genetic predisposition interacts with *social factors*, for example overactivity is more frequent among children brought up in institutions and those living in poor social conditions. Many *other aetiological factors* have been suggested including prematurity, perinatal complications, fetal exposure to alcohol and drugs taken by the mother, and exposure to environmental lead, and certain food additives. The role of these factors is as yet uncertain.

Prognosis

Overactivity improves as the child grows older, especially when it is mild and not present in every situation. Impulsiveness, inattention, and the associated learning difficulties persist into adolescence in about one-half of children with attention deficit hyperactivity disorder; and about half of the adolescent cases persist into adult life. Affected individuals are also at risk for substance abuse, antisocial behaviour, and other psychiatric disorders.

Management

Care is usually shared between the general practitioner and a specialist who evaluates the problems and plans the management and provides some of the treatment.

Assessment Since the problem behaviours vary in different settings (see above), information should be obtained from teachers as well as from the parents and the child. Evidence should be sought for a co-morbid disorder that may be contributing to the overall problems and may be treatable. Assessment by an educational psychologist may be needed to establish the extent of the learning difficulties.

Support for parents and family Parents and family are helped to understand the nature of the condition and supported in their efforts to contain and live with the overactivity. In *behavioural parent training*, parents are helped to reinforce positive behaviour, avoid punitive responses to problem behaviours, and find alternative ways of dealing with defiant or disruptive behaviour.

Support for teachers Teachers also need to understand the condition and to be supported. Some schools are able to make special arrangements for teaching that take account of these children's short attention span, and shield other children from the disruptive effects of the restless behaviour.

Medication For unknown reasons, *stimulant drugs* such as methylphenidate and amphetamine have the paradoxical effect of reducing the overactivity in many cases. The treatment is generally reserved for the more severe cases because there may be the side effects of loss of appetite, insomnia, headaches, and stomach pains. Growth may be slowed although adult stature does not seem to be affected. When possible, a specialist opinion should be obtained before prescribing. It appears that hyperactive children treated in this way do not become addicted to the stimulant drug. About two-thirds of children improve in the short term, and even partial improvement may help the child to cope better at school. However, school grades do not always improve and the long-term benefits of the treatment are uncertain. Symptoms return soon after the drug is withdrawn.

Other treatments Parents may ask advice about special diets and dietary supplements. There is no convincing evidence that treatments of this kind are effective, though some parents report benefits and others wish to try them.

Conduct disorder

This disorder is characterized by severe and persistent antisocial behaviour clearly greater than ordinary mischievousness and rebellion. Extreme cases are easy to define but the dividing line between normal and abnormal conduct is sometimes difficult to draw. It is the most common type of psychiatric disorder among older children and adolescents, but the exact prevalence is difficult to estimate because there is no clear and objective dividing line between conduct disorder and normal bad behaviour, and because children with conduct disorder often have co-morbid disorders, including attention deficit hyperactivity disorder and depression.

Clinical features

In the *pre-school period* the disorder usually manifests as aggressive behaviour to other children, and rebelliousness with the parents, often accompanied by overactivity.

TABLE 20.14	Clinical features of conduct disorder
◆ Disobedience	
◆ Lying	
◆ Aggressive behaviour	
◆ Problems at school	
◆ Truanting	
◆ Stealing	
◆ Vandalism and fire-setting	
◆ Disapproved sexual behaviour	
◆ Alcohol and drug abuse	

TABLE 20.15	Management of conduct disorder
◆ Treat any co-morbid condition	
◆ Explain the problem to the parents and child	
◆ Help the child to describe his concerns and worries	
◆ If possible reduce or avoid any stressors	
◆ Discuss management with the parents, and consider parent training	
◆ Consider anger management for the child	
◆ Consider remedial teaching	
◆ (Rarely) residential placement when problems are severe and the is family extremely disruptive	
◆ (Occasionally) medication (see text)	

The clinical features in *later childhood* are listed in Table 20.14. It should be noted that: (i) repeated stealing is less significant in young children than at older ages because children below about 7 years do not usually have a full appreciation of what constitutes the ownership of property; (ii) disapproved sexual behaviour in younger children includes frequent masturbation and intrusive sexual curiosity; and (iii) alcohol and drug abuse may begin in older children and adolescents.

Aetiology

Environmental factors are important. Conduct disorder is more frequent among children from unstable, insecure, and rejecting families living in deprived areas. It is more frequent also among children from broken homes, and those who have been in residential care in early childhood. Conduct disorder is related also to adverse factors in the wider social environment, such as overcrowding and high crime rates. *Genetic factors* have not been shown to be important in the majority of cases.

Prognosis

Mild conduct disorders generally improve but more severe cases usually run a prolonged course in childhood and adolescence, and some persist into adult life. There are no good indicators of outcome for the individual child, except that the behaviour is more likely to persist when it is severe and when the quality of personal relationships is poor.

Management

Any co-morbid disorder should be treated (Table 20.15). Treatment of the conduct disorder is directed to the family as well as the child, although some families are difficult to help. Mild disorders often recover with time and can be managed by the general practitioner with advice to the parents on setting consistent limits to the child's behaviour. More severe disorders generally require specialist management, which has the following steps:

1. *Explain and discuss* the problem with the parents and the child.

2. *Reduce or avoid any stressful circumstances*, if this is possible.

3. *Discuss how the parents manage the behaviour.* Consider *behavioural parent training* to reduce any unwitting reinforcement of the child's undesirable behaviour, and to help the parents to respond positively to normal behaviour.

4. *Arrange remedial teaching* if there are reading or other educational difficulties.

5. *Consider anger management* a form of cognitive behaviour therapy, which is sometimes helpful for older children and adolescents.

6. *Consider residential placement.* In a very few cases, when the disorder is severe and intractable and the home is disruptive, the child may be placed in a foster home, residential home, or special school. This is done exceptionally and only after thorough discussion between all those involved with the child.

7. *Medication* may be used to treat associated attention deficit hyperactivity disorder, and risperidone is sometimes tried when the conduct disorder is severe.

Although these measures may reduce the immediate difficulties, there is no convincing evidence that any treatment affects the long-term course of conduct disorder. However, when adverse social and family factors improve for any reason, the disorder may improve.

Repeated absence from school

Repeated and prolonged absence from school has four causes:

1. Repeated or prolonged physical illness.

2. Parents who keep the child at home to help with domestic work or for other reasons.

3. **Truancy**, where the child rebels against going to school.

4. **School refusal**, where a physically healthy child wishes to go to school—and the parents support this—but is unable to do so because of emotional problems.

Of these four causes, truancy requires brief discussion and school refusal a longer account.

Truancy

Truancy is a form of rebellion and requires a direct and energetic approach agreed by the parents and teachers. Strong pressure should be brought to bear on the child to return to school, while an attempt should be made to resolve any educational or other problems at school. If these steps fail, legal proceedings may be initiated by the educational authorities.

School refusal

The child shows mounting signs of unhappiness and anxiety when it is time to go to school and is reluctant to leave home. The child may complain of feeling ill, and especially of unexplained physical symptoms such as headache, abdominal pain, diarrhoea, or sickness. These complaints occur on school days but not at other times. Some children leave home to go to school but become increasingly distressed as they approach it. The final refusal to go to school can arise:

- *gradually* after a period of increasing difficulty of the kind just described;

- *after an enforced absence*, usually due to minor physical illness;

- *after an upsetting event* either *at school*, such as bullying, or failure *in the family*, such as discord between the parents, or illness in a parent or grandparent.

Whatever the final sequence of events, these children are extremely resistant to efforts to return them to school, and their evident distress makes it hard for the parents to insist that they go.

Associated disorder In younger children *separation anxiety* is important. In older children there may be a *phobic* or *depressive disorder*. In the remaining cases there is no disorder and the refusal is an understandable but

TABLE 20.16	Management of school refusal
Exclude a primary disorder	Physical illness
	Separation anxiety
	Other anxiety disorders
	Depressive disorders
Identify stressors at home	Marital problems
	Threats of separation
	Illness of family member
Identify stressors at school	Criticism
	Failure
	Bullying
Modify stressors if possible	Advice for parents
	Discussion with teachers
Return to school	Firm approach
	Sympathetic support
Psychiatric opinion if the above fail	

exaggerated *response to problems at school or at home* of the kind noted above.

Outcome Most younger children eventually return to school. A few severely affected adolescents cannot be returned to school before the age at which compulsory school attendance ends.

Management (Table 20.16) General practitioners are often asked for help with these problems. They can usually assist all but the severe cases and early intervention may prevent worsening of the condition. The plan of management is shown in Table 20.16. The doctor should explain sympathetically but firmly to the parents and the child the nature of the condition and the need to achieve an early return to school. The arrangements should be agreed with both parents, with the teachers, and if possible with the child. The doctor's role is to support the parents in carrying out the plan. If the parents find it difficult to adopt a firm approach, a nurse or social worker may accompany the child to school on the first few occasions.

If these simple measures fail, referral to a child psychiatrist is appropriate. The psychiatrist will look again for a possible primary psychiatric disorder, explore the causes for the child's distress in more detail, and employ the greater resources of the psychiatric team to help the child overcome the fear of going to school. Occasionally, admission to hospital is arranged to separate the child from particularly stressful circumstances at home or provide intensive treatment for anxiety or depression. Very occasionally the problems improve after a change of school.

Juvenile delinquency: children who break the law

Delinquency is the failure of a young person to obey the law. It is not a psychiatric disorder but its causes include psychiatric disorder, usually conduct disorder. Also, parents often ask for advice from doctors about their delinquent children. Delinquency is most common at the age of 15–16 years. It is much more common in boys than girls. When asked about their own conduct, most adolescent boys admit having broken the law at some time, often with minor acts of shoplifting. Up to a fifth of adolescent boys are found to have carried out an offence, usually a trivial one. Of these only a few continue to offend in adult life. Parents can usually be reassured that a single act, especially if carried out with a group of others, is not of serious significance. (See pp. 295–6.)

Disorders of development

Disorders of development are divided into **specific disorders** in which only a single function is involved and **pervasive disorders** in which a wide range of aspects of psychological development are affected. Autism is the least rare of the pervasive development disorders and the only one discussed here. Others are discussed in *The Shorter Oxford Textbook of Psychiatry*.

Disorders of the development of intellectual function are not included in this diagnostic group. They are classified as learning disability, and are discussed in Chapter 21. Specific disorders of development are more common than pervasive disorders, but the latter are more serious. It is important to detect all these disorders at an early stage and arrange specialist assessment.

Specific developmental disorders

These circumscribed developmental delays are of the four kinds shown in Table 20.17. As explained above, the disorders do not involve general intellectual development; nor do they involve general social development (which occurs in autism).

TABLE 20.17 Specific developmental disorders in childhood

- Reading disorder
- Arithmetic disorder
- Motor disorder
- Language disorder

Specific reading disorder (dyslexia)

This condition is also known as **developmental reading disorder**. The child's reading age is significantly (two standard deviations) below the level expected from age and IQ and this is not due solely to inadequate education. Writing and spelling are also impaired but other aspects of development are not, although the child's conduct may be disordered as a reaction to frustrating experiences at school or for other reasons. Compared with children with general backwardness at school, those with specific reading disorder are more often boys and are more likely to have minor neurological abnormalities; they are less likely to come from disadvantaged families.

Aetiology The frequent occurrence of reading disorder in family members suggests a genetic aetiology and several loci for dyslexia have been reported. Genetic heterogeneity can be expected because several complex processes are involved in reading.

Prognosis When the disorder is mild, about a quarter of the children read normally by adolescence. When the disorder is severe, most children still have severe problems in adolescence and later. Prognosis is worse when there is a co-morbid conduct disorder.

Management Special education in reading is required, the important first step being to reawaken the interest of the child after what has often been a long experience of failure. For this reason early detection is important.

Other specific developmental disorders

Three other conditions parallel specific reading disorder in their form, unknown aetiology, and management through special training. Mild cases generally improve gradually with time; severe cases may persist into adult life.

Specific arithimetic disorder resembles specific reading disorder except that the problem is with arithmetic.

Specific motor disorder Children with this disorder have delayed motor development and poor coordination without general intellectual impairment or a specific neurological cause. They are late in developing the skills of feeding, walking, and dressing. They are clumsy, tending to break things, and are not good at games. Some have difficulty in writing and drawing.

Specific developmental language disorder Children with this disorder have delayed speech in the absence of general learning disability or another cause such as deafness, cerebral palsy, or autism. On starting school, 5 per cent of children have difficulty in making themselves understood by strangers and 1 per cent are seriously retarded in speech. Serious delays in the production or understanding of speech has obvious consequences for education and social development and may be associated with behavioural problems. Hence early detection is important. Management is with speech therapy and remedial teaching.

Childhood autism

Although rare, autism is important because it is a serious disorder. All doctors should be able to recognize the possibility that it is present, although positive diagnosis usually requires a specialist opinion.

Epidemiology

Autism occurs in about 0.75 per 1000 children, and is four times more common in boys than in girls. An additional 1.2 per 1000 have features that are similar but do not meet the full diagnostic criteria for autism (atypical autism) giving an overall rate for 'autism spectrum disorders' of about 2 per 1000 children. Some recent studies have reported rates twice as high for both autism and spectrum disorders. At the time of writing it is not certain whether these higher figures indicate an increasing incidence or more complete ascertainment of cases.

Clinical features

Autism is characterized by the early onset of difficulties in social interaction and communication, together with restricted and repetitive behaviours and interests. The abnormal behaviour starts in early childhood after a period of normal development. The clinical features (Table 20.18) include the following, though many children do not show all of them.

Inability to relate Autistic children do not respond to affectionate behaviour by smiling or cuddling, and may be no more responsive to their parents than to

strangers. They lack interest in other children and avoid eye contact ('gaze avoidance'). In some, these difficulties diminish as the child grows older; in others they persist into adult life.

Disorders of speech and language Speech may develop normally and then decline, or develop late. These children have difficulty in two-way conversations, and some ask a string of questions instead. Some use language in unusual ways, referring to themselves as he or she, echoing what they have heard earlier, or inventing words. Occasionally, speech never develops.

Impaired non-verbal communication These children do not point at objects, nod, or imitate or use play to communicate in the way that normal children do.

Resistance to change Some autistic children are distressed by changes in their daily routine. They prefer the same food, insist on wearing the same clothes, or engage in the same repetitive games.

Repetive interests and behaviours are common. These children have narrow and often eccentric interests, for example lists of dates or facts. They may make stereotyped hand movements, often within the peripheral part of the field of vision, or rock repeatedly from side to side.

Seizures About a quarter of autistic children develop epileptic seizures, usually at about the time of adolescence.

Other features Some are *emotionally labile*, suddenly becoming angry or fearful without apparent reason. They may be *overactive* and *distractible*. They may *sleep badly* and they may *wet or soil* themselves.

Aetiology

The cause of autism is unknown and likely to be heterogeneous.

Genetic factors Twin and family studies indicate that genetic factors are of major importance. There appear to be multiple interacting genes, though at the time of writing no definitely confirmed linkages have been reported. The phenotype associated with the genetic predisposition appears to include cases that do not meet all the diagnostic criteria for autism (autistic spectrum disorders).

Organic brain disorder The occurrence of seizures in about 20 per cent of patients at the time of adolescence (see above) suggests an organic brain disorder, at least in some cases. However, so far neuropathological, brain imaging, and neurochemical findings are inconsistent.

TABLE 20.18 Clinical features of childhood autism
◆ Inability to relate and gaze avoidance
◆ Speech and language disorder
◆ Impaired non-verbal communication
◆ Resistance to change
◆ Odd behaviour and mannerisms
◆ Seizures
◆ Emotional lability, overactivity, poor concentration

Cognitive abnormalities involve, in particular, symbolic thinking and language. An important deficit, present in many but not all of these children, is the inability to judge correctly what other people are thinking and to use this knowledge to predict their behaviour (lack of a 'theory of mind').

Abnormal parenting has not been shown to be a cause. This is an important point for families to understand since many blame themselves for the child's problems.

Prognosis

About half of the children who meet the criteria for autism acquire some useful speech, although serious impairments usually remain. Those who improve may continue to show emotional coldness and odd behaviour. As mentioned already, about 20 per cent develop epilepsy in adolescence. Between 10 and 20 per cent of children with autism are eventually able to attend an ordinary school and then obtain work. A further 10–20 per cent cannot work but can live at home and attend a training centre. The remainder are unable to lead an independent life. The prognosis of autistic spectrum disorder is generally rather better though it too may persist into adult life.

Differential diagnosis

Childhood autism has to be distinguished from several other disorders.

1. **Asperger's syndrome**. This is characterized by severe and sustained abnormalities of social and other behaviour, similar to those of autism, but without the impairements of language and cognition found in autism. Its cause is unknown. The abnormalities usually persist into adult life.

2. **Deafness**. This can be excluded by appropriate tests of hearing.

3. **Specific developmental language disorder** (see p. 291), in which the child usually responds normally to people.

4. **Learning disability**, in which there is general intellectual retardation with relatively less language impairment than in autism and a more normal response to other people.

5. **Other developmental disorders**. There are other rare and poorly understood disorders of development that may be identified by specialists.

Treatment

The advice of a specialist should be obtained. There is no specific treatment and management has three aspects.

Management of abnormal behaviour Usually a *behavioural approach* is used. Factors are identified that appear to be reinforcing the problem behaviour; for example, increased attention from the parents at times when behaviour is abnormal than at other times. The reinforcing factors are reduced if possible and the child's response is monitored. These procedures lead to short-term improvement in some cases but may not produce lasting benefit.

Special schooling Most autistic children require special schooling to help them achieve their remaining potential for development. Lessons are brief, the teacher to pupil ratio is high, and classes are small. Under these conditions, autistic children can progress in their school work and in their social behaviour. Residential schooling may be needed for the most severely affected children.

Help for the family The primary care team has an important role in working with the specialist services to explain the nature of the disorder, support the parents, and help them to establish as normal a life as possible for the affected child and for the rest of the family. Many parents find it helpful to join a group of other parents of autistic children where they can discuss common problems. Respite care is also helpful.

Other disorders affecting speech

It is convenient at this point to consider two other disorders in which speech is affected without general intellectual retardation or autism. These are **stammering** and **elective mutism**.

Stammering

Stammering is a disturbance of the rhythm and fluency of speech. It is not a psychiatric disorder, nor is it usually associated with psychiatric disorder although may cause distress. Stammering may take the form of repetitions of syllables or words, or of pauses in the production of speech. Stammering is four times more frequent in boys than girls. It usually begins in the early stages of language development, and in most cases does not last long. About 1 per cent of children suffer from stammering after starting school.

Aetiology The aetiology of stammering is not known.

Prognosis Most children improve with time but a minority persist into adult life.

Treatment is by *speech therapy*; this may help in the short term but its long-term value is uncertain.

Selective mutism

In this rare condition, a child refuses to speak in some circumstances but speaks normally in others. Usually, speech is lacking outside the home and is normal at home. Often, there is other negative behaviour such as refusing to sit down or to play when asked to do so. The condition usually begins between 3 and 5 years of age, after normal speech has been acquired.

Aetiology The cause is unknown.

Prognosis About half improve after 5 years; the course after that is uncertain.

Treatment There is no specific treatment of proven effectiveness. Parents should be told what little is known about the condition. Any stressful circumstances at home or at school should be modified if possible, although this will not necessarily lead to improvement in the mutism.

Gender identity disorder

Some boys consistently prefer girls' games, enjoy dressing in girls' clothes, and prefer the company of girls. Some of these boys also have an effeminate manner and say they want to be girls—they have a disorder of gender identity. Some girls show corresponding masculine behaviours and preferences.

Aetiology The cause of this disorder is unknown. Some parents encourage feminine behaviour in boys (or tomboyish behaviour in girls), but most children brought up in these ways develop normally. Therefore, there may be innate causes but none has been identified with certainty.

Prognosis Some children with gender identity problems grow up normally. Others become either homosexual, bisexual, or, less often, transsexual.

Management When the behaviour is not extreme parents should be reassured and helped to encourage behaviour appropriate to the child's gender. When the behaviour is extreme, the child should be assessed by a child psychiatrist who may offer counselling to the parents and child, and may use a behavioural approach to reinforce more appropriate behaviour. It is not known whether such treatment alters the long-term outcome.

Psychological disorders of physically ill children

Most children adapt well to the experience of physical illness. When there are psychological problems these generally resemble those of physically ill adults, discussed in Chapter 11. Most of the points made there also apply also to children, so only a few special issues will be considered in this section.

Children's reactions to physical illness

Acute physical illness is more likely to cause delirium in children than in adults. A familiar example is delirium caused by febrile illness. *Chronic physical illness* and its treatment can affect self-esteem and social development. These problems are particularly common with neurological disorders including epilepsy, diabetes, leukaemia, and other life-threatening conditions.

Reactions of the parents

Although all parents are distressed when their child develops a chronic physical illness, some react more severely. Some parents *deny* the seriousness of the condition, some *reject* the child, and some are *overprotective*. With time, most parents regain a satisfactory, loving relationship with their ill child, and cope successfully with the difficulties. The family doctor can help parents to achieve a satisfactory adjustment.

Reactions of siblings

The brothers and sisters of children with serious physical illness or handicap generally manage well, and some even acquire increased abilities to cope with stress. However, some siblings feel neglected, or resent having to spend time helping to care for the ill or handicapped child. A few develop a psychiatric disorder, usually an anxiety or depressive disorder. When a child is seriously ill, the family doctor should always consider the needs of the siblings and the parents.

Admission to hospital

Many children cope well with admission to hospital but some become anxious or depressed, or regress in behaviour. Usually, these consequences are short lived, but repeated admission to hospital, especially in the early or middle years of childhood, may be followed by lasting emotional or behavioural disturbances. This result is more likely when there are poor family relationships or social problems. It is now general policy to encourage parents to visit their child in hospital frequently, to stay in hospital if the child is severely ill, and to take part in the child's care. Primary care and hospital staff can prepare children for admission to hospital by explaining what will happen in terms appropriate to the child's age, and by guiding the parents in how to reinforce this explanation.

Chronic fatigue syndrome

This disorder occurs occasionally in childhood. The clinical picture and management resemble those for the same condition in adults (see p. 94).

Disorders of adolescence

There are no psychiatric disorders specific to this period of life. Younger adolescents may develop the disorders of childhood, older adolescents may develop some of the disorders of adult life. For this reason, the subject will be considered briefly, drawing attention to the main conditions that are encountered at this age, but not repeating information presented elsewhere in this or other chapters. Juvenile delinquency is not a psychiatric disorder although it is associated with such a disorder. Since it occurs mainly in the adolescent period, it is described in this section, after the review of psychiatric disorders.

Adjustment disorders

These are common in adolescence, often with depressive symptoms.

Emotional disorders

Anxiety disorders

Social phobia often begins in early adolescence, and a few cases of agoraphobia begin in late teenage years. Some phobic disorders that started in childhood persist into adolescence. **Obsessional disorders** may begin in adolescence. **School refusal** and **truancy** are common between 14 years of age and the end of compulsory schooling.

Depressive disorders

Depressive disorders in adolescence are generally characterized by loss of energy, difficult relationships at home, withdrawal from other social contacts, and underachievement at school. Profound depressive mood and extreme guilt are less common; when present, these features suggest that the depressive disorder is the first phase of a manic-depressive disorder (see below).

Manic-depressive disorder (bipolar disorder)

This is rare before puberty but increases in incidence during adolescence. The clinical features of the **depressive phase** are similar to those in adults (see p. 98) except that delusions and hallucinations are less frequent. Among adolescents **mania** presents most often with increased energy, reduced sleep, irritability, and disinhibited behaviour.

The treatment of manic-depressive disorder in adolescence resembles that for adults (see p. 115) except that: (i) drug doses are lower, according to age; (ii) lithium is used less often; and (iii) electroconvulsive therapy (ECT) is used only very occasionally and then for very severe, drug-resistant depression in older adolescents.

Deliberate self-harm

This important problem among adolescents is discussed on p. 181.

Eating disorders

Bulimia nervosa and **anorexia nervosa** often begin in adolescence and are among the more common disorders at this age. These disorders are described in Chapter 12.

Conduct disorders

About half of adolescent conduct disorders begin in childhood. In adolescence the most common features are truancy, offences against property (including the taking and driving of cars), abuse of alcohol and drugs, and, among girls, promiscuity.

Schizophrenia

Schizophrenia sometimes begins in adolescence, more commonly in boys than girls. The clinical picture is like that of schizophrenia in young adults (see p. 123). Treatment is also similar, though with appropriate reductions in drug doses and even greater emphasis on work with the family. The prognosis is poor.

Substance abuse

Many adolescents take drugs, especially cannabis, and drink alcohol—but only a minority abuse these substances. The factors leading from use to abuse are complex and not fully understood. They include family and wider social adversity, drug use by parents, depressive disorder, and conduct disorder. The association with conduct disorder is particularly important. Treatment is similar to that for adults with similar problems, usually with an emphasis on family problems and any associated conduct or depressive disorder.

Juvenile delinquency

Parents sometimes ask general practitioners for advice about their delinquent adolescents. Delinquency is the failure of a young person to obey the law—it is not a psychiatric disorder, although psychiatric disorder, usually conduct disorder, is one of its causes.

Delinquency is most common at the age of 15–16 years. It is much more common in boys than girls. Up to a fifth of adolescent boys are found to have carried out an offence, albeit usually a trivial one. However, when asked about their own conduct, 9 out of 10 adolescent boys admit to behaviour that broke the law, often with minor acts of shoplifting. Of these adolescents, only a few continue to offend in adult life and parents can usually be reassured that a single act, especially if carried out as part of a group, is not likely to be of serious significance.

Causes As well as the association with *conduct disorder*, noted above, delinquency is related to low *social class*, *poverty*, *poor housing*, and *poor education*, so that rates are greater in areas of social deprivation. Delinquency is more frequent in children from *broken homes*, *families with discord*, and *very large families*. Repeated offending is associated with several interrelated factors:

* *personal factors* including school underachievement, and hyperactivity;

* *family factors* including criminality in the parents, family discord, and lack of supervision;

* *psychiatric disorder* is present in about a third of 16–18-year-olds who have been sentenced;

* *other factors* including substance abuse and unfavourable peer group pressure.

Management Delinquency is dealt with by the courts who generally obtain a *social report* about the young person's family and social and material environment, an *educational report*, and, in certain cases, a *psychiatric report* (see p. 327). The arrangements vary in different countries and readers should find out about the arrangements in the country in which they are training. Usually, the emphasis is on secondary prevention rather than punishment, with involvement of social, educational, and sometimes psychological or psychiatric services in an attempt to:

* treat any associated psychiatric disorder;

* improve the family environment;

* help the offender to develop better skills for resisting peer group pressure, solving problems, and managing anger;

* improve educational and vocational accomplishments.

Although such measures are helpful for the majority, a minority offend repeatedly. Additional resources for this minority include youth treatment centres and (residential) young offenders' institutions.

TABLE 20.19　Forms of child abuse
◆ Physical abuse
◆ Sexual abuse
◆ Emotional abuse
◆ Fetal abuse
◆ Neglect
◆ Munchausen syndrome by proxy

Disorders of parent–child relationships

Breakdown of the normal caring relationship between adults in the parental role and small children can result in the conditions listed in Table 20.19. The term **child abuse** refers to **physical**, **emotional**, and **sexual abuse**, and is sometimes used to include the other conditions. **Fetal abuse** is behaviour detrimental to the fetus, such as physical assault on the pregnant mother or the taking, by the mother, of substances likely to harm the fetus. It alone is not discussed further in this section.

Physical abuse (non-accidental injury)

These terms refers to deliberate infliction of injury on a child, usually by one of the parents, a co-habitee of the mother, or, occasionally, by a paid carer. Each year about 1 per 1000 children receive injuries of such severity that there is evidence of bone fracture or bleeding around the brain. Less severe injury is more frequent, but its frequency is uncertain because it does not always come to professional attention.

Detecting abuse

Since parents seldom reveal the condition directly, clinicians have to be *alert to indirect indications*. Particular vigilance is needed when the family has features associated with a high risk for abuse (see below). The problem may

TABLE 20.20　Injuries caused by physical abuse
◆ Multiple bruising
◆ Abrasions
◆ Bites
◆ Burns
◆ Torn lips
◆ Fractures
◆ Retinal haemorrhage
◆ Subdural haemorrhage

become apparent when the parents bring a child to the doctor with an injury said to have been caused accidentally. Alternatively, relatives, neighbours, teachers, or other people may become concerned and report the problem to the police, social workers, or voluntary agencies. Suspicion of physical abuse should be aroused by:

- the *nature* of the injuries (Table 20.20);

- *previous suspicious injury*;

- *unconvincing explanations* of the way in which the injury was sustained;

- *delay* in seeking help;

- *incongruous reactions* to the injury by the carers;

- *fearful responses of the child* to the carers ('frozen watchfulness')

- *other evidence of distress* such as social withdrawal, regression, low self-esteem, or aggressive behaviour.

Aetiology

There are three sets of aetiological factors relating to the parents, the child, and the social circumstances (Table 20.21). The common factor is a failure of the normal emotional bonding between the parent or other carer and the infant. Knowledge of these risk factors assists in the detection of child abuse.

Management

Assessment of the injuries When abuse is suspected a specialist assessment should be arranged, giving a full account of the reasons for suspicion (see above). Usually, the child will be admitted to a paediatric ward for assessment, which includes taking *photographs* of the injuries and a *radiological examination*, which may show evidence of previous fracture. Occasionally, the examination will reveal a bone disorder such as osteogenesis imperfecta suggesting that the fractures were caused accidentally. *Computerized tomography* is performed if subdural haemorrhage is suspected. All findings should be *documented fully* since evidence may be needed at subsequent legal proceedings.

Subsequent action If it appears that non-accidental injury is probable, an experienced senior doctor and social worker should *talk to the parents*. Arrangements should be made to *examine other children* without delay, to ensure their safety. The procedure varies with local administrative arrangements: in the UK social services play an important role. The primary care team will be involved with the specialist team in the immediate and long-term plans for the child and the other members of the family.

Returning the child Sometimes the abused child can return home if support and close supervision are provided for the parents. When abuse has been severe or prolonged, however, the child may need to move to foster care while help is given to the parents. Sometimes permanent separation is necessary. These very difficult decisions are usually made by a paediatrician or child psychiatrist and a social worker, both experienced in such problems, after discussion with the family doctor. Since children returning to their parents may suffer further serious injury or even death, it is vitally important that a very careful assessment be made before a physically abused child is returned to the parents, and that there is close supervision of the child after return.

Prognosis

Children who have been subjected to physical abuse are at high risk of delayed development, learning difficulties, and emotional and behavioural disorders extending into adult life. As adults, former victims of abuse may have difficulties in rearing their own children and some abuse them.

TABLE 20.21 Risk factors for physical abuse
In the parent
◆ Very young age
◆ Abnormal personality
◆ Unsatisfactory or broken marriage
◆ Social isolation
◆ Former victim of abuse
◆ Criminal record
◆ Psychiatric disorder
In the child
◆ Premature
◆ Separated in early life
◆ Needing special neonatal care
◆ Congenital malformation
◆ Chronic illness
◆ Difficult temperament
In the environment
◆ Poor housing
◆ Family violence
◆ Little feeling of community
◆ Other stressful living conditions

Sexual abuse

The term sexual abuse refers to the involvement of children in sexual activities to which they cannot give legally informed consent, or which violate generally accepted cultural rules, and which they may not fully comprehend. The term covers various forms of sexual contact, some involving violence, as well as activities such as posing for pornographic photographs or films. The abuser is usually known to the child and is often a member of the family.

Prevalence

The prevalence of sexual abuse is difficult to determine; more cases have been reported to doctors in recent years but it is not certain whether this indicates a true increase in the problems, or more complete reporting.

Clinical features

The children are more often female and the offenders usually male. Sexual abuse may be reported directly by the child or by a relative or other person. Children are more likely to report abuse when the offender is a stranger than when he is a family member. Sometimes, sexual abuse is discovered during the investigation of other conditions; for example, symptoms in the urogenital or anal area, behavioural or emotional disturbance, inappropriate sexual behaviour, or pregnancy. In adolescent girls, running away from home or unexplained suicidal attempts should raise the suspicion of sexual abuse. When abuse occurs within the family, relationship problems are common.

The *immediate consequences* of sexual abuse include anxiety, depression, and anger; inappropriate sexual behaviour; and unwanted pregnancy. *Long-term effects* include low self-esteem, mood disorder, self-harm, difficulties in relationships, and sexual maladjustment.

Assessment

It is important to be alert to the possibility of sexual abuse, and to give serious attention to any complaint made by a child of being abused in this way. It is also important not to make the diagnosis without adequate evidence from a thorough social investigation of the family, and from physical and psychological examinations of the child. If the general practitioner suspects sexual abuse, he should obtain the advice of a child psychiatrist and a social worker experienced in these problems.

It is essential that information from children is obtained carefully. The child should be encouraged sympathetically to describe what has happened. Drawings or toys may help younger children to give a description, but great care should be taken not to suggest answers to the child. When the circumstances make it appropriate a physical examination is carried out by a paediatrician, including inspection of the genitalia and anal region. If intercourse may have taken place in the past 72 hours, specimens should be collected from the genital and any other relevant regions.

Management

The initial management and the measures to protect the child are similar to those for physical abuse. In families where sexual abuse has occurred, the members may deny the seriousness of the abuse and the existence of other family problems. Sometimes a family member has engaged in other deviant sexual behaviour. The discovery of abuse may lead to family conflict that adds to the child's distress. Decisions about treatment and removal from home are taken only after the most careful consideration of all the implications. The sexual development of the abused child is often abnormal requiring help long after the event.

Late reports of sexual abuse

Some adults report sexual abuse that occurred when they were children. Sometimes the adults have always been aware of the abuse but have been previously unable to confide in a doctor or other person. At other times adults report the recall of sexual abuse that they had not previously remembered. When this latter experience takes place during a course of counselling it sometimes transpires that the 'memory' is false and is a response to repeated questioning or interpretations from the therapist (**false memory syndrome**). The problem is discussed further on p. 67.

Emotional abuse

The term emotional abuse refers usually to severe and persistent emotional neglect, verbal abuse, or rejection sufficient to impair a child's physical or psychological development. Emotional abuse often accompanies other forms of child abuse but may occur alone. Management resembles that for cases of physical abuse: the parents require help for their own emotional problems, the child needs counselling, and, in severe cases, a period of separation from the parents.

Neglect

Child neglect includes neglect of the child's physical or emotional needs, upbringing, safety, or medical care, all of which may lead to physical or psychological harm. Child neglect is associated with adverse social circumstances, and is a common reason for foster care.

Neglect of a child's emotional needs and nutrition may lead to failure to thrive physically in the absence of a detectable organic cause. In children under 3 years, this condition is called **non-organic failure to thrive**; in older children it is called **deprivation dwarfism**. At both ages, height and weight are reduced and development is delayed. The children are irritable and unhappy. Given adequate care and nutrition most recover.

Munchausen syndrome by proxy

In this rare disorder, a parent (usually the mother) takes her child repeatedly to a doctor with false accounts of symptoms and sometimes with fabricated signs of illness such as haematuria. She seeks repeated investigations and treatment for the child. The parent has a personality disorder and sometimes a factitious disorder herself. She may be experiencing stressful circumstances but it is usually unclear why these should result in this unusual behaviour. This disorder is rare and some even question its existence. The diagnosis should be made only after the most careful investigation by a specialist. Treatment is with general measures of counselling and help with social problems. The prognosis is poor for the child and the mother.

Some ethical problems in child psychiatry

Conflicts of interest

Usually the interests of the child are the same as those of the parents. When they are not, those of the child generally take precedence—most obviously in cases of child abuse. Occasionally, the decision is less obvious, for example when a depressed mother is neglecting her child but is likely to become more depressed if substitute care is arranged. If the problems are anticipated, they can usually be resolved by discussion with the parents and between the professionals caring for the mother and child.

Confidentiality

The care of children often involves the sharing of information with non-medical agencies that do not have identical policies about the confidentiality of records. Careful thought should be given to the information that it is essential to share, and the need should be discussed with the parents and, if they are old enough, with the children concerned.

Consent

Consent to treatment Children develop psychologically at different speeds, but the law has to set a single age for consent. For this and other reasons, the age below which it is the parents who consent to treatment for their child, differs in different legislations. Even below the age of consent, the child's agreement should be obtained whenever possible since without it treatment will be more difficult. Parents also have the right to *refuse* treatment for a child below the age of consent though only when this does not conflict with their duty to protect the child. If the parents' refusal seems not to be in the interests of the child, most countries provide for a decision by a court of law. In English law, when a 16- or 17-year-old refuses treatment to which the parents have consented, the outcome is decided by the court on the circumstances of the individual case.

Consent for psychiatric research poses similar problems for other medical research with subjects below the age of consent. Parents may find it difficult to balance the risks to their child against the benefits there will usually be for other children treated in the future. It is important therefore to discuss the issues thoroughly, and usually with a person additional to the person requesting consent; and to allow the parents plenty of time to reach their decision.

Further reading

Goodman, R. & Scott, S. (2005). *Child Psychiatry*. 2nd edn. Blackwell, Oxford.
A clear account of child psychiatry that links research finding to practical advice about management.

Appendix 20.1 A comprehensive scheme for history taking and examination in child psychiatry

The format and extent of an assessment will depend on the nature of the presenting problem. The following scheme is taken from the book by Graham (1990), which should be consulted for further information. *Graham suggests that clinicians with little time available should concentrate on items in bold type.*

1. Nature and severity of presenting problems(s). Frequency. Situations in which it occurs. Provoking and ameliorating factors. Stresses thought by parents to be important.

2. *Presence of other current problems or complaints.*

   (a) Physical. Headaches, stomach aches. Hearing, vision. Seizures, faints, or other types of attacks.

   (b) Eating, sleeping, or elimination problems.

   (c) **Relationship with parents and siblings. Affection, compliance.**

   (d) Relationships with other children. Special friends.

   (e) Level of activity, attention span, concentration.

   (f) Mood, energy level, sadness, misery, depression, suicidal feelings. General anxiety level, specific fears.

   (g) Response to frustration. Temper tantrums.

   (h) Antisocial behaviour. Aggression, stealing, truancy.

   (I) **Educational attainments, attitude to school attendance.**

   (j) Sexual interest and behaviour.

   (k) Any other symptoms, tics, etc.

3. *Current level of development.*

   (a) Language: comprehension, complexity of speech.

   (b) Spatial ability.

   (c) Motor coordination, clumsiness.

4. *Family structure.*

   (a) Parents: ages, occupations. **Current physical and emotional state.** History of physical or psychiatric disorder. Whereabouts of grandparents.

   (b) Siblings: ages, presence of problems.

   (c) Home circumstances: sleeping arrangements.

5. *Family function.*

   (a) **Quality of parental relationship. Mutual affection. Capacity to communicate about and resolve problems. Sharing of attitudes over child's problem.**

   (b) **Quality of parent–child relationship. Positive interaction: mutual enjoyment. Parental level of criticism, hostility, rejection.**

   (c) Sibling relationship.

   (d) Overall pattern of family relationships. Alliance, communication. Exclusion, scapegoating. Intergenerational confusion.

6. *Personal history.*

   (a) Pregnancy—complication. Medication. Infectious fevers.

   (b) Delivery and state at birth. Birthweight and gestation. Need for special care after birth.

   (c) Early mother–child relationship. Postpartum maternal depression. Early feeding patterns.

   (d) Early temperamental characteristics. Easy or difficult, irregular, restless baby and toddler.

   (e) Milestones. Obtain exact details only if outside range of normal.

   (f) **Past illnesses and injuries. Hospitalizations.**

   (g) Separations lasting a week or more. Nature of substitute care.

   (h) Schooling history. Ease of attendance. Educational progress.

Appendix 20.1 *Cont'd.*

7. *Observation of child's behaviour and emotional state.*

 (a) **Appearance. Signs of dysmorphism. Nutritional state. Evidence of neglect, bruising, etc.**

 (b) **Activity level. Involuntary movements. Capacity to concentrate.**

 (c) **Mood. Expression or signs of sadness, misery, anxiety, tension.**

 (d) **Rapport, capacity to relate to clinician. Eye contact. Spontaneous talk. Inhibition and disinhibition.**

 (e) **Relationship with parents. Affection shown. Resentment. Ease of separation.**

 (f) Habits and mannerisms.

 (g) Presence of delusions, hallucinations, thought disorder.

 (h) Level of awareness. Evidence of minor epilepsy.

8. *Observation of family relationships.*

 (a) Patterns of interaction—alliances, scapegoating.

 (b) Clarity of boundaries between generations: enmeshment.

 (c) Ease of communication between family members.

 (d) Emotional atmosphere of family. Mutual warmth. Tension, criticism.

9. *Physical examination of child.*

10. *Screening neurological examination.*

 (a) Note any facial asymmetry.

 (b) Eye movements. Ask child to follow a moving finger and observe eye movement for jerkiness, incoordination.

 (c) Finger–thumb apposition. Ask the child to press the tip of each finger against the thumb in rapid succession. Observe clumsiness, weakness.

 (d) Copying patterns. Drawing a man.

 (e) Observe grip and dexterity in drawing.

 (f) Observe visual competence when drawing.

 (g) Jumping up and down on the spot.

 (h) Hopping.

 (i) Hearing. Capacity of child to repeat numbers whispered 2 m behind him.

(From Graham P. J. (1999). *Child Psychiatry: a Developmental Approach*, 3rd edn. Oxford University Press, Oxford.)

CHAPTER 21

Learning disability (mental retardation)

Chapter contents

Terminology *303*

Epidemiology *304*

Clinical features *304*

Emotional and behavioural problems *305*

Physical disorders among people with learning disability *305*

Effects of learning disability on the family *305*

Causes of learning disability *305*

Causes of behaviour problems *309*

Assessment of learning disability *309*

Prevention and early detection *310*

Services for people with learning disability *311*

Psychiatric disorder in people with learning disability *313*

Ethical problems in the care of people with learning disability *314*

Appendix: Notes on some causes of learning disability *316*

The term **learning disability** and the alternative term **mental retardation**, denote an irreversible impairment of intelligence originating early in life (as opposed to dementia, which develops later) with associated limitations of social functioning. Although not reversible, much can be done to enable people with this condition to live as normally as possible. To achieve this, the main requirements are educational and social rather than medical: special schooling, sheltered work and housing, and support for the affected person and for the family. Nevertheless, general practitioners are involved in important aspects of the care of people with learning disability: they may be the first to identify the problem, they help the family to come to terms with the condition, and they provide general medical services throughout the person's life. And whatever their specialty, all doctors will see people with learning disability who are seeking help for a medical or surgical condition. Therefore, all doctors need to be able to interview people with learning disability and understand their special needs. They need to know in general terms the causes of learning disability and, in more detail, the features of two of the most frequent genetic conditions: **Down's syndrome** and **fragile-X syndrome**. They need also a broad understanding of the range of services available for these patients and when to refer to a psychiatrist.

Terminology

Several terms are used to describe people with intellectual impairment originating early in life. In the UK, the term **learning disability** is generally used. In many other countries the term is **mental retardation** and this is the one used in the classification systems ICD-10 and DSM-IV. In the past the condition has been known at various times as mental deficiency, mental subnormality, and mental handicap. We use the term learning disability.

The term learning disability implies more than intellectual impairment. The word disability draws attention to what the DSM definition refers to as 'concurrent deficits and impairments in adaptive behaviour, taking into account the person's age'. It therefore separates those who cannot lead a near normal life from people of the same IQ level who can. Despite this emphasis on disability, the degree of intellectual impairment is still important and learning disability is divided into subgroups based on IQ: mild (IQ 50–70), moderate (IQ 35–49), severe (IQ 24–34), and profound (IQ < 20).

Epidemiology

Between 2 and 3 per cent of the population have an IQ < 70, but only about 1 per cent have learning disability (i.e. IQ < 70 together with impairment of functioning). The rate of moderate or severe learning disability is 3–4 per 1000 of the population aged 15–19 years, or 6–8 people in a general practitioner's average list of 2000 patients. This *prevalence* has changed little since the 1930s even though the *incidence* of severe mental retardation has fallen by one-third to one-half in the same period, partly as a result of improved antenatal and neonatal care. The reason that the prevalence has not changed despite the lower incidence, is that people with learning disability are living longer.

Clinical features

People with learning disability perform badly on all kinds of intellectual task including learning, short-term memory, the use of concepts, and problem solving. Sometimes, one specific function is impaired more than the rest; for example, the use of language. The clinical features are described best by reference to the subgroups of mild, moderate, severe, and profound disability (Fig. 21.1; Table 21.1).

Mild learning disability (IQ 50–70)

About 80 per cent of people with learning disability fall into this group. Their appearance is usually normal and any sensory or motor deficits are slight. Most develop more or less normal language abilities and social behaviour during the pre-school years, so that in the least severe cases the learning disability may not be identified until the child starts school. In adult life most can

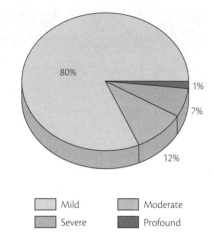

Fig. 21.1 Degrees of learning disability found in the general population.

TABLE 21.1 Levels of learning disability
Mild (IQ 50–70)
This group accounts for 80% of all those affected
◆ Specific causes uncommon
◆ Many need practical help and special education
◆ Few need special psychiatric or social services
Moderate (IQ 35–49)
This group accounts for 12% of all those affected
◆ Most can manage some independent activities
◆ Require special education, sheltered occupation, and supervision
Severe (IQ 20–34)
This group accounts for 7% of all those affected
◆ Specific causes usual
◆ Social skills severely limited
◆ Require close supervision and much practical help
Profound (IQ below 20)
This group accounts for 1% of all those affected
◆ Specific causes usual
◆ Physical problems usual: severely disabled
◆ Require help with basic self-care

live independently, although some need help with housing and employment, and support when they are experiencing stress.

Moderate learning disability (IQ 35–49)

Individuals in this group account for about 12 per cent of those with learning disability. Most have enough language development to communicate, and most can learn to care for themselves albeit with supervision. As adults most continue to do this and are able to undertake simple routine work.

Severe learning disability (IQ 20–34)

About 7 per cent of the people with learning disability are in this group. In the pre-school years their development is greatly slowed, and so is their learning when they go to school. With special training, many can eventually look after themselves under supervision and they can communicate albeit in simple ways. As adults most are able to undertake simple tasks and limited social activities. Many have associated physical disorders (see below).

A small number of these people have a single highly developed cognitive ability of a kind normally associated with superior intelligence, such as the ability to carry out feats of mental arithmetic or memory. Such people are called **idiots savants**.

Profound learning disability (IQ below 20)

About 1 per cent of those with learning disability are in this group. Few learn to care for themselves completely. A few achieve some simple speech and social behaviour. Physical disorders are very frequent.

Emotional and behavioural problems

As well as the direct effects of intellectual impairment, children with learning disability may show any of the common behavioural problems of childhood (see Chapter 20). These problems tend to occur at a later age than in a child of normal intelligence, and to last longer, although they usually improve slowly with time. A minority show severely disordered behaviour such as self-injury or aggression that threatens the well-being of the patient or the carers. Such behaviour is referred to as **challenging behaviour**.

Problem behaviours may be reactions to stressful events or to physical illness, secondary to psychiatric disorder, associated non-specifically with the underlying brain disorder, or specifically related to the genetic cause of the learning disability. These associations are considered further on p. 309.

Sexual problems

Some people with learning disability show a child-like curiosity about other people's bodies, which can be misunderstood as sexual. Many need sympathetic help in understanding sexual feelings at and after puberty. Concern is sometimes expressed that people with learning disability may give birth to children with learning disability. However, many of the causes of

learning disability are not inherited; and most of those that are inherited are associated with infertility. A more important concern is that people with severe learning disability are unlikely to be able to function well as parents. If termination of pregnancy or sterilization are considered, difficult ethical and legal problems can arise relating to consent, and specialist advice is usually necessary.

Physical disorders among people with learning disability

Physical disorders are most frequent among those with severe and profound learning disability, many of whom have sensory or motor disabilities, or epilepsy. Impaired hearing or vision may add an important additional obstacle to normal cognitive development. Motor disabilities, which are frequent, include spasticity, ataxia, and athetosis. Only a third of such people are continent and ambulant; and a quarter are highly dependent on other people.

Effects of learning disability on the family

When a newborn child is found to have learning disability, the parents are distressed and some reject the child at first, although this rejection seldom lasts long. More often the diagnosis is not made until after the first year of life. When this happens, the parents have to abandon their earlier hopes and expectations, and many experience a period of depression, guilt, shame, or anger. A few parents reject the child while others become overinvolved in the child's care to the detriment of their other children. Most parents eventually achieve a satisfactory adjustment but however well they adjust psychologically, they are faced with the prospect of prolonged hard work, and social problems. If the child also has a physical handicap, these problems are the greater. For these reasons, the parents of a child with learning disability need long-term support.

Causes of learning disability

Mild learning disability is usually due to a combination of genetic and adverse environmental factors, such as extreme prematurity and damage to the brain during birth. *Severe and profound learning disability* is usually due to specific pathological conditions, most of which can be diagnosed in life and about two-thirds of which can be diagnosed before birth. The causes of *moderate learning disability* are varied.

General causes (Box 21.1)

Genetic causes Much mild learning disability represents the lower end of the normal distribution curve of intelligence, which is mainly determined by polygenic inheritance. Specific genetic abnormalities are responsible for many of the metabolic and other disorders that cause severe learning disability. (Some of these causes are discussed further below.)

Antenatal damage is caused by *intrauterine infection* (such as rubella or syphilis) or toxic substances (such as *lead poisoning* or *excessive alcohol* use by the mother). In some developing countries, *hypothyroidism* due to iodine deficiency is important.

Perinatal damage This damage arises from birth injury, kernicterus, and intraventricular haemorrhage, and other less frequent conditions.

Postnatal damage is due to injury or resulting from child abuse, infections (encephalitis and meningitis), and lead intoxication.

Social factors include associations with lower social class, poverty, poor housing, and an unstable family environment.

Malnutrition is a common cause of learning disability in developing countries. It is much less frequent in Western countries.

Specific causes

Many specific causes of learning disability have been identified, many of which are abnormalities of chromosomes or genes, some associated with specific biochemical abnormalities. Because most of these causal conditions are rare they are not described fully in this chapter. For more information, the reader should consult the *New Oxford Textbook of Psychiatry*, a similar work of reference, or a textbook of paediatrics.

Genetic causes fall into five main groups of which only two of the more frequent, **Down's syndrome** and **fragile-X syndrome**, will be described further here. Brief explanatory notes on some of the others are provided in Appendix 21.1. The numbers in brackets refer to these notes.

1. **Dominant conditions**. Neurofibromatosis (*9*) and tuberose sclerosis (*10*) are examples of these rare conditions.

2. **Recessive conditions**. This is the largest group of specific genetic disorders. It includes most of the inherited metabolic conditions, such as phenylketonuria (*3*), homocystinuria (*4*), and galactosaemia (*5*).

3. **Chromosome abnormalities**. The most common chromosome abnormality is Down's syndrome (described below). Abnormalities in the number of sex chromosomes, as in Klinefelter's syndrome (XXY) and Turner's syndrome (XO), sometimes lead to learning disability as well as to physical abnormalities.

4. **X-linked conditions**. Specific genes on the X chromosome cause rare syndromes including the Lesch–Nyhan syndrome (*8*). Rett's syndrome is an X-linked dominant disorder in which affected girls develop normally in the first year and then regress. The causation of the more common fragile-X syndrome is described below.

5. **Genomic imprinting** is gene expression dependent on the parent of origin. Prader–Willi syndrome and Angelman's syndrome are both due to an abnormality in the 15q11-13 region. Altered paternal expression of genes in this region causes the Prader–Willi syndrome with hypotonia, hyperphagia, obesity, and daytime sleepiness. Altered maternal expression of a gene in this region leads to Angelman's syndrome with characteristic abnormal movements and a sociable disposition.

6. Conditions known to be inherited but in a less well understood way include microcephaly (*17*).

Down's syndrome

This condition used to be reported in about 1 in 600 births. As a result of prenatal screening and, if the mother wishes, termination of pregnancy the rate is now about 1 in every 1000 births.

Clinical features (Table 21.2)

External abnormalities The clinical picture is made up of features any one of which can occur in a normal person. When four of these features occur together, there is strong evidence for the syndrome.

1. The *head*: the occiput is flat.

2. The *eyes*: there are oblique palpebral fissures and epicanthic folds.

3. The *mouth*: the mouth and teeth are small, the tongue is furrowed, and the palate is high-arched.

4. The *hands*: these are short and broad, with a curved fifth finger, and a single transverse palmar crease.

5. The *joints*: these are hyperextensible or hyperflexible and the *muscles* are hypotonic.

Internal abnormalities, which are common, include *congenital heart disease*, especially septal defects (in about

BOX 21.1 CAUSES OF LEARNING DISABILITY*

Genetic

- *Dominant genes* (causing gross brain disease):

  neurofibromatosis (9);

  tuberose sclerosis (10).

- *Recessive genes* causing metabolic disorder involving:

  amino acids (e.g. phenylketonuria (3), homocystinuria (4));

  the urea cycle (e.g. citrullinuria, aminosuccinic aciduria);

  lipids (Tay–Sachs (6), Gaucher, and Niemann–Pick diseases);

  carbohydrate (galactosaemia);

  mucopolysaccharidoses (e.g. Hurler's syndrome (7)).

- *Chromosome abnormalities*:

  Down's syndrome (see p. 306);

  Klinefelter's syndrome;

  Turner's syndrome;

- *X-linked disorders*:

  Lesch–Nyhan syndrome;

  fragile-X syndrome (see p. 308);

  cranial malformations;

  hydrocephaly (16)

  microcephaly (17).

- **Polygenic factors**:

  influencing the normal distribution of intelligence.

Antenatal damage

- *Infections*: rubella (12), cytomegalovirus (14), syphilis, toxoplasmosis (13).
- *Intoxications*: lead, certain drugs, alcohol.
- *Physical damage*: injury, radiation, hypoxia.
- *Endocrine disorders*: hypothyroidism (20), hypoparathyroidism.

Perinatal damage

- Birth asphyxia.
- Kernicterus.
- Intraventricular haemorrhage.

BOX 21.1 CAUSES OF LEARNING DISABILITY* *(continued)*

Postnatal damage

- *Injury*: accidental, child abuse.
- *Infection*: encephalitis, meningitis.
- *Lead intoxication*.

Malnutrition

* Numbers in brackets refer to the numbered paragraphs in Appendix 21.1 (see p. 316) where brief additional information is provided. For more information about any of the conditions in this table, see a textbook of paediatrics.

TABLE 21.2	Abnormalities found in Down's syndrome

External abnormalities

- Flat occiput
- Oblique palpebral fissures
- Epicanthic folds
- Small mouth, high-arched palate
- Furrowed tongue
- Short, broad hands
- Single transverse palmer crease
- Curved fifth finger
- Hypotonia and extensive joints

Internal abnormalities

- Congenital heart disease
- Intestinal abnormalities
- Impaired hearing

20 per cent), and *intestinal abnormalities*, especially duodenal obstruction. *Hearing* may be *impaired*.

Learning disability In Down's syndrome the degree of learning disability varies considerably from person to person; usually the IQ is between 20 and 50, but in 15 per cent it is greater than 50.

Temperament The temperament of children with Down's syndrome is usually affectionate and easy-going, and many show an interest in music.

Behaviour problems are less frequent than in most other forms of learning disability; nevertheless about a quarter of children with Down's syndrome are chaotic and difficult to engage.

Ageing In the past, many people with Down's syndrome died in infancy but with improved medical care

about a quarter now live beyond the age of 50. Signs of ageing appear prematurely and *Alzheimer-like neuropathological changes* are found in the brain of most of those dying at the age of 40 years or more. However, for unknown reasons, survivors do not show signs of dementia until later, with a mean age of onset of about 50 years.

Aetiology

In about 95 per cent of cases there is trisomy of chromosome 21 (i.e. three chromosomes 21 instead of the usual two). These cases, which result from *failure of dysjunction* during meiosis, are more frequent in the children of older mothers and the risk of recurrence in a subsequent child is about 1 in 100.

The remaining 5 per cent of cases of Down's syndrome are attributable to *translocation* involving chromosome 21. The tendency to translocation is often inherited and the risk of recurrence, about 1 in 10, is higher than that in non-disjunction cases.

When non-disjunction takes places during a cell division after fertilization, normal and trisomic cells occur together in the same person, a condition known as **mosaicism**. In this 1 per cent of cases, the effects on cognitive development are particularly variable.

Fragile-X syndrome

The condition is so-called because a break is seen in an X chromosome of a proportion of cells when cultured in a medium deficient in folate. The basis of this abnormality is a region of CGG repeats in the gene *FMR1*. The repeats accumulate with successive copying, and affect the function of the gene when their number excedes 200. Men and women with 50–200 repeats are carriers, though men are unlikely to pass on the condition as *FMR*, which is found active mainly in the brain and testis, probably modifies the activity of other genes. Testing can identify heterozygous females who are clinically normal, and identify males who are carriers.

The disorder occurs in about 1 in 1200 males and in a milder form in 1 in 2000 females. The condition is the second most frequent cause of mental retardation (Down's syndrome is the first), accounting for about 7 per cent of moderate and about 4 per cent of mild learning disability among males, and about 3 per cent of moderate and mild mental retardation among females.

Affected children have *characteristic features*, none of which is diagnostic. These are a high forehead, prominent supraorbital ridges, and large ears. After puberty, the testes are enlarged. These children also have increased rates of abnormalities of speech and language, social impairment, and disorders of attention. Speech is often rapid and disorganized with frequent repetition of words and phrases (a disorder known as **cluttering**). However, the clinical picture varies greatly from one affected person to another.

Since absence of these physical characteristics does not exclude the diagnosis it is appropriate to test for the disorder in all unexplained cases of mental retardation.

Causes of behaviour problems

Behavioural problems among people with mental retardation have several causes, summarized in Table 21.3.

Reactions to stressful events When people with learning disability react to stress, they often display their distress through behaviour rather than words; for example in agitation, fearfulness, irritability, and dramatic behaviours. Stressful events include family tensions, or losses due to bereavement or changes of staff.

Frustration This may be caused by disability, difficulty in communication, inability to acquire social skills, and educational failure.

Over- or understimulation An overstimulating environment may cause problems such as agitation or aggression, while an understimulating environment may lead to withdrawal, self-stimulation, or self-injury.

Reactions to undiagnosed physical illness It is important to consider this possibility whenever behaviour becomes more disturbed.

Psychiatric disorder When people with learning disability develop psychiatric disorder, the first evidence is often a change of behaviour (see below, p. 313).

Brain damage Behaviour problems may be associated non-specifically with the learning disability, presumably through the underlying damage to the brain. Many children with learning disability are distractible and overactive. A few have more severe behaviour problems including repeated self-injury and autistic behaviours, including stereotyped repetitive and apparently purposeless activities such as rocking to and fro, head banging, and mannerisms. Self-injury and autistic behaviours are more frequent among people with severe learning disability: they occur in about 40 per cent of children and 20 per cent of adults.

Associated with epilepsy Epilepsy is strongly associated with behaviour disorder, especially hyperkinetic behaviour. (Some behaviour disorder associated with epilepsy is caused by the anticonvulsant drugs.)

Associated with specific genetic causes (behavioural phenotypes) Some genetic causes of learning disability also cause a specific pattern of behaviour problems. for example, children with the rare Prader–Willi syndrome have a voracious appetite, pick and scratch their skin, and show outbursts of unprovoked rage; while children with the rare Lesch–Nyhan syndrome injure themselves seriously by biting their lips and fingers. Such genetically determined behaviours are particularly difficult to modify. The term behavioral phenotype is sometimes used to include also psychiatric disorders that are strongly associated with a genetically determined condition, for example Alzheimer's disease in patients with Down's syndrome (see p. 308).

Assessment of learning disability

Severe learning disability is usually diagnosed in infancy, as it is often associated with physical abnormalities or with delayed motor development. It is more difficult to diagnose less severe learning disability, which has to be done on the basis of delays in psychological development. A full assessment includes history taking,

TABLE 21.3 Causes of behaviour disorder in people with learning disability

- ◆ Stressful events
- ◆ Frustration
- ◆ Over- or understimulation
- ◆ Undiagnosed physical illness
- ◆ Psychiatric illness
- ◆ Brain damage
- ◆ Epilepsy
- ◆ Behavioural phenotypes

interviewing, physical examination, behavioural assessment, developmental testing, and examination of the mental state.

This section is concerned mainly with assessment in childhood since this is when assessment usually takes place. A similar scheme is used when adolescents or adults are assessed and the following account includes some advice on interviewing such people.

Suggestibility among people with learning disability

When interviewing people with learning disability, the interviewer should remember that some are unusually suggestible. There are several reasons for this increased suggestibility:

- a strong wish to please others, especially people in authority;

- reliance on cues from the interviewer when deciding what answer to give, rather than reliance on factual information;

- a tendency to reply 'yes' rather than 'no' to yes/no questions, regardless of the appropriateness of this response.

Interviewing people with learning disability

The procedure is generally similar to those described in Chapter 2 for interviewing people of normal intelligence, but some special points should be noted:

1. Ask *simple questions* avoiding subordinate clauses, passive verb constructions, figures of speech, and other complexities of grammar.

2. *Allow adequate time* for the patient to respond and do not appear impatient.

3. *Check answers to closed questions* (e.g. 'do you feel sad?'), which may have to be used because the patient cannot volunteer information. A positive answer can be checked by asking the opposite (e.g. 'do you feel happy?').

4. *Avoid leading questions and check responses.* Because some people with learning disability are suggestible (see above), it is especially important to avoid leading questions. Some people with learning disability repeat the interviewer's last words. For example, interviewer: 'Do you feel sad?'; patient: 'Sad'.

5. *Check with an informant.* People with learning disabilities often have difficulty in timing the onset or describing the sequence of symptoms. Whenever possible these and other important points should be checked with an informant.

History taking

Particular attention is given to any *family history* suggesting an inherited disorder, and to *abnormalities in the pregnancy or delivery*. Dates of passing *developmental milestones* should be ascertained, and a full account obtained of any *behaviour disorders*. The parents or another informant should be interviewed in every case; patients who have reasonable language ability should be interviewed as well.

Physical examination

The physical examination should include the recording of *head circumference*, *height*, and *weight*. Abnormal physical signs may indicate one of the rare specific syndromes. The *neurological examination* should include attention to vision and hearing.

Behavioural assessment

This is based on the account given by the parents or other informants and on observations of: (i) the child's *ability to communicate*; (ii) *sensorimotor skills*; (iii) any *unusual behaviour*; and (iv) at an appropriate age, ability for *self-care*.

Developmental testing

This is a complex procedure, which is performed usually in a specialist unit. Clinical observation is combined with standardized measurements of *intelligence*, *language development*, *motor performance*, and *social skills*.

Overall assessment

The overall assessment begins by distinguishing learning disability from other conditions, such as delayed development, blindness, deafness, and childhood autism. The last three may coexist with learning disability and worsen the behaviour problems. Any medical and social factors contributing to the overall handicaps are recorded, together with the attitudes of people who may be involved in the patient's care.

Prevention and early detection

Prevention

Primary prevention depends mainly on genetic screening and counselling, together with good antenatal and obstetric care (Table 21.4). In some developing countries, correction of iodine deficiency and malnutrition is important. **Secondary prevention** aims to reduce the effect of the primary disorder; for example by providing 'enriching' education.

TABLE 21.4 Prevention and early detection of learning disability

Prevention

♦ Before pregnancy:

   rubella immunization

   genetic counselling

♦ During pregnancy:

   avoid excess alcohol

♦ During and after delivery:

   care of premature infants

Early detection

♦ During pregnancy:

   ultrasound screening

   amniocentesis

   fetoscopy

♦ After delivery:

   screening for phenylketonuria

   screening for hypothyroidism

   galactosaemia

Genetic screening and counselling Most parents seek advice only after the birth of a first child with learning disability. Those asking for advice before or during the first pregnancy usually do so because there is a person with learning disability in the extended family. Specialist advice is usually needed to assess the risk that an abnormal child will be born, and to explain this risk to the parents so that they can make their own decision whether to start or continue the pregnancy.

Antenatal care *Immunization against rubella* should be provided for girls who lack immunity, before the age at which they could become pregnant. Women already pregnant should be advised on the *harmful effects of excessive alcohol* consumption.

Perinatal care *Improved care for premature and low birthweight infants* can prevent learning disability in some infants who would otherwise have suffered brain damage. However, the same methods enable the survival of disabled children who, without these methods, would have died.

Early detection

Prenatal care *Ultrasound scanning* of the fetus, *amniocentesis*, and *fetoscopy* can reveal disorders due to chromosomal abnormalities, most open neural tube defects, and about half of inborn errors of metabolism. Because amniocentesis carries a small but definite risk, it is usually offered only to women who have carried a previous abnormal fetus, women with a family history of congenital disorder, and those over 35 years of age.

Postnatal care Phenylketonuria, hypothyroidism, and galactosaemia can be detected by routine testing of infants.

Services for people with learning disability

Principles of service provision

Services for people with learning disability should aim to achieve the following goals (Table 21.5):

1. Provide a pattern of life that is as similar as possible to that of other people ('**normalization**').

2. Recognize that each person with learning disability has individual needs.

3. Develop abilities as well as compensate for disability.

4. Offer a choice of services and involve the disabled person in the choice.

Most learning disability is detected by family doctors and paediatricians. However, the wide range of needs of people with learning disability can be met only by a care teams that include psychiatrists, psychologists, nurses, residential care staff, teachers, occupational therapists, physiotherapists, and speech therapists. Self-help groups for parents are useful, and volunteers can play a valuable part in the arrangements.

Care for people with mild and moderate learning disability

Few people with mild learning disability need specialist services. Most live with their families, cared for when necessary by the family doctor. When specialist treatment is needed it is usually for associated physical disability or illness, emotional disorder, or psychiatric illness. When placement away from home is needed it

TABLE 21.5 Goals of service provision for a person with learning disability

♦ 'Normalize' the person's life

♦ Recognize individual needs

♦ Develop abilities

♦ Offer choice

TABLE 21.6 Components of a service for people with learning disability

- Support for family at home; respite admissions
- Education, training, and occupation
- Social activities
- Accommodation
- Help with financial and other problems
- General medical services

is usually because of difficulties in the family, or physical problems. In these cases fostering or boarding school placement for children or residential care for adults is arranged. Adults with mild learning disability may need extra support when they are facing problems with housing and employment, or with the problems of growing old (Table 21.6).

Help for families

Parents need help as soon as the diagnosis of learning disability is made. It is seldom enough to explain the problem once; most parents need to hear the information several times before they can take in all its implications. Adequate time is needed to explain the prognosis, indicate what help can be provided, and discuss the part the parents can play in helping their child achieve his full potential. As explained above, parents need continuing psychological support and help with practical matters such as day care during school holidays, babysitting, or arrangements for family holidays. These provisions are needed in particular at times of change for the patient, especially leaving school, and at times when there are additional problems in the family such as the illness of another child.

Education

Education and training should begin early. Extra education and training before school age (**compensatory education**) helps children with learning disability to realize their potential. When the normal school age is reached, the least disabled children can be educated in a special class in an ordinary school. More disabled children benefit more from attendance at a school for children with learning difficulties. For intermediate levels of disability a choice has to be made between education in an ordinary school or a special school. The former offers the advantages of more normal social surroundings and greater expectations of progress; it has the disadvantages of lack of special teaching skills and the risk that the child may not be accepted by more able children. Since learning is slow, education may need to extend into adult life.

Leaving school

The period after leaving school is difficult for people with learning disability and they need a lot of help from their general practitioner and the specialist services. It is important to review the prospects for employment, suitability for further training, and requirements for day care. At this stage of life, it may be difficult for the parents to look after a young person with severe learning disability and residential care may be required. Wherever the person is living, there is a need for sheltered work or other occupation after leaving school.

Training and work

Most people with mild learning difficulties are capable of work and benefit from appropriate training. However, except at times of full employment, suitable work may not be available and sheltered occupation is needed. Most school-leavers with moderately severe learning disability need sheltered work or further training when they leave school. Most need these special provisions throughout their lives, although some do progress to normal employment.

Social activities

People with learning disability need to develop leisure activities appropriate to their age, ability, and interests. Whenever possible this should be achieved by joining activities arranged for able people, but clubs and day centres for the disabled are also needed. For the most disabled, leisure activities need to be arranged as part of the programme of the training centres that provide sheltered work.

Accommodation

Many people with learning disability live with their families. For the rest, a variety of accommodation is required ranging from ordinary housing to staffed hostels. A useful intermediate level of supervision is provided in a 'core and cluster' system in which several group homes are sited near to a central staffed unit. When parents grow old and can no longer care for their disabled son or daughter, special accommodation is required. In most places the supply of such accommodation has not kept pace with the increasing life expectancy of people with learning disability.

Help with financial and other practical problems

People with learning disability may need help in managing their money, dealing with forms, regulations, and other problems of daily life.

General medical services

People with learning disability sometimes receive substandard medical care because doctors do not detect their needs or do not provide the extra support needed to enable these patients to cooperate with treatment. It is good practice to keep a register of these patients and arrange regular health checks.

Care for people with severe learning disability

A general practitioner with 2000 patients will care for, on average, only two children with severe learning disability. In two-thirds of cases, the severely disabled child can remain at home provided that the parents are helped to deal with behavioural problems, epilepsy, physical disability, or incontinence. This help may be day care or respite care—short stays in residential care or hospital when the parents need a holiday, or when another member of the family is ill. When the child attends school, there is often a need for help with transport and for support in the school holidays. As well as these practical provisions, parents need information and psychological support.

The remaining one-third of children with severe learning disability need residential care, often because of physical disability, behavioural problems, or incontinence too great for the parents to manage.

Care for elderly people with learning disability

As people with learning disability live longer, provision is needed increasingly for the later years of their lives. At this stage, parents are no longer able to provide care and physical illness or dementia may add to the person's disability. It is important to recognize these problems when planning services.

Psychiatric disorder in people with learning disability

Diagnosis

There are several reasons why psychiatric diagnosis is difficult in people with learning disability.

1. Patients may have *insufficient verbal ability* to describe abnormal experiences accurately (the level of ability corresponds to an IQ level of about 50).

2. Some people with learning disability are *suggestible* (see p. 310) and may answer positively to a question about a symptom when they have not in fact experienced it.

3. For the above reasons, diagnosis often has to be *based on reports by others* of changes in the patient's behaviour. These informants may know little about patients' past history, may not have spent much time with them recently, or may not be observant.

TABLE 21.7 Systematic assessment of a patient with learning disability
◆ Severity of the learning disability
◆ Cause of the learning disability
◆ Developmental disorder
◆ Other psychiatric disorder
◆ Personality disorder
◆ Problem behaviours
◆ Other (e.g. medical) disorders

4. *Some causes of learning disability also cause abnormal behaviour* (see p. 309). Behaviour problems due to psychiatric disorder may be wrongly ascribed to this other cause, or vice versa.

5. Learning disability is *associated with autism* (see p. 291), and some of the symptoms of autism can be mistaken for those of another psychiatric disorder, for example obsessive-compulsive disorder. Psychiatric disorder should be diagnosed only after deciding whether autism—or another pervasive developmental disorder (see p. 291)—is present.

6. *Physical illness* or *stressful events* can cause changes in behaviour, and both should be considered before the diagnosis of mental disorder is made.

The stages of a systematic assessment of a patient with learning disability are shown in Table 21.7.

Prevalence of psychiatric disorder

Among people with learning disability the prevalence of mental disorder is generally rather greater than in people within the normal range of intelligence. All types of mental disorder may occur at any degree of learning disability, but at the severe level the most frequent are **autism, hyperkinetic syndrome, stereotyped movements, pica,** and **self-mutilation**. Some people with learning disability have **epilepsy**, and this in turn may be associated with mental disorder (see p. 146).

Specific psychiatric disorders

Delirium and dementia

These disorders are common among people with learning disability. Sometimes, disturbed behaviour resulting from delirium is the first indication of physical illness. As with people of normal intelligence, delirium is more common among children and the elderly. Dementia causes a progressive decline in intellectual and social functioning from the previous level. Among the causes of dementia (see p. 141), Alzheimer's disease is more common in patients with Down's syndrome than in the general population (see p. 308).

Autism

Autism is more common in people with learning disability than in the rest of the population, with a prevalence of about 1–2 per cent in all children with learning disability, and about 5 per cent in people with severe learning disability. Looked at in another way, about two-thirds of children with autism also have some degree of learning disability.

Schizophrenia

Among schizophrenic people with learning disability, delusions are less elaborate than they are among schizophrenics of normal intelligence, and hallucinations have a simple and repetitive content. 'First rank' and other typical symptoms of schizophrenia are uncommon, and often the main features are a further impoverishment of a person's already limited thinking, and an increased disturbance of behaviour and social functioning. When the IQ is below 45, it is difficult to make a definite diagnosis of schizophrenia. When the diagnosis of schizophrenia is probable but not certain, a trial of treatment with antipsychotic drugs may be carried out.

Mood disorder

When people with learning disability develop a **depressive disorder** they are less likely than people of normal intelligence to complain of low mood or to express depressive ideas. Diagnosis has to be made mainly on observable features such as an appearance of sadness, reduction of appetite, disturbance of sleep, retardation, or agitation. A severely depressed patient with adequate verbal abilities may describe depressive ideas, delusions, or hallucinations. A few of these patients make attempts at suicide, although these are usually poorly planned. **Mania** has to be diagnosed mainly on overactivity and behavioural signs indicating excitement and irritability.

Stress-related and anxiety disorders

Stress-related and **adjustment disorders** occur commonly among people with mild and moderate learning disability, especially when they are facing changes in the routine of their lives. **Phobic disorders** are common, while conversion and dissociative symptoms are more conspicuous than in the corresponding disorders of people of normal intelligence. Treatment of all these conditions is directed mainly to: (i) reducing stressors by effecting improvements in the patient's environment; and (ii) if verbal skills are sufficient, counselling.

Personality disorder

Personality disorders are common among people with learning disability and sometimes lead to greater problems in management than the learning problems. Because psychological development is delayed, the diagnosis is not generally made until the age of 20 years. There is no specific treatment and management has to be directed to finding an environment as suitable as possible to the patient's temperament. If verbal skills are sufficient, counselling may be helpful.

Attention deficit hyperactivity disorder

This disorder occurs more commonly among children with learning disability than among those of normal intelligence. The clinical picture and treatment are the same as those among children of normal intelligence (see p. 288).

Challenging behaviour

Challenging behaviour (that is, behaviour that threatens the safety of the patient or other people) may be caused by psychiatric disorder but it has many other causes including:

- *pain and discomfort* due to associated physical conditions;
- *frustration* due to difficulty in communication;
- epilepsy;
- side effects of medication.

Treatment of psychiatric disorder

Treatment of mental disorder among people with learning disability is similar to that of the same disorder in a patient of normal intelligence. Because patients are less likely to report the side effects of drugs, particular care is needed in adjusting dosage. In the more serious cases, admission to hospital is often needed.

Treatment of challenging behaviour

If possible, the cause of the challenging behaviour is treated. If the behaviour persists, behavioural treatment may be tried, directed to changing any factors that appear to be reinforcing the behaviour.

Ethical problems in the care of people with learning disability

Most of the ethical problems encountered in the care of people with learning disability are similar in kind to those in the care of other patients. Two problems will be mentioned further.

Normalization, autonomy, and conflicts of interest

If people with learning disability are to live as normally as possible, they require support. Often this support comes from their family and arrangements that were entered into willingly at one time may become unduly burdensome if the needs of the disabled person increase, other children have additional needs, or the carers grow older. The problem can usually be resolved by discussion between the disabled person, the carers and other members of the family, and professionals with a duty of care for the various people involved. Comparable conflicts of interest may arise also when deciding whether a disabled child should be educated in an ordinary school or a special school for handicapped children.

Consent to treatment and research

Most learning disabled people can give informed consent provided that explanations are in clear and simple language, and adequate time is set aside for discussion. In the UK, when an adult with (usually severe) learning disability cannot give informed consent, no one can consent for him and the doctor has to decide what is in his best interests. (The law differs in some other countries.) The problem should be discussed with the family or a professional who knows the patient well. If there is time and the problem is particularly difficult—for example, termination of pregnancy—it may be appropriate to seek a ruling from the courts. If the condition is urgent and life-threatening it may be possible to proceed under common law, although expert medicolegal advice should be obtained first.

Further reading

Fraser, W. & Kerr, M. (eds) (2003). *The Psychiatry of Learning Disability*, 2nd edn. Gaskell, London.
Written as a basic text for psychiatric trainees, the book is a useful source of further information for non-specialist readers.

Appendix 21.1 Notes on some causes of learning disability

Syndrome	Aetiology	Clinical features	Comments
Chromosome abnormalities			
(Down's syndrome and X-linked retardation are described in the text)			
1. Triple X	Trisomy X	No characteristic feature	Mild retardation
2. Cri du chat	Deletion in chromosome 5	Microcephaly, hypertelorism, typical cat-like cry, failure to thrive	
Inborn errors of metabolism			
3. Phenylketonuria	Autosomal recessive causing lack of liver phenylalanine hydroxylase. Commonest inborn error of metabolism	Lack of pigment (fair hair, blue eyes), retarded growth. Associated epilepsy, microcephaly, eczema, and hyperactivity	Detectable by postnatal screening of blood or urine. Treated by exclusion of phenylalanine from the diet during early years of life
4. Homocystinuria	Autosomal recessive causing lack of cystathione synthetase	Ectopia lentis, fine fair hair, joint enlargement, skeletal abnormalities similar to Marfan's syndrome. Associated with thromboembolic episodes	Retardation variable. Sometimes treatable by methionine restriction
5. Galactosaemia	Autosomal recessive causing lack of galactose-1-phosphate uridyl transferase	Presents after the introduction of milk into the diet. Failure to thrive, hepatosplenomegaly, cataracts	Detectable by postnatal screening for the enzymic defect. Treatable by galactose-free diet. Toluidine blue test on urine
6. Tay–Sachs disease	Autosomal recessive resulting in increased lipid storage (the earliest form of cerebromacular degeneration)	Progressive loss of vision and hearing. Spastic paralysis. Cherry red spot at macula of retina. Epilepsy	Death at 2–4 years
7. Hurler's syndrome (gargoylism)	Autosomal recessive affecting mucopolysaccharide storage	Grotesque features. Protruberant abdomen. Hepatosplenomegaly. Associated cardiac abnormalities	Death before adolescence
8. Lesch–Nyhan syndrome	X-linked recessive leading to enzyme defect affecting purine metabolism. Excessive uric acid production and excretion	Normal at birth. Development of choreoathetoid movements, scissoring position of legs, and self-mutilation	Can be diagnosed prenatally by culture of amniotic fluid and estimation of relevant enzyme. Postnatal diagnosis by enzyme estimation in a single hair root. Death in second or third decade from infection or renal failure. Self-mutilation may be reduced by treatment with hydroxytryptophan
Other inherited disorders			
9. Neurofibromatosis (Von Recklinghausen's syndrome)	Autosomal dominant inheritance	Neurofibromata, *café au lait* spots, vitiligo. Associated with symptoms determined by the site of neurofibromata. Astrocytomas, meningioma	Retardation in a minority
10. Tuberose sclerosis (epiloia)	Autosomal dominant (very variable penetrance)	Epilepsy, adenoma sebaceum on face, white skin patches, shagreen skin, retinal phakoma, periungual fibromata. Associated multiple tumours in kidney, spleen, and lungs	Retardation in about 70%
11. Lawrence–Moon–Biedl syndrome	Autosomal recessive	Retinitis pigmentosa, polydactyly, sometimes with obesity and impaired genital function	Retardation usually not severe

Appendix 21.1 *Cont'd*

Syndrome	Aetiology	Clinical features	Comments
Infection			
12. Rubella embryopathy	Viral infection of mother in first trimester	Cataract, microphthalmia, deafness, microcephaly, congenital heart disease	If mother infected in first trimester, 10–15% of infants are affected (infection may be subclinical)
13. Toxoplasmosis	Protozoal infection of mother	Hydrocephaly, microcephaly, intracerebral calcification, retinal damage, hepatosplenomegaly, jaundice, epilepsy	Wide variation in severity
14. Cytomegalovirus	Virus infection of mother	Brain damage. Only severe cases are apparent at birth	
15. Congenital syphilis	Syphilitic infection of mother	Many die at birth. Variable neurological signs. 'Stigmata' (Hutchinson teeth and rhagades often absent)	Uncommon since routine testing of pregnant women.
Cranial malformations			
16. Hydrocephalus	Sex-linked recessive. Inherited developmental abnormality (e.g. atresia of aqueduct, Arnold–Chiari malformation. Meningitis. Spina bifida)	Rapid enlargement of head in early infancy, symptoms of raised CSF pressure. Other features depend on aetiology	Mild cases may arrest spontaneously. May be symptomatically treated by CSF shunt. Intelligence can be normal
17. Microcephaly	Recessive inheritance, irradiation in pregnancy, maternal infections	Features depend on aetiology	Evident in up to a fifth of institutionalized patients with learning disability
Miscellaneous			
18. Spina bifida	Aetiology multiple and complex	Failure of vertebral fusion. Spina bifida cystica is associated with meningocele or, in 15–20%, myelomeningocele. Latter causes spinal cord damage, with lower limb paralysis, incontinence, etc.	Hydrocephalus in four-fifths of those with myelomeningocele. Retardation in this group
19. Cerebral palsy	Perinatal brain damage. Strong association with prematurity	Spastic (commonest), athetoid and ataxic types. Variable in severity	Majority are below average intelligence. Athetoid are more likely to be of normal IQ
20. Hypothyroidism (cretinism)	Iodine deficiency or (rarely) atrophic thyroid	Appearance normal at birth. Abnormalities appear at 6 months. Growth failure, puffy skin, lethargy	Now rare in Britain. Responds to early replacement treatment
21. Hyperbilirubinaemia	Haemolysis, rhesus incompatibility, and prematurity	Kernicterus. Choreoathetosis, opisthotonus, spasticity, convulsions	Prevention by antirhesus globulin. Neonatal treatment by exchange transfusion

CHAPTER 22

Psychiatry and the law

Chapter contents

Psychiatry and civil law *320*

Psychiatry and criminal law *322*

The relationship of psychiatry and the law is of importance to all doctors for five reasons:

1. Laws, regulations and official guidelines provide backing to some aspects of ethical medical care—examples are given throughout this book.

2. The law regulates the circumstances under which treatment can be given without patients' consent and the compulsory admission of psychiatric patients to hospital. Primary care practitioners and hospital doctors may encounter situations in which patients refuse essential treatment and may have to decide whether to invoke powers of compulsory admission (since the details of mental health law varies among countries only general principles are described in this chapter).

3. There are other situations in which doctors may be asked for reports used in legal decisions: the capacity to make a will or to care for property, and claims for compensation for injury. They may be asked for reports that set out the relationship between any psychiatric disorder and criminal behaviour.

4. A minority of patients behave in ways which break the law. Doctors need to understand legal issues as part of their management of care.

5. Victims of crime may suffer immediate and long-term psychological consequences

This chapter considers these issues and ends with advice on writing reports for the courts and other medicolegal purposes.

Psychiatry and civil law

Laws concerning consent to treatment, compulsory admission, and treatment

Consent to treatment

In general, the law requires that patients cannot be treated unless they first consent. This consent must be given:

• *voluntarily*, without undue influence;

• *by the patient*; no one can consent on his behalf, although he may obtain advice from relatives or others whom he trusts;

• by the patient who has been *informed* of the likely benefits, side effects, and possible adverse outcomes of the treatment.

Except for minor procedures, the patient's consent should be *documented*. Important examples are covered elsewhere in this book. Table 22.1 summarizes key situations in which issues of consent are likely to arise.

Informed consent and mental illness

There are special problems about informed consent for treatment in those who are mentally ill. Some patients, by reason of their illness, are not capable of informed consent; others do not recognize that they are ill and require treatment. To be capable of consent, patients need to be able to:

• **understand** the information provided about the treatment;

• **retain** this information;

• **evaluate** the information to arrive at a decision.

Patients with delirium or dementia may be unable to consent to treatment *because they cannot understand, retain, or evaluate information.* (Dementia does not inevitably lead to these consequences and each patient should be evaluated carefully.)

TABLE 22.1 Situations in which problems of consent to treatment are likely to arise

• Emergency life-threatening situations

• Increasing or severe cognitive impairment

• Mental disorder impairing ability to give informed consent to treatment of physical disorder

• Amongst children

• Amongst people with learning disability

• Unwilling or unable to give consent to treatment of major mental disorder

Other psychiatrically ill people are capable of consent but *do not recognize that they are unwell or in need of psychiatric treatment.* This arises particularly with schizophrenia and manic-depressive disorders.

Compulsory admission and treatment of mental illness

All countries have laws covering the circumstances in which compulsory psychiatric treatment can be given to patients with psychiatric disorder who do not consent. In general, compulsory treatment can be initiated only in hospital.

Mental health laws regulate the circumstances in which people with mental illness can be admitted to hospital and treated without their consent. These laws have three purposes, which are shown in Table 22.2. They ensure essential treatment for mentally ill people who do not recognize that they are ill, and refuse treatment. Three criteria are used to decide whether treatment is essential:

1. The **safety of the patient**—usually from suicidal impulses.

2. The **safety of others**—for example, from the violent impulses of a paranoid patient.

3. The need for urgent measures to **prevent deterioration** that will lead to one of the two previous criteria.

The details of mental health law vary in different countries; even within the UK, the laws in England and Wales differ in certain ways from those in Scotland and Northern Ireland. The most widely used sections of the Mental Health Act for England and Wales (at the time of writing) are shown in Box 22.1 as an illustration of the general principles discussed below. Readers should seek advice about local legislation. However, there are important common features of most systems of law (Table 22.3).

Joint decisions The patient's refusal to have treatment cannot be overturned by a single doctor except in situations of extreme urgency. For example, in England and Wales two doctors and a social worker are required to agree about the decision.

Defined periods of detention The law sets strict limits on the period of involuntary detention and treatment.

TABLE 22.2 Purposes of mental health law

• To ensure essential treatment

• To protect other people

• To protect from wrongful detention

BOX 22.1 MENTAL HEALTH ACT 1983 FOR ENGLAND AND WALES: THE MOST WIDELY USED SECTIONS

Section number	Order	Duration	Authorization
2	Assessment order	28 days	Recommendation of two doctors (one approved) plus application by nearest relative or social worker
3	Treatment order	6 months	As for Section 2 initially, and renewable
4	Emergency order	72 hours	Recommendation by one doctor plus application by nearest relative or social worker
5 (2)	Holding order	72 hours	One doctor
5 (4)	Holding order	6 hours	One registered mental nurse
58	'Hazardous treatment'		Consent or second opinion
136	Police order	72 hours	Police officer

TABLE 22.3 Role of mental health law in relation to criminal behaviour

- Police powers to detain for medical assessment
- Emergency treatment by doctors
- Urgent admission procedures for patient with mental disorders who are not in hospital
- Emergency procedures for compulsory detention of patients already in hospital (general or psychiatric)
- Longer term procedures for chronic mental disorder

If longer periods of detention are needed, further orders must be made.

Appeal against detention An important safeguard against misuse of the power to detain is a system of independent review. The detailed arrangements vary in different countries; for example in England and Wales patients can appeal first to members of the board of management of the hospital to which they have been admitted. If this appeal fails, they can appeal to a mental health tribunal consisting of a lawyer, a doctor, and a layperson.

Early discharge from detention Some patients recover so quickly that compulsory detention is no longer needed at a time before the original detention period has elapsed. In these circumstances the original order can be terminated.

Provision for detention of patients already in hospital The provisions described so far apply to patients who are not inpatients at the time when the order is made. Sometimes a patient enters hospital voluntarily and then demands to leave. Normally, he is free to do

this but, in some circumstances, discharge would endanger his own life or health or endanger other people. If there is evidence of mental disorder, mental health laws provide that the patient can be held in hospital for a brief period sufficient to arrange a full assessment for detention.

Detention by the police Police officers sometimes encounter people apparently suffering from mental disorder. Mental health laws generally contain provision for the police to detain such persons until they can be assessed.

Consent to certain treatments Generally, the legal authority to detain the patient carries with it the authority to give basic treatment, even without the patient's consent (e.g. sedation). However, in some countries additional authority has to be obtained before certain treatments can be given without consent. In England and Wales, these treatments are electroconvulsive therapy and medication continued for more than 3 months for patients subject to mental health law orders.

Patients who have offended People with psychiatric illness who have been convicted of offences may need to be transferred to hospital either from the court or after a period in prison. Mental health laws contain provisions for the compulsory detention in hospital of such people, either on terms similar to those of detained patients who have not offended or with restrictions on the consultant psychiatrist's usual powers of discharge. These provisions, which are complex and mainly of concern to psychiatrists, are not detailed here.

Other aspects of civil law

Patients' ability to manage their affairs

Some patients, most often those who are demented, become incapable of managing their affairs by reason of mental disorder and are vulnerable to exploitation. When this happens, legal arrangements exist to enable another responsible person to act for the patient. The doctor should advise the close relatives when this circumstance arises, explain the risks to property, and outline the legal provisions. If the relatives decline to take action the doctor can initiate proceedings himself. In English law there are two procedures: power of attorney and receivership. Comparable procedures are available in other countries.

Power of attorney requires the person to give written authorization for someone else to act for him. It is, of course, essential that the person giving authority is able to understand what he is doing and be able to judge the suitability of the person chosen to act for him.

Receivership is a more complex procedure with the greater safeguards needed for a person who is unable to make the judgement required in authorizing a power of attorney. An application is made to a legal body (in England and Wales the Court of Protection), which decides for the patient whether to appoint someone (a 'receiver') to act on his behalf.

Making a will

Doctors are sometimes asked to advise whether a patient is capable of making a will; that is, whether he has 'testamentary capacity'. The requirements are that the person:

- understands what a will is;

- knows the nature and extent of his property (although not in detail);

- knows who his close relatives are and can assess their claims to his property;

- does not have any mental abnormality that might distort his judgement (e.g. delusions about the actions of his relatives).

Most patients with mental disorder are wholly capable of making a will.

Fitness to drive

Questions about fitness to drive arise quite often in relation to psychiatric disorder. Patients may drive recklessly if they are manic, depressed and suicidal, or aggressive; or if they abuse alcohol or drugs. Concentration on driving may be impaired in many kinds of psychiatric disorder, and also by the sedative side effects of drugs used in treatment. The issue should be considered in all cases in which a patient drives a motor vehicle. Advice to stop driving should be given if necessary and the patient reminded of his duty to report illnesses to the licensing authority. Particular caution is required for patients who drive public service vehicles or goods vehicles.

Compensation for personal injury

Doctors are often asked to write medical reports about disability following accidents or other trauma and in relation to claims of medical negligence. Such reports are concerned mainly with the nature and outlook of physical disability, but they should include any psychiatric consequences directly attributable to the trauma or induced by the physical disability. It may be necessary to comment on the possibility of exaggeration or even simulation. The conclusions should summarize the psychological and social consequences of the trauma and the extent to which they appear to be attributable to it.

In many cases there is evidence that there were psychological problems or social difficulties before the event and it is important to decide how far the psychological and social changes found after the trauma are a continuation of these previous difficulties rather than new developments. Evidence from a close relative or other informant, interviewed separately, should be obtained whenever possible. Acute stress disorder and post-traumatic stress disorder are considered on pp. 63–6.

Giving evidence in court

Doctors who are required to give verbal evidence in court should speak beforehand to a lawyer involved in the case to find out what points are likely to be raised in court. The doctor should prepare by reading any available documents including witness statements and social reports. If necessary, he should consult medical works of reference. Doctors should remember that their role is to use their special knowledge to assist the court to reach its own decision, not to tell the court what to do. When replying to questions in court, answers should be brief, clear, and restricted to the medical evidence. Speculation should be avoided.

Psychiatry and criminal law

Figures for the prevalence of crime must be viewed cautiously as they depend on reporting and upon

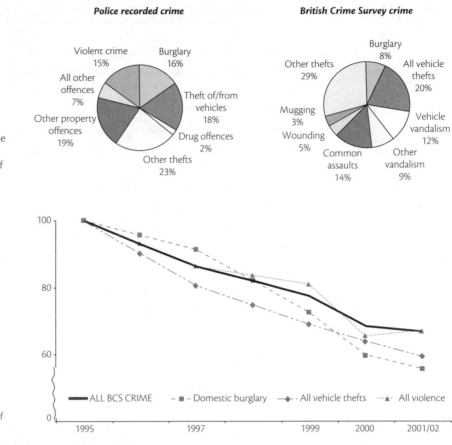

Fig. 22.1 Types of crime as recorded by the police and the British Crime Survey, 2001/02. (Reproduced by permission of The Home Office.)

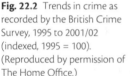

Fig. 22.2 Trends in crime as recorded by the British Crime Survey, 1995 to 2001/02 (indexed, 1995 = 100). (Reproduced by permission of The Home Office.)

definitions of crime. In most countries property offences are the most common type of crime. However, much criminal behaviour is unreported and this is especially true of violence within the home. Figure 22.1 illustrates the difference between patterns of police-recorded and self-reported crime. There are large national differences in rates and patterns. Figure 22.2 shows that in the UK, contrary to public belief, rates of most types of crime have been decreasing in recent years as assessed by self-report.

In all cultures, crime is predominantly the activity of young men. Social studies have drawn attention to social and economic causes of crime in the family, peer group, and subculture, and in conditions of poverty, poor schooling, and unemployment. It is widely held that such social causes of crime are more important than individual psychological factors such as genetics and psychological traits. However, doctors are most likely to be involved in relation to possible psychological risk factors.

Few psychiatric patients break the law and when they do, it is usually in minor ways. Although serious violent offences by psychiatric patients receive much publicity, they are infrequent and committed by an extremely small minority of patients. It is, however, important that doctors are aware of the risk of criminal behaviour amongst those who are mentally ill. Threats of violence to self or to others should be taken seriously, as should the possibility of unintended harm resulting from disinhibited, reckless, or ill-considered behaviour. Specialist advice should always be sought where there is concern and doubt about appropriate action.

Associations between specific psychiatric disorders and types of offence

Box 22.2 summarizes the associations between psychiatric disorders and offending. There are also some associations between particular offences and psychiatric disorder. Most offences have predominantly social causes and few are associated specifically with psychiatric disorder. Since categories of offence are defined for legal purposes, it is not surprising that there is no close correspondence between these categories and

BOX 22.2 ASSOCIATIONS BETWEEN PSYCHIATRIC DISORDERS AND OFFENDING

Schizophrenia	Crime is uncommon and usually minor. Persecutory delusion or hallucinations may lead to violent offences. Threats of violence should be taken seriously.
Depressive disorder	Some depressive delusions may lead to attempts at homicide to spare the victims from what is seen as an intolerable future. Infanticide within 12 months of birth.
Mania	Exuberant, unpredictable behaviour may result in fraud, theft, or, rarely, violence.
Organic mental disorder	Dementia may result in shoplifting or disinhibited minor sexual offences.
Personality disorder	Common characteristic of serious offenders. Link between antisocial personality and violent offences.
Alcohol abuse	Common association includes family and other violence, and dangerous driving.
Drug abuse	Particularly associated with theft to obtain or pay for drugs.
Learning disability	Usually minor crimes by individuals lacking understanding of the legal implications of their actions.

categories of psychiatric disorder. Any offence can be associated with several kinds of psychiatric disorder.

Crimes of violence

Figure 22.3 shows the relative proportions of types of violent crime.

Homicide In the UK, less than a third of homicides are by mentally disordered people. In countries with higher homicide rates the proportion is lower. The victims are usually family members or close acquaintances. The disorders most often associated with homicide are: schizophrenia, personality disorder, severe depressive disorder, and alcoholism—many murderers are intoxicated with alcohol at the time of the crime. Pathological jealousy (see p. 133), which may be associated with any of these conditions, is particularly dangerous.

Infanticide, the killing of a child below the age of 12 months by the mother, is of two kinds. When the killing is within 24 hours of birth, the baby is usually unwanted, and the mother is often young, distressed, and ill-equipped to deal with the child, but not usually suffering from psychiatric disorder. When the killing is more than 24 hours after the birth, the mother usually has a puerperal psychosis. About a third of mothers in this second group try to kill themselves after killing the child.

Family violence short of homicide is common but often undetected. It is strongly associated with excessive consumption of alcohol. It may affect children (child abuse is considered on p. 296), the spouse, or an elderly relative living in the house. Wife battering is associated with aggressive personality, alcohol abuse, and sexual jealousy. Marital therapy may be attempted to reduce factors provoking the violence, but often alternative safe accommodation has to be found for the woman and any children.

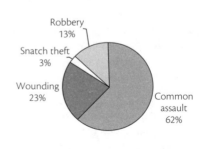

Fig. 22.3 Types of violent crime as reported by the police and the British Crime Survey, 2001/02. (Reproduced by permission of The Home Office.)

Police recorded crime

Homicide 0.1%
Other violence 6%
Robbery 15%
Sexual offences 5%
Common assault 32%
Harassment 14%
Wounding 28%

British Crime Survey crime

Robbery 13%
Snatch theft 3%
Wounding 23%
Common assault 62%

BOX 22.3 SEXUAL OFFENCES

Indecent exposure	Indecent exposure of the genitalia is mainly an offence of men between 25 and 35 years of age. The offence is usually a result of the psychiatric disorder known as exhibitionism (see p. 212), although in a minority exposure is a prelude to a sexual assault.
Rape	Rape is forceful sexual intercourse with an unwilling partner. The degree of force varies: in some cases force is threatened either verbally or with a weapon, in others there is extreme brutality. Few rapists have a psychiatric disorder.
Unlawful intercourse	This is sexual intercourse with a child under the age at which legal consent can be given. The sexual acts vary from minor indecency to seriously aggressive penetrative intercourse, but most do not involve violence. The offence is common. An adult who repeatedly commits sexual offences against children is known as a **paedophile**. Most are male. Some are timid and sexually inexperienced, some mentally retarded, and some have difficulty in finding a sexual partner of their own age. Others prefer intercourse with children to that with adults. Although most offences do not involve major assault and most convicted offenders do not reoffend, an important minority persist in their behaviour and a few progress to more serious and damaging forms of sexual behaviour with children.
Incest	Incest is sexual activity between members of the same family, most often between father and daughter, or between siblings. Child sexual abuse is described in Chapter 20. When incest has been discovered the family needs much specialist support to deal with guilt and recriminations. *The effects of sexual abuse on children are described on p. 297.*

Sexual offences (Box 22.3) Most sexual offences are committed by men. The most frequent offences are indecent exposure, rape, and unlawful intercourse. The common sexual offence among women is prostitution.

Other offences

Shoplifting Most shoplifters act for gain but a minority do so when mentally disordered. Patients with alcoholism, drug dependence, and chronic schizophrenia may shoplift because they lack money, and patients with dementia may forget to pay. Patients with depressive disorder or anorexia nervosa may shoplift with less obvious motives when they do not need what they have stolen. Among middle-aged, female shoplifters it is common to find family and social difficulties and depression.

Arson is setting fire to property, an act that may also endanger life. Most arsonists are male. Usually there is no obvious motive for the act and many arsonists are referred for a medical opinion. However, few have a psychiatric disorder.

Repeated gambling ('pathological gambling') This term is used to describe a condition in which a person describes an intense urge to gamble and a preoccupation with thoughts about gambling. Gambling is not, in itself, an offence but large debts can accumulate and may result in stealing or fraud. Some psychiatrists regard this condition as a disorder akin to addiction to alcohol, and offer treatment similar to that used for substance abuse. The results of such treatment are uncertain.

The role of doctors

Apart from providing factual medical reports, doctors may be asked to advise on certain legal issues (Box 22.4). Most are the province of the specialist psychiatrist but general practitioners and other doctors may be asked for advice and asked to prepare a formal report (Box 22.5).

It is an important ethical principle that both doctors and those they are assessing are clear that *acting for a third party*, such as a court, involves different obligations and responsibilities to usual clinical practice where the relationship is between the doctor and patient.

Assessment of criminal responsibility

In deciding whether a person is guilty of an offence against the law, emphasis is placed, in the legal system,

BOX 22.4 THE ROLE OF DOCTORS IN RELATION TO CRIME

- Advice to the police when they are deciding whether to proceed with charges against mentally ill people.

- Fitness to plead. To be fit to plead, a person must be able to: understand the nature of the charge and the difference between a plea of guilty and a plea of not guilty, instruct lawyers and challenge jurors, and follow evidence presented in court. A person can suffer from severe mental disorder and still be fit to plead. A person judged unfit to plead is not tried but detained in a hospital until fit to plead, at which time (if it comes) the case is tried.

- Assessment of responsibility.

- Advice on sentencing.

- Treatment of offenders:

  in a penal institution,

  in hospital,

  in the community.

- Assessment of dangerousness (see p. 31).

on the person's intentions at the time of the offence and on his ability to control his actions at that time— the concept of **responsibility**.

For most offences, a person is not regarded as culpable unless he was able to choose whether or not to perform the unlawful action, and unless he was able to control his behaviour at the time. The doctor has to make a judgement about the mental state at the time of the offence. This is difficult because it can only be based on the mental state at the time of a medical assessment made after (sometimes long after) the event, together with the offender's account and that of any witnesses. A doctor who was treating the person before the offence will have knowledge of their mental state at that time but can still only make a judgement about the mental state when the offence was carried out.

In English law, questions about **diminished responsibility** are most often raised in relation to a charge of murder: if the plea is upheld and the person is found guilty, it is of manslaughter not murder.

Advice relevant to sentencing

The court may ask for medical advice that will assist in deciding the appropriate sentence after a person has been found guilty. This advice may be about the prognosis of any mental disorder that is present, the likely effects of psychiatric treatment, and the probability of the person offending again.

Treatment of mentally abnormal offenders

The courts take psychiatric evidence into account when sentencing mentally disordered offenders, and this evidence includes advice about psychiatric treatment. The treatment of mental disorder in an offender is not different from that of the same disorder in a person who has not offended, but treatment may need to given in a more secure place.

Usually, appropriate treatment can be given within the ordinary psychiatric services, as an outpatient or as an inpatient. However, when there is a continuing risk to other people of aggression, arson, or sexual offences, treatment is arranged in a unit providing greater security to ensure the protection of society. Mental health legislation is generally used to detain these patients. Severe personality disorders are common among offenders but few are amenable to treatment.

Victims of crime

There is increasing worry about the risks of crime, especially violent crime to individuals and in particular to children. Figure 22.4 shows the main reported worries in the UK. Doctors are sometimes asked to assist the victims of crime. Many suffer from one of the persistent reactions to stress described in Chapter 5, and require the forms of treatment outlined there.

The British Crime Survey 2001/02 found that 75 per cent of victims of domestic burglaries reported they had been emotionally affected, 28 per cent reported themselves very much upset, and 27 per cent quite a lot upset. The commonest emotions were anger, shock, loss of confidence, and feeling vulnerable and scared. A few develop a depressive disorder, anxiety disorder, or post-traumatic stress disorder (see p. 65) in response to the stressful events and are treated in the ways described in the chapters dealing with these conditions.

Victims require immediate support and practical help from doctors in primary care or from emergency department staff. They also need to be told that they can obtain later help if required by consulting doctors

BOX 22.5 PREPARING A MEDICAL REPORT

When a doctor is asked for a written medical report on a person he should avoid as far as possible technical language, he should explain any technical terms that are essential, and he should not use jargon. The report should be concise, have a clear structure, and be limited to matters relevant to the reason for the report. The following headings are recommended.

Report for criminal proceedings

1. *The doctor's particulars*: full name, qualifications, and present appointment.

2. *When the interview was conducted* and whether any third person was present.

3. *Sources of information* including any documents that have been examined.

4. Relevant points from the *family and personal history* of the defendant. Usually these can be brief, especially if a social report is available to the court.

5. The accused person's *account of the events of the alleged offence*: whether he admits to the offence or has another explanation of the events; and if he admits to it, his attitude and expressed degree of remorse.

6. *Other relevant behaviour* such as the abuse of alcohol or drugs, the quality of relationships with other people, general social competence, and behaviour indicating ability to tolerate frustration.

7. *Mental state at the time of the assessment*, mentioning only positive findings or specifically relevant negative ones.

8. A *diagnosis* in terms of relevant legal categories: in Britain the categories of *mental illness*, *mental impairment*, and *psychopathic disorder* are used in the Mental Health Act. A more specific diagnosis can be added (such as dementia or schizophrenia) but the court is unlikely to be helped by the finer nuances of diagnosis.

9. *Mental state at the time of the alleged offence*. As explained above, this question is highly important in law but difficult to answer on medical evidence. A judgement is made on the points set out above: in summary, present mental state, diagnosis, the accused person's account, and accounts from any witnesses. If the person has a chronic mental illness (such as dementia) it is less difficult to infer his mental state at the time of the alleged offence than it is if he has a depressive disorder, which could have been more or less severe at the former time than it was at the assessment. To add to the difficulty, the court does not simply require a general statement about the mental state at the time, but a specific judgement about the accused person's intentions.

10. *Fitness to plead* is referred to when this is relevant (see p. 326 for further advice on this point).

11. *Advice on further treatment* is likely to be particularly helpful to the court. Any recommendations should be feasible and to ensure this the person making the report will need to consult colleagues if he cannot himself carry out the whole of the recommended procedures. It is not the doctor's role to advise the court about sentencing, although sometimes it is helpful to indicate the likely psychiatric consequences of different forms of sentence that might be considered by the court (e.g. custodial vs. non-custodial).

Reports for compensation and other civil proceedings

The general principles are similar to those described above. It is essential to provide information about the circumstances of the event and the immediate and later reactions to it.

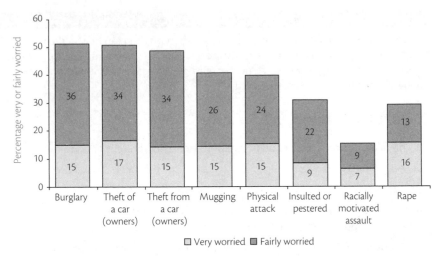

Fig. 22.4 Principal worries about crime as reported by the British Crime Survey, 2001/02. (Reproduced by permission of The Home Office.)

or one of the police and community schemes that provide counselling and practical help.

Victims of rape and other sexual assault often suffer severe immediate distress, and many experience post-traumatic stress disorder and sexual dysfunction. In some regions, special services have been set up to help rape victims deal with the immediate psychological effects of the experience and to identify persistent symptoms that may require specialist treatment.

Further reading

Stone, J. H., Roberts, M., O'Grady, J., Taylor, A. V., and O'Shea, K. (2000). *Faulk's basic forensic psychiatry.* Blackwell, Oxford.
A useful medium length reference work.

Index

acceptance 68
acute distress 154
acute illness 151-2, 153
acute stress disorder 63-5
adjustment reactions 67-8, 154
adolescents 277, 295-6
 suicide in 172
 see also child and adolescent
  psychology
adoption studies 43, 105, 126
aetiology 39-48
aggression 133
agitated depression 100
agitation 99
agoraphobia 82-3
Al-Anon 194
alcohol abuse 171, 177, 184-95
 alcohol consumption 184-5
 alcohol-related harm 185-8
  fetal alcohol syndrome 186
  physical effects 186
  prevention of 188-9
  psychiatric disorders 186-7
  social damage 187-8
 detoxification 193
 elderly patients 228-9
 safe level of consumption 184
 self-help groups 194
 terminology 184
 treatment 192-3, 194
alcohol dependence syndrome 188
Alcohol Use Disorders Identification
 Test (AUDIT) 189-91
alcohol withdrawal syndrome 188
alcoholic dementia 187
alcoholic hallucinosis 187
Alcoholics Anonymous 194
Alzheimer's disease 220-2
amenorrhoea 162
amnesia 95, 143-4
anhedonia 2, 99
anorexia nervosa 162-5, 295
anterograde amnesia 10
anticipatory anxiety 3

antidepressants 57, 79, 81, 85, 110-11,
 132, 158, 235, 242-8
 see also individual drugs
antiepileptic drugs 117, 118
antiparkinsonian drugs 242
antipsychotics 57, 117, 118, 130-1, 158,
 235, 238-42
antisocial personality disorder 54
anxiety 26, 86
 abnormal 74
 appearance 2
 normal 73
 pathological 3
 related to physical illness 151, 154
anxiety disorder 74-85, 86, 104
 adolescents 295
 children 283
 elderly patients 227-8
anxiolytics 57, 79, 81, 83, 88, 235,
 236-8
 abuse 200-1
 see also individual drugs
appearance 24-5
appetite, loss of 100
Asperger's syndrome 293
assertiveness training 260
assessment 30-2
association studies 44
attention deficit hyperactivity disorder
 11, 287-8, 314
atypical depression 101
auditory hallucinations 4, 27, 121
autism 292-3, 314
aversion therapy 261

baby blues 103, 114
Beck suicide intent scale 173-4
behaviour 24-5
Behaviour therapy 280-1
behavioural model 41-2

benzodiazepine withdrawal syndrome
 201
benzodiazepines 236-7
beta-blockers 81, 237
binge eating 162
biochemical studies 43-5
bipolar disorder 101, 108, 114, 116, 117
blunting of mood 3, 26, 120
body dysmorphic disorder 91
breast-feeding 158, 234
breath-holding 282
bulimia nervosa 162, 165-6, 262, 263,
 295
buspirone 237

CAGE questionnaire 191, 192
cancer, psychological impact 156
cannabis 202
carbamazepine 57, 250, 252
care plan 35
case notes 32
catatonia 122
cerebral tumours 146
cerebrovascular disease 145-6
challenging behaviour 305, 314
child abuse 286-7
child and adolescent psychiatry
 275-301
 assessment 277-9
 causes of psychiatric disorder 279-80
 ethical issues 299
 psychological disorders of physically
  ill children 294-5
 suicide 172
 treatment 280-1
child development 276-7
childhood sex abuse 66, 298
chloral hydrate 238
choreiform movements 10
chronic fatigue syndrome 94
chronic illness 152, 153, 154

classic conditioning 45
classification of mental disorders 13–14
clozapine 239, 241
cluttering 309
co-morbidity 14
cognitive behaviour therapy 166, 258–60
cognitive distortions 106
cognitive enhancers 235, 252
cognitive processes 46
cognitive therapy 65, 78, 81–2, 83, 85, 88, 111, 114
communication 35, 36
community mental health care 267–74
compliance with drug therapy 233
compulsive rituals 9–10, 26
concentration 11, 28
concordance 233
concrete thinking 121
conduct disorder 288–91
confabulation 10
confidentiality 33, 36
confusion 11, 29
consciousness, abnormalities of 11
contingency management 261
conversion disorders 94–5, 100
coping strategies 46, 62, 64
counselling 256
countertransference 257
couple therapy 266
couvade syndrome 157
crisis intervention 67–8
cyclothymia 52, 103
cytogenetic studies 44

dangerous severe personality disorder 54
deliberate self-harm 169–70, 176–82
    factors predicting suicide 175
delirium 11, 124, 137, 138–40, 313–14
    aetiology 138
    causes of 139
    clinical features 138
    elderly patients 220
    management 138–40
delirium tremens 188
delusional disorders 6–8, 26–7, 100, 119, 123, 124, 133
delusional memory 7
delusional mood 7
delusional perception 4, 7
dementia 76, 104, 105, 124, 137, 140–3, 220–6, 313–14
    aetiology 141
    causes of 142
    clinical features 140–1
    differential diagnosis 142–3

management 141–2
    see also individual types of dementia
denial 63, 68
dependence syndrome 183
dependency 68, 256–7
depersonalization 3, 100
depression 26
    appearance 2
    elderly patients 226–7
    masked 98
    related to physical illness 151, 154
    suicide 171
depressive disorder 66, 86–7, 98–101
    adolescents 295
    children 284
    mild 98
    moderate 99–100
    severe 100–1
depressive pseudodementia 99
depressive stupor 101
depressive thinking 99
derealization 3
detoxification
    alcohol 193
    opioids 200
developmental disorders 291–4
diagnosis 11–14
Diagnostic and Statistical Manual (DSM) 13
dialectical behaviour therapy 53
disablement 16
disorientation 28
displacement 63, 68
dissociative disorders 94–5
dissociative symptoms 64
dopamine system stabilizers 239
Down's syndrome 306, 308
drug interactions 232
drug overdose 170, 177
drugs causing psychiatric symptoms 152
dynamic psychotherapy 111, 263–5, 281
dyslexia 291
dyspareunia 209–10
dysthymia 103
dystonia 10

eating disorders 161–7, 295
Edinburgh Postnatal Depression Scale 115
elation 2, 3
elderly, psychiatric disorders in 215–29
    alcohol and drug abuse 228–9
    anxiety disorders 227–8
    delirium 220
    dementia 220–6
    depression 226–7

mania 227
    normal ageing 216
    paranoia 227, 228
    physical abuse 229
electroconvulsive therapy 111, 117, 131, 227, 252
electrophysiology 45
emotional abuse 298
emotional incontinence 3
emotional response to stress 64
encopresis 286–7
endocrine abnormalities 107
endocrinology 45
enuresis 285–6
epidemiology 42, 149–51
epilepsy 137, 146–7
erectile dysfunction 208–9
ethical issues
    assessment 32, 33
    children and adolescents 299
    learning disability 314–15
ethology 46
evidence-based medicine 47–8
exhibitionism 212
explanation 40
exposure 260

factitious disorder 95–6
false memory syndrome 11, 67
family history 22–3
family risk studies 43
family studies 126
family therapy 266, 280
fatigue 151
fetal alcohol syndrome 186
fetishism 211
fetishistic transvestism 211–12
flashbacks 64
flattening of mood 3, 26
flight of ideas 5, 101
folie à deux 7, 134
food refusal 282
formal thought disorder 121
formication 201
formulations 16, 17, 36
fragile-X syndrome 306, 308–9
frontotemporal dementia 142
fugue 95
functional symptoms 89–96, 104

gender identity disorder (transsexualism) 213, 294
generalized anxiety disorder 75–9, 81

genetic counselling, psychological impact 156, 157
genetics 42-3, 44
grandiose delusions 7
grief 70-1
group therapy 265-6

hallucinations 4-5, 27, 100, 102
hallucinogens 202
head injury 145
heredity 279
homicidal ideas 100
homosexuality 214
Huntington's chorea 142
hydrocephalus, normal pressure 144-5
hyperemesis gravidarum 157
hypersomnia 167-8
hyperventilation 75-6, 78
hypnagogic hallucinations 4
hypnopompic hallucinations 4
hypnotics 235, 238
    abuse 200-1
hypochondriacal delusions 8, 100
hypochondriasis 91
hypomania 101

identification 63
idetic imagery 3
idiopathic hypersomnia 168
illness behaviour 67-8
illusions 4, 27
imagery 3
imipramine 85
insight 11, 29, 102, 121, 123
insomnia 167, 282
intelligence tests 29, 30
International Classification of Diseases (ICD) 13
interpersonal psychotherapy 111, 166
interviewing
    cultural differences 19-20
    patient 16-19
    problems with 20
    relatives and informants 19
intoxication 186
intrusive thoughts 10
irritable bowel syndrome 93

jamais vu 10
jealousy, pathological 133-4
juvenile delinquency 295-6

knight's move thinking 5
Korsakov's syndrome 144, 187

labile mood 3, 26
learning disability (mental retardation) 303-17
    assessment 309-10
    causes 305-9
        behavioural problems 309
    clinical features 304-5
    effects on family 305
    emotional and behavioural problems 305
    epidemiology 304
    ethical issues 314-15
    and physical illness 305
    prevention and early detection 310-11
    and psychiatric disorder 313-14
    services available 311-13
    terminology 303-4
legal aspects 319-28
    civil law 320-2
    criminal law 322-8
    victims of crime 8, 10
Lewy body disease 222
liaison service 155
libido, loss of 100
life charts 34, 35-6
life events 114, 128
linkage studies 44
lithium 57, 117, 132, 158, 248-50, 251
lysergic acid diethylamide (LSD) 202

malingering 94, 96
mania 101-2, 116-17
    elderly patients 227
manic stupor 102
mannerisms 122
maternity 'blues' 158
medical model 41
memory 28-9
memory loss 10-11
menopause 159
menstrual disorders 159
Mental Health Act (1983) 321
mental state examination 24, 161
Mini Mental State Examination 37
miscarriage 157-8
mode of inheritance 43
monoamine oxidase inhibitors 79, 245-8

mood 26
    and appearance 2, 24-5
    variability of 2, 3
mood congruent 100
mood disorders 97-118, 314
    see also depressive disorder; mania
mood stabilizers 235, 248
multiple causes 40
multiple chronic functional symptoms 94
multiple personality 95
multiple sclerosis 146
Munchausen syndrome 96
    by proxy 96, 299
musculoskeletal pain 93-4
mutism 26

narcolepsy 167-8
neglect 298-9
neuroleptic malignant syndrome 241
neuropathology 45
neuropsychological tests 30
neurosis 12
nightmares and night terrors 282, 285
nihilistic delusions 7, 100
non-reductionist models 41
numbing 62

obesity 166-7
obsessional doubts 86
obsessional images 86
obsessional impulses 86
obsessional personality 59, 86
obsessional phobias 3, 9, 86
obsessional rituals 86
obsessional ruminations 86
obsessional slowness 86
obsessional symptoms 100
obsessional thoughts 26, 86
obsessive-compulsive disorder 9, 85-8
    children 284-5
obsessive-compulsive symptoms 8-10
obstetrics and gynaecology, psychiatric aspects 156-9
    loss of fetus and stillbirth 157-8
    menstrual disorders 159
    postpartum mental disorders 103-4, 108, 114, 158-9
    pregnancy 156-7
    see also pregnancy
older children 282-91
operant conditioning 45
opioids 199-200

organic delusional disorder 144
organic mental states 138
organic mood disorder 144
organic personality disorder 144
orientation 27–8
overactive patients 29
overvalued ideas 8

paedophilia 212
pain disorder 91
panic attacks 76
panic disorders 83–5
paranoia 227, 228
paranoid delusions 7
paraphilias 211
parasomnias 168
parent-child relationship disorders
    296–9
Parkinson's disease 142
pathological depression 2
perception 3–4, 27
perceptual disturbances 100
perpetuating factors 41
persecutory delusions 100
perseveration 5–6
personal history 23–4
personality assessment 50–2
personality disorders 49–60, 171, 314
    aetiology 55
    definition of 50
    epidemiology 54–5
    management 55–8
    prognosis 55
    specialist classifications 59–60
    types of 52–4
personality tests 30
pharmacological dependence 196
pharmacology 45
phencyclidine 202
phobias 3, 79–80, 100
phobic anxiety disorders 79–83
phobic disorder 66
    children 283–4
physical abuse
    children 286–7
    elderly patients 229
physical disorders, psychological impact
    151–4
    acutely distressed patients 154
    children 294–5
    determinants of 152
    examples
        cancer 156
        genetic counselling 156
        screening procedures 156
        surgical treatment 156

high risk of psychiatric problems 152
    management of 153–4
    psychiatric assessment 153
    psychiatric disorders related to
        physical illness 152
    psychiatric emergencies 154–5
    refusal of consent to treatment 154
physical examination 29–30
physical/psychiatric disorders,
    association of 149–59
physician-assisted suicide 171–2
pica 282
post-traumatic stress disorder 64, 65–6
postnatal depression 103, 114, 159
poverty of thought 5
pre-school children 281–2
precipitating factors 41
predisposing factors 41
pregnancy 156–7
    drugs used in 158
    opioid dependence 199
    prescribing in 234
    termination of 158
    unwanted 157
    see also obstetrics and gynaecology,
        psychiatric aspects
premature ejaculation 210
premenstrual syndrome 159
pressure of thought 5
prion disease 142
problem lists 32–3
problem-solving techniques 257–8
projection 63
pseudocyesis 157
pseudodementia 142–3, 226
pseudohallucinations 4
psychiatric assessment 153
psychiatric emergencies 154–5
psychiatric history 20–4
psychiatric services in general hospitals
    155–6
psychoactive substance abuse 195–203
    anxiolytics and hypnotics 200–1
    hallucinogens 202
    opioids 199–200
    organic solvents 202–3
    stimulants 201
psychological dependence 196
psychological tests 30
psychological treatment 255–66
psychomotor retardation 99
psychosis 12
psychosomatic diseases 151
psychosurgery 253–4
psychotherapy 57, 256
psychotic depression 100
psychotropic drugs 231–3
puerperal psychosis 103–4, 108, 114,
    158–9
rapid cycling 102
rating-scales of behaviour 30

rational suicide 171
rationalization 63
reaction formation 63
reductionist models 41
referral letter 36
refusal of treatment 154, 181–2
regression 63
relaxation training 78, 259–60
religious delusions 8
remote causes 40
repression 62, 63
response prevention 260
retarded depression 100
retarded ejaculation 210
retrograde amnesia 10

sadomasochism 212
schizoaffective disorder 124–5
schizophrenia 7, 76, 81, 87, 104, 105,
    119–35, 314
    adolescents 295
    aetiology 125–7
    course and prognosis 127–8
    diagnosis and clinical features 119–25
    epidemiology 125
    ICD-10 criteria 135
    management 128–33
    suicide 171
schizotypal personality 52
Schneider's 'first rank' symptoms 123,
    124
school refusal 290
screening procedures, psychological
    impact 156
seasonal affective disorder 104, 253
second person hallucinations 27
selective mutism 294
selective noradrenaline reuptake
    inhibitors 244
selective serotonin reuptake inhibitors
    79, 85, 243–4
self-control 260–1
self-injury 177–8
self-laceration 182
separation anxiety disorder 284
serial 7s test 28
sexual behaviour 206–7
sexual delusions 8
sexual dysfunction 207–11
sexual preference 211–13
sexual response 206
sexuality and gender 205–14
sleep apnoea 168
sleep disorders 75, 99–100, 167–8
sleep-wake schedule disorder 168
sleep-walking 285

social anxiety disorder 284
social inadequacy 81
social isolation 171
social phobia 80–2
sociology 46–7
solvent abuse 202–3
somatic symptoms 64
somatization 91, 284
somatoform disorders 92
speech 25–6
stammering 293
stillbirth 157–8
stimulant abuse 201
stimulants 235
stress response 61–71
   adjustment reactions 67–8
   components of 62
   normal 62–3
   special situations 67
study designs 42
stupor 11, 95, 122, 143
   depressive 101
   manic 102
sublimation 63
substance abuse 104–5
   adolescents 295
   see also psychoactive substance abuse
suicidal ideas 26, 100
suicide 108, 169–76
   causes of 171–2

epidemiology 170
help following 176
incidence of 170
management of at-risk patients
   175–6
risk assessment 172–5
suicide note 170
suicide pacts 172
suicide prevention 176
surgery, psychological impact 156

tactile hallucinations 4
temper tantrums 282
terminal illness 68–70, 152
thiamine deficiency 144
thinking 26
   abnormalities of 5
third person hallucinations 27
thought blocking 5
thought broadcasting 8
thought insertion 8
thought stopping 260
thought withdrawal 8
tics 10
transference 257
transient global amnesia 146
transsexualism 213

tricyclic antidepressants 79, 242–3
truancy 290
twin studies 43, 105, 126

understanding 40
undifferentiated somatoform disorder
   91
unresponsive patients 29

vaginismus 209
vascular dementia 222
violent behaviour 155
visual hallucinations 4, 121
voyeurism 212

waxy flexibility 122
weight loss 100
Wernicke-Korsakov syndrome 144
Wernicke's encephalopathy 144, 187
word salad 121